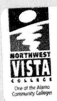
NATIONAL SAFETY COUNCIL

INJURY FACTS®

FORMERLY
ACCIDENT FACTS®

The National Safety Council, chartered by an act of Congress, is a nongovernmental, not-for-profit, public service organization. The mission of the National Safety Council is to save lives by preventing injuries and deaths at work in homes and communities, and on the roads through leadership, research, education and advocacy.

Injury Facts®, the Council's annual statistical report on unintentional injuries and their characteristics and costs, was prepared by:

Research and Statistical Services Group:
Mei-Li Lin, Executive Director
Kenneth P. Kolosh, Manager, Statistics Department
Kevin T. Fearn, Sr. Statistical Associate

Publications Department:
Jennifer Yario, Production Manager
Ian Palmer, Senior Graphic Designer
Tracy Haas, Editorial Assistant

Questions or comments about the content of *Injury Facts* should be directed to the Research and Statistics Department, National Safety Council, 1121 Spring Lake Drive, Itasca, IL 60143, by phone at (630) 775-2322, fax to (630) 285-0242, or E-mail *rssdept@nsc.org*.

For price and ordering information, visit *www.nsc.org* or write Customer Service, National Safety Council, 1121 Spring Lake Drive, Itasca, IL 60143, by phone (800) 621-7619, or fax (630) 285-0797.

Acknowledgments
The information presented in *Injury Facts* was made possible by the cooperation of many organizations and individuals, including state vital and health statistics authorities, state traffic authorities, state workers' compensation authorities, trade associations, Bureau of the Census, Bureau of Labor Statistics, Consumer Product Safety Commission, Federal Highway Administration, Federal Railroad Administration, International Labour Office, National Center for Health Statistics, National Fire Protection Association, National Highway Traffic Safety Administration, National Transportation Safety Board, National Weather Service, Mine Safety and Health Administration, and the World Health Organization. Specific contributions are acknowledged in footnotes and source notes throughout the book.

Visit the National Safety Council's website:

www.nsc.org

You may be an elected official. You may represent a company. You may be an active member of your community. Whoever you are, if you are reading this Foreword, you care about saving lives.

The National Safety Council has set a goal of saving 10,000 lives and preventing 1 million injuries between 2009 and 2014, the Council's 100th anniversary. This goal will be accomplished through leadership, research, education and advocacy in the workplace, on the roads, and in homes and communities.

Injury Facts® is used by people like you who care about saving lives to make better, more informed decisions and to help accurately communicate safety risks in an intuitive and appealing manner. Information on topics such as distracted driving, teen driving, workplace safety, and injuries in the home and community can be found in these pages.

However, unless the information in *Injury Facts* is put to use, the data within this publication provides little value. The Council encourages businesses and individuals to get involved. There are many ways to work with the Council to help save lives. Visit: *www.nsc.org/get_involved/Pages/Home.aspx* to start working with the Council today.

Overall, unintentional injury deaths were up 1.9% in 2009 compared with the revised 2008 total. Unintentional injury deaths were estimated to total 128,200 in 2009 and 125,800 in 2008.

The resident population of the United States was 306,803,000 in 2009, an increase of 1% from 2008. The unintentional injury death rate in 2009 was 41.8 per 100,000 population—up 1.0% from 2008 and 23% greater than the lowest rate on record, which was 34.0 in 1992.

The graph on page v shows the overall trends in the number of unintentional injury deaths, the population, and the death rate per 100,000 population. A more complete summary of the situation in 2009 and recent trends is given on page 2.

Changes in the 2011 Edition
Editions of *Injury Facts* prior to 2011 included estimates of disabling injuries. Starting with the 2011 edition, the Council has adopted the concept of "medically consulted injury" in place of "disabling injury." This new defintion is adopted from the National Center for Health Statistics.

A medically consulted injury as defined by NCHS is an injury serious enough that a medical professional was consulted. Moving *Injury Facts* estimates from disabling injuries to medically consulted injuries provides several advantages. First and foremost, a medically consulted injury is a more inclusive definition that allows for more comprehensive estimates of the true burden of unintentional injuries. Second, medically consulted injury estimates are updated each year by NCHS, allowing the Council to provide the most timely and accurate data possible. Finally, the previous definition of disabling injury often was misinterpreted as a workers' compensation injury. Medically consulted injuries should help eliminate this confusion. For more information on medically consulted injuries, please see the Technical Appendix on page 197.

Look for **new** data on…

• Work injuries by nature of injury
• Traumatic brain injury
• Workplace falls
• Off-the-job injuries
• Workplace Safety Index
• Injury rates by region of the world

and **updated** or **expanded** data on…

• General mortality
• Occupational injury and illness incidence rates by industry
• Occupational injury and illness profile data by industry sector
• Workers' compensation claims and costs
• Disasters
• Comparing safety of transportation modes
• Traffic safety issues (alcohol, occupant protection, speeding, etc.)
• Consumer product-related injuries
• Accidental deaths by state

For more information on this and other products, visit the Council's website (*www.nsc.org*), call Customer Service at (800) 621-7619, or contact your local Chapter.

Comments and suggestions to improve *Injury Facts* are welcome. Contact information is given on page ii.

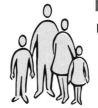

FOREWORD (CONT.)

UNINTENTIONAL INJURY DEATHS, DEATH RATES AND POPULATION, UNITED STATES, 1903-2009

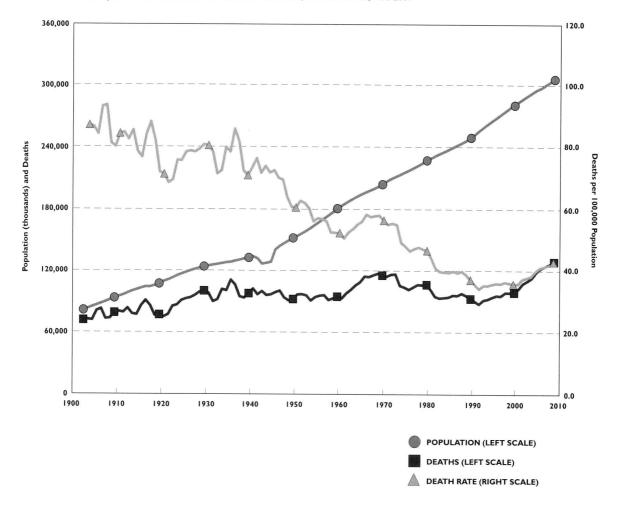

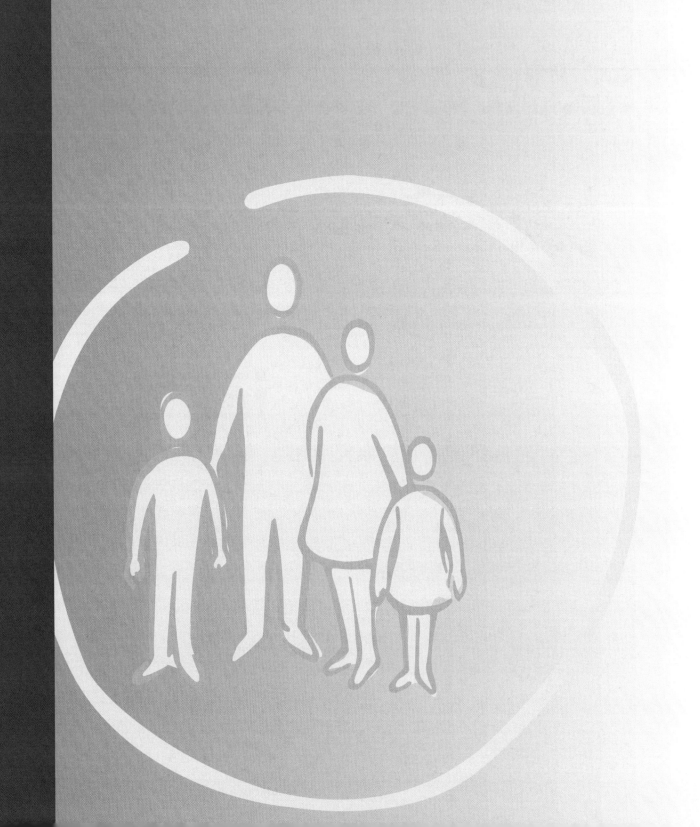

OVERVIEW OF ALL INJURY DEATHS, 2007

World:
Deaths From Injuries
4,000,000

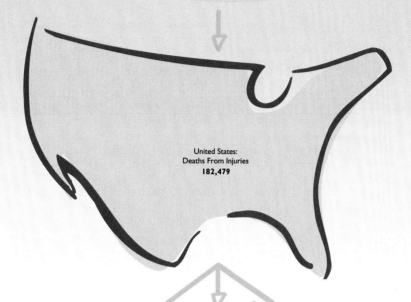

United States:
Deaths From Injuries
182,479

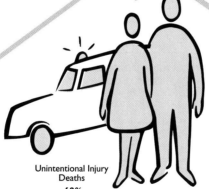

Intentional Injury
Deaths
29%

Unintentional Injury
Deaths
68%

Undetermined
Injury Deaths
3%

Work Deaths
(non-motor-vehicle)
2%

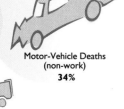

Motor-Vehicle Deaths
(non-work)
34%

Motor-Vehicle Work Deaths
2%

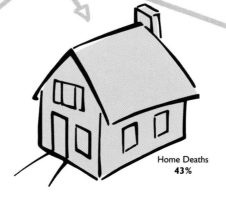

Home Deaths
43%

Public Deaths
19%

Unintentional injury deaths were up 1.9% in 2009 compared with the revised 2008 estimate. Unintentional injury deaths were estimated to total 128,200 in 2009 and 125,800 in 2008. The 2009 estimate, the highest on record, is 47% greater than the 1992 total of 86,777 (the lowest annual total since 1924).

The death rate in 2009 was 41.8 per 100,000 population—23% greater than the lowest rate on record, which was 34.0 in 1992. The 2009 death rate was up about 1% from the 2008 revised rate of 41.4.

Comparing 2009 with 2008, motor vehicle and work deaths decreased while public and home deaths increased. The population death rate in the motor vehicle, public, and work classes declined, but the home rate increased.

The motor vehicle death total was down 9.6% in 2009. The 2009 mileage death rate of 1.21 per 100 million vehicle miles, the lowest on record, was down 10% from the revised 2008 rate of 1.34. The 2009 rate was down 16% from the revised 2007 rate of 1.45.

According to the latest final data (2007), unintentional injuries continued to be the fifth leading cause of death, exceeded only by heart disease, cancer, stroke, and chronic lower respiratory diseases.

Nonfatal injuries also affect millions of Americans. In 2009, 38.9 million people—about 1 out of every 8—sought medical attention. In 2008, about 27.9 million people were treated in hospital emergency departments.

The economic impact of these fatal and nonfatal unintentional injuries amounted to $693.5 billion in 2009. This is equivalent to about $2,300 per capita, or about $5,900 per household. These are costs that every individual and household pays whether directly out of pocket, through higher prices for goods and services, or through higher taxes.

Between 1912 and 2009, unintentional injury deaths per 100,000 population were reduced 49% (after adjusting for the classification change in 1948) to 38.8 from 82.4. The reduction in the overall rate during a period when the nation's population tripled resulted in 5.6 million fewer people being killed due to unintentional injuries than there would have been if the rate had not been reduced.

ALL UNINTENTIONAL INJURIES, 2009

Class	Deaths	Change from 2008	Deaths per 100,000 persons	Medically consulted injuries[a]
All classes[b]	128,200	+1.9%	41.8	38,900,000
Motor vehicle	35,900	−10%	11.7	3,500,000
Public non-work	34,293			3,300,000
Work	1,407			200,000
Home	200			(c)
Work	3,582	−19%	1.2	5,100,000
Non-motor vehicle	2,175			4,900,000
Motor vehicle	1,407			200,000
Home	65,200	10%	21.3	21,100,000
Non-motor vehicle	65,000			21,100,000
Motor vehicle	200			(c)
Public	25,100	3%	8.2	9,400,000

Source: National Safety Council estimates (rounded) based on data from the National Center for Health Statistics, state departments of health, and state traffic authorities (except for the work figures, which are from the Bureau of Labor Statistics, Census of Fatal Occupational Injuries [CFOI]). The National Safety Council adopted the CFOI count for work-related unintentional injuries beginning with 1992. See the Glossary for definitions and the Technical Appendix for estimating procedures. Beginning with 1999 data, deaths are classified according to the 10th revision of the International Classification of Diseases. Caution should be used when comparing data classified under the two systems.
[a]Totals shown are approximations based on the National Safety Council's analysis of National Health Interview Survey results, which is conducted by the National Center for Health Statistics. The totals are the best estimates for the current year. They should not, however, be compared with totals shown in previous editions of this book to indicate year-to-year changes or trends. See the Glossary for definitions and the Technical Appendix for estimating procedures.
[b]Deaths and injuries for the four separate classes add to more than the "All classes" figures due to rounding and because some deaths and injuries are included in more than one class. For example, 1,407 work deaths involved motor vehicles and are in both the work and motor vehicle totals, and 200 motor vehicle deaths occurred on home premises and are in both home and motor vehicle. The total of such duplication amounted to about 1,607 deaths and 200,000 injuries in 2009.
[c]Less than 10,000.

ALL UNINTENTIONAL INJURIES, 2008
(CONT.)

3

UNINTENTIONAL INJURY DEATHS BY CLASS, UNITED STATES, 2009

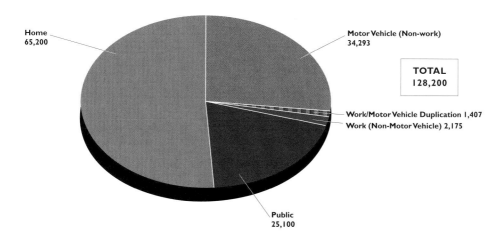

Home
65,200

Motor Vehicle (Non-work)
34,293

TOTAL
128,200

Work/Motor Vehicle Duplication 1,407
Work (Non-Motor Vehicle) 2,175

Public
25,100

UNINTENTIONAL MEDICALLY CONSULTED INJURIES BY CLASS, UNITED STATES, 2009

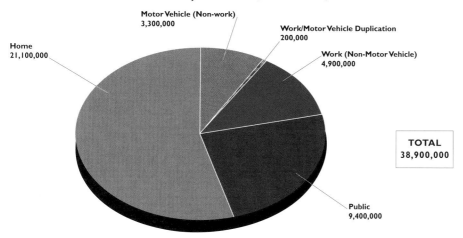

Motor Vehicle (Non-work)
3,300,000

Work/Motor Vehicle Duplication
200,000

Home
21,100,000

Work (Non-Motor Vehicle)
4,900,000

TOTAL
38,900,000

Public
9,400,000

COSTS OF UNINTENTIONAL INJURIES BY CLASS, 2009

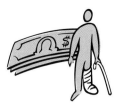

The total cost of unintentional injuries in 2009, $693.5 billion, includes estimates of economic costs of fatal and nonfatal unintentional injuries together with employers' uninsured costs, vehicle damage costs, and fire losses. Wage and productivity losses, medical expenses, administrative expenses, and employers' uninsured costs are included in all four classes of injuries. Cost components unique to each class are identified below.

Motor vehicle crash costs include property damage from motor vehicle accidents. Work costs include the value of property damage in on-the-job motor vehicle accidents and fires. Home and public costs include estimated fire losses, but do not include other property damage costs.

Besides the estimated $693.5 billion in economic losses

from unintentional injuries in 2009, lost quality of life from those injuries was valued at an additional $3,421.3 billion, making the comprehensive cost $4,114.8 billion in 2009.

Several cost benchmarks were updated for the 2005-2006 edition, making 2004 and later costs not comparable to previous years. The method used to estimate the number of medically attended injuries by class was revised to use the latest National Health Interview Survey data. Estimated property damage costs in motor vehicle crashes were rebenchmarked using National Highway Traffic Safety Administration data. The value of a statistical life also was updated, which affects only the comprehensive cost mentioned in the paragraph above.

CERTAIN COSTS OF UNINTENTIONAL INJURIES BY CLASS, 2009 ($ BILLIONS)

Cost	Total[a]	Motor vehicle	Work	Home	Public non-motor vehicle
Total	$693.5	$244.7	$168.9	$192.2	$108.2
Wage and productivity losses	357.4	83.1	82.4	126.4	69.2
Medical expenses	147.3	41.9	38.3	42.2	27.0
Administrative expenses[b]	117.2	78.3	33.1	11.1	7.0
Motor vehicle damage	39.4	39.4	2.0	(c)	(c)
Employers' uninsured costs	19.7	2.0	10.3	4.6	3.2
Fire loss	12.5	(c)	2.8	7.9	1.8

Source: National Safety Council estimates. See the Technical Appendix. Cost-estimating procedures were revised extensively for the 1993 edition of Accident Facts®. In general, cost estimates are not comparable from year to year. As additional data or new benchmarks become available, they are used from that point forward. Previously estimated figures are not revised.
[a]Duplication between work and motor vehicle, which amounted to $20.5 billion, was eliminated from the total.
[b]Home and public insurance administration costs may include costs of administering medical treatment claims for some motor vehicle injuries filed through health insurance plans.
[c]Not included, see comments above.

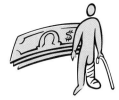

COSTS OF UNINTENTIONAL INJURIES BY CLASS, 2009

TOTAL COST
$693.5 BILLION

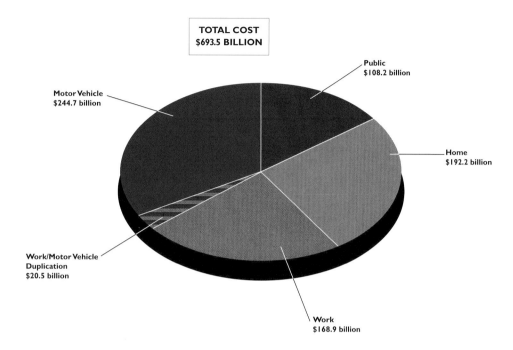

Public
$108.2 billion

Motor Vehicle
$244.7 billion

Home
$192.2 billion

Work/Motor Vehicle
Duplication
$20.5 billion

Work
$168.9 billion

COSTS OF UNINTENTIONAL INJURIES BY COMPONENT

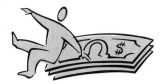

Wage and productivity losses

A person's contribution to the wealth of the nation usually is measured in terms of wages and household production. The total of wages and fringe benefits, together with an estimate of the replacement cost value of household services, provides an estimate of this lost productivity. Also included is travel delay for motor vehicle accidents.

Medical expenses

Doctor fees; hospital charges; the cost of medicines; future medical costs; and ambulance, helicopter, and other emergency medical services are included.

Administrative expenses

Includes the administrative cost of public and private insurance, and police and legal costs. Private insurance administrative costs are the difference between premiums paid to insurance companies and claims paid out by them. It is their cost of doing business and is part of the cost total. Claims paid by insurance companies are not identified separately, as every claim is compensation for losses such as wages, medical expenses, property damage, etc.

Motor vehicle damage

Includes the value of damage to vehicles from motor vehicle crashes. The cost of normal wear and tear to vehicles is not included.

Employers' uninsured costs

This is an estimate of the uninsured costs incurred by employers, representing the dollar value of time lost by uninjured workers. It includes time spent investigating and reporting injuries, administering first aid, hiring and training replacement workers, and the extra cost of overtime for uninjured workers.

Fire loss

Includes losses from structure fires and nonstructure fires such as vehicles, outside storage, crops, and timber.

Work—Motor vehicle duplication

The cost of motor vehicle crashes that involve people in the course of their work is included in both classes, but the duplication is eliminated from the total. The duplication in 2009 amounted to $20.5 billion and consisted of $3.7 billion in wage and productivity losses, $2.1 billion in medical expenses, $12.3 billion in administrative expenses, $2.0 billion in vehicle damage, and $0.4 billion in employers' uninsured costs.

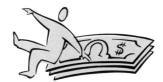

COSTS OF UNINTENTIONAL INJURIES BY COMPONENT, 2009

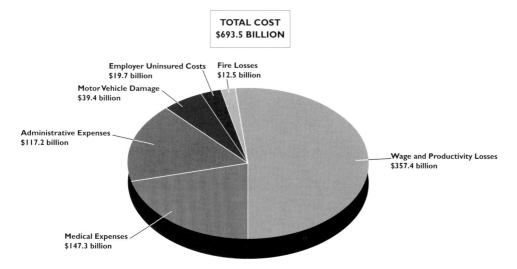

TOTAL COST
$693.5 BILLION

Employer Uninsured Costs
$19.7 billion

Fire Losses
$12.5 billion

Motor Vehicle Damage
$39.4 billion

Administrative Expenses
$117.2 billion

Wage and Productivity Losses
$357.4 billion

Medical Expenses
$147.3 billion

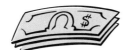

COST EQUIVALENTS

The costs of unintentional injuries are immense—billions of dollars. Because figures this large can be difficult to comprehend, it is sometimes useful to reduce the numbers to a more understandable scale by relating them to quantities encountered in everyday life. The table below shows how the costs of unintentional injuries compare to common quantities such as taxes, corporate profits, or stock dividends.

COST EQUIVALENTS, 2009

The cost of ...	Is equivalent to ...
...All injuries ($693.5 billion)	...84 cents of every dollar paid in federal personal income taxes **or** ...50 cents of every dollar spent on food in the United States
...Motor vehicle crashes ($244.7 billion)	...purchasing 400 gallons of gasoline for each registered vehicle in the United States **or** ...more than $1,200 per licensed driver
...Work injuries ($168.9 billion)	...29 cents of every dollar of corporate dividends to stockholders **or** ...12 cents of every dollar of pre-tax corporate profits **or** ...exceeds the combined profits reported by the 32 largest Fortune 500 companies
...Home injuries ($192.2 billion)	...a $369,500 rebate on each new single-family home built **or** ...46 cents of every dollar of property taxes paid
...Public injuries ($108.2 billion)	...a $11.7 million grant to each public library in the United States **or** ...a $95,000 bonus for each police officer and firefighter

Source: National Safety Council estimates

DEATHS DUE TO UNINTENTIONAL INJURIES, 2009

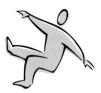

TYPE OF EVENT AND AGE OF VICTIM

All unintentional injuries

The term "unintentional" covers most deaths from injury and poisoning. Excluded are homicides (including legal intervention), suicides, deaths for which none of these categories can be determined, and war deaths.

	Total	Change from 2008	Death rate[a]
Deaths	128,200	+1.9%	41.8

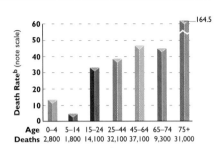

Age	0–4	5–14	15–24	25–44	45–64	65–74	75+
Deaths	2,800	1,800	14,100	32,100	37,100	9,300	31,000

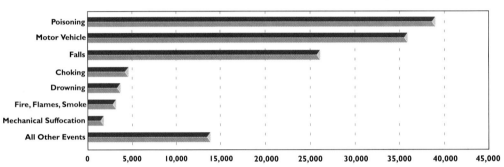

Poisoning

Includes deaths from drugs, medicines, other solid and liquid substances, and gases and vapors. Excludes poisonings from spoiled foods, salmonella, etc., which are classified as disease deaths.

	Total	Change from 2008	Death rate[a]
Deaths	39,000	+13%	12.7

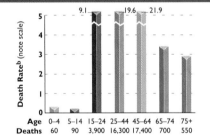

Age	0–4	5–14	15–24	25–44	45–64	65–74	75+
Deaths	60	90	3,900	16,300	17,400	700	550

Motor vehicle accidents

Includes deaths involving mechanically or electrically powered highway transport vehicles in motion (except those on rails), both on and off the highway or street.

	Total	Change from 2008	Death rate[a]
Deaths	35,900	-10%	11.7

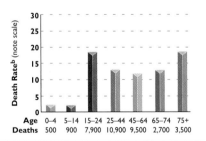

Age	0–4	5–14	15–24	25–44	45–64	65–74	75+
Deaths	500	900	7,900	10,900	9,500	2,700	3,500

Falls

Includes deaths from falls to another level or on the same level. Excludes falls in or from transport vehicles, or while boarding or alighting from them.

	Total	Change from 2008	Death rate[a]
Deaths	26,100	+7%	8.5

See footnotes on page 9.

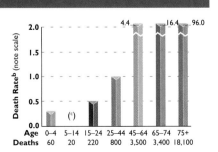

Age	0–4	5–14	15–24	25–44	45–64	65–74	75+
Deaths	60	20	220	800	3,500	3,400	18,100

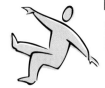

TYPE OF EVENT AND AGE OF VICTIM

Choking

Includes deaths from unintentional ingestion or inhalation of food or other objects resulting in the obstruction of respiratory passages.

	Total	Change from 2008	Death rate[a]
Deaths	4,600	(c)	1.5

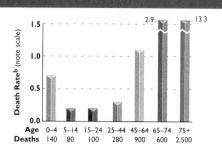

Drowning

Includes nontransport-related drownings such as those resulting from swimming, playing in the water, or falling in. Excludes drownings in floods and other cataclysms, which are classified to the cataclysm, and boating-related drownings.

	Total	Change from 2008	Death rate[a]
Deaths	3,700	+6%	1.2

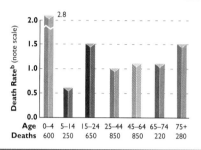

Fires, flames, and smoke

Includes deaths from exposure to fires, flames, and smoke and from injuries in fires, such as falls and struck by falling objects. Excludes burns from hot objects or liquids.

	Total	Change from 2008	Death rate[a]
Deaths	3,200	(c)	1.0

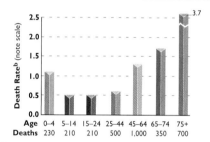

Mechanical suffocation

Includes deaths from hanging and strangulation, and suffocation in enclosed or confined spaces, cave-ins, or by bed clothes, plastic bags, or similar materials.

	Total	Change from 2008	Death rate[a]
Deaths	1,800	+6%	0.6

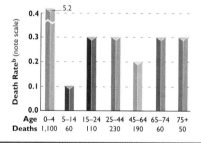

All other types

Most important types included are natural heat and cold; firearms; struck by or against object; machinery; electric current; and air, water, and rail transport.

	Total	Change from 2008	Death rate[a]
Deaths	13,900	–4%	4.5

Note: Category descriptions have changed due to adoption of ICD-10. See the Technical Appendix for comparability.
[a]Deaths per 100,000 population.
[b]Deaths per 100,000 population in each age group.
[c]Change less than 0.5%.

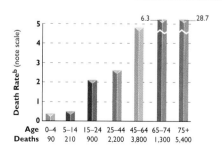

LEADING CAUSES OF DEATH

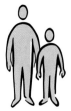

Unintentional injuries are the fifth leading cause of death overall and first among people 1 to 44 years old. By single years, unintentional injuries are the leading cause from age 1 to 42.

Causes are ranked for both sexes combined. Some leading causes for males and females separately may not

be shown. Beginning with 1999 data, deaths are classified according to the 10th revision of the International Classification of Diseases. See the Technical Appendix for comparability.

DEATHS AND DEATH RATES BY AGE AND SEX, 2007

Cause	Number of deaths			Death rates[a]		
	Total	Male	Female	Total	Male	Female
All ages[b]						
All causes	**2,423,712**	**1,203,968**	**1,219,744**	**804.4**	**810.9**	**798.1**
Heart disease	616,067	309,821	306,246	204.5	208.7	200.4
Cancer (malignant neoplasms)	562,875	292,857	270,018	186.8	197.3	176.7
Stroke (cerebrovascular disease)	135,952	54,111	81,841	45.1	36.4	53.6
Chronic lower respiratory diseases	127,924	61,235	66,689	42.5	41.2	43.6
Unintentional injuries	**123,706**	**79,827**	**43,879**	**41.1**	**53.8**	**28.7**
Motor vehicle	*43,945*	*31,102*	*12,843*	*14.6*	*20.9*	*8.4*
Poisoning	*29,846*	*19,644*	*10,202*	*9.9*	*13.2*	*6.7*
Falls	*22,631*	*11,597*	*11,034*	*7.5*	*7.8*	*7.2*
Choking[c]	*4,344*	*2,294*	*2,050*	*1.4*	*1.5*	*1.3*
Drowning	*3,443*	*2,681*	*762*	*1.1*	*1.8*	*0.5*
All other unintentional injuries	*19,497*	*12,509*	*6,988*	*6.5*	*8.4*	*4.6*
Alzheimer's disease	74,632	21,800	52,832	24.8	14.7	34.6
Diabetes mellitus	71,382	35,478	35,904	23.7	23.9	23.5
Influenza and pneumonia	52,717	24,071	28,646	17.5	16.2	18.7
Nephritis and nephrosis	46,448	22,616	23,832	15.4	15.2	15.6
Septicemia	34,828	15,839	18,989	11.6	10.7	12.4
Under 1 year						
All causes	**29,138**	**16,293**	**12,845**	**681.8**	**745.0**	**615.6**
Congenital anomalies	5,785	3,066	2,719	135.4	140.2	130.3
Short gestation, low birth weight, n.e.c.	4,857	2,677	2,180	113.7	122.4	104.5
Sudden infant death syndrome	2,453	1,422	1,031	57.4	65.0	49.4
Maternal complications of pregnancy	1,769	1,008	761	41.4	46.1	36.5
Unintentional injuries	**1,285**	**715**	**570**	**30.1**	**32.7**	**27.3**
Mechanical suffocation	*889*	*510*	*379*	*20.8*	*23.3*	*18.2*
Motor vehicle	*124*	*57*	*67*	*2.9*	*2.6*	*3.2*
Choking[c]	*70*	*38*	*32*	*1.6*	*1.7*	*1.5*
Drowning	*57*	*31*	*26*	*1.3*	*1.4*	*1.2*
Fires and flames	*38*	*20*	*18*	*0.9*	*0.9*	*0.9*
All other unintentional injuries	*107*	*59*	*48*	*2.5*	*2.7*	*2.3*
Complications of placenta, cord, membranes	1,135	630	505	26.6	28.8	24.2
Bacterial sepsis	820	466	354	19.2	21.3	17.0
Respiratory distress	789	472	317	18.5	21.6	15.2
Circulatory system disease	624	354	270	14.6	16.2	12.9
Neonatal hemorrhage	597	367	230	14.0	16.8	11.0
1 to 4 years						
All causes	**4,703**	**2,634**	**2,069**	**28.6**	**31.3**	**25.7**
Unintentional injuries	**1,588**	**987**	**601**	**9.6**	**11.7**	**7.5**
Motor vehicle	*551*	*309*	*242*	*3.3*	*3.7*	*3.0*
Drowning	*458*	*310*	*148*	*2.8*	*3.7*	*1.8*
Fires and flames	*201*	*130*	*71*	*1.2*	*1.5*	*0.9*
Choking[c]	*77*	*61*	*16*	*0.5*	*0.7*	*0.2*
Mechanical suffocation	*72*	*42*	*30*	*0.4*	*0.5*	*0.4*
All other unintentional injuries	*229*	*135*	*94*	*1.4*	*1.6*	*1.2*
Congenital anomalies	546	286	260	3.3	3.4	3.2
Homicide	398	213	185	2.4	2.5	2.3
Cancer (malignant neoplasms)	364	191	173	2.2	2.3	2.2
Heart disease	173	82	91	1.1	1.0	1.1
Influenza and pneumonia	109	55	54	0.7	0.7	0.7
Septicemia	78	44	34	0.5	0.5	0.4
Certain conditions originating in the perinatal period	70	34	36	0.4	0.4	0.4
Benign neoplasms	59	28	31	0.4	0.3	0.4
Chronic lower respiratory diseases	57	30	27	0.3	0.4	0.3

See source and footnotes on page 12.

LEADING CAUSES OF DEATH (CONT.)

DEATHS AND DEATH RATES BY AGE AND SEX, 2007 (Cont.)

Cause	Number of deaths			Death rates[a]		
	Total	Male	Female	Total	Male	Female
5 to 14 years						
All causes	**6,147**	**3,585**	**2,562**	**15.3**	**17.5**	**13.1**
Unintentional injuries	**2,194**	**1,346**	**848**	**5.5**	**6.6**	**4.3**
Motor vehicle	*1,285*	*765*	*520*	*3.2*	*3.7*	*2.7*
Drowning	*224*	*157*	*67*	*0.6*	*0.8*	*0.3*
Fires and flames	*211*	*116*	*95*	*0.5*	*0.6*	*0.5*
Poisoning	*81*	*50*	*31*	*0.2*	*0.2*	*0.2*
Mechanical suffocation	*72*	*50*	*22*	*0.2*	*0.2*	*0.1*
All other unintentional injuries	*321*	*208*	*113*	*0.8*	*1.0*	*0.6*
Cancer (malignant neoplasms)	959	499	460	2.4	2.4	2.3
Congenital anomalies	374	194	180	0.9	0.9	0.9
Homicide	346	210	136	0.9	1.0	0.7
Heart disease	241	133	108	0.6	0.6	0.6
Suicide	184	131	53	0.5	0.6	0.3
Chronic lower respiratory diseases	118	78	40	0.3	0.4	0.2
Influenza and pneumonia	103	52	51	0.3	0.3	0.3
Benign neoplasms	84	47	37	0.2	0.2	0.2
Stroke (cerebrovascular disease)	83	37	46	0.2	0.2	0.2
15 to 24 years						
All causes	**33,982**	**25,316**	**8,666**	**80.1**	**116.1**	**42.1**
Unintentional injuries	**15,897**	**11,905**	**3,992**	**37.5**	**54.6**	**19.4**
Motor vehicle	*10,568*	*7,667*	*2,901*	*24.9*	*35.2*	*14.1*
Poisoning	*3,159*	*2,430*	*729*	*7.4*	*11.1*	*3.5*
Drowning	*630*	*555*	*75*	*1.5*	*2.5*	*0.4*
Falls	*233*	*197*	*36*	*0.5*	*0.9*	*0.2*
Fires and flames	*194*	*124*	*70*	*0.5*	*0.6*	*0.3*
All other unintentional injuries	*1,113*	*932*	*181*	*2.6*	*4.3*	*0.9*
Homicide	5,551	4,829	722	13.1	22.2	3.5
Suicide	4,140	3,481	659	9.8	16.0	3.2
Cancer (malignant neoplasms)	1,653	987	666	3.9	4.5	3.2
Heart disease	1,084	700	384	2.6	3.2	1.9
Congenital anomalies	402	241	161	0.9	1.1	0.8
Stroke (cerebrovascular disease)	195	113	82	0.5	0.5	0.4
Diabetes mellitus	168	98	70	0.4	0.4	0.3
Influenza and pneumonia	163	91	72	0.4	0.4	0.3
Complicated pregnancy	160	0	160	0.4	0.0	0.8
Human immunodeficiency virus infection	160	88	72	0.4	0.4	0.3
Septicemia	160	85	75	0.4	0.4	0.4
25 to 34 years						
All causes	**42,572**	**29,792**	**12,780**	**105.4**	**144.8**	**64.5**
Unintentional injuries	**14,977**	**11,384**	**3,593**	**37.1**	**55.3**	**18.1**
Motor vehicle	*7,087*	*5,413*	*1,674*	*17.5*	*26.3*	*8.4*
Poisoning	*5,700*	*4,171*	*1,529*	*14.1*	*20.3*	*7.7*
Drowning	*381*	*330*	*51*	*0.9*	*1.6*	*0.3*
Falls	*334*	*288*	*46*	*0.8*	*1.4*	*0.2*
Fires and flames	*222*	*137*	*85*	*0.5*	*0.7*	*0.4*
All other unintentional injuries	*1,253*	*1,045*	*208*	*3.1*	*5.1*	*1.0*
Suicide	5,278	4,281	997	13.1	20.8	5.0
Homicide	4,758	4,019	739	11.8	19.5	3.7
Cancer (malignant neoplasms)	3,463	1,692	1,771	8.6	8.2	8.9
Heart disease	3,223	2,177	1,046	8.0	10.6	5.3
Human immunodeficiency virus infection	1,091	653	438	2.7	3.2	2.2
Diabetes mellitus	610	359	251	1.5	1.7	1.3
Stroke (cerebrovascular disease)	505	252	253	1.2	1.2	1.3
Congenital anomalies	417	243	174	1.0	1.2	0.9
Chronic liver disease and cirrhosis	384	261	123	1.0	1.3	0.6
35 to 44 years						
All causes	**79,606**	**50,105**	**29,501**	**184.8**	**232.2**	**137.2**
Unintentional injuries	**16,931**	**12,022**	**4,909**	**39.3**	**55.7**	**22.8**
Poisoning	*7,575*	*4,947*	*2,628*	*17.6*	*22.9*	*12.2*
Motor vehicle	*6,370*	*4,702*	*1,668*	*14.8*	*21.8*	*7.8*
Falls	*593*	*476*	*117*	*1.4*	*2.2*	*0.5*
Drowning	*417*	*334*	*83*	*1.0*	*1.5*	*0.4*
Fires and flames	*307*	*198*	*109*	*0.7*	*0.9*	*0.5*
All other unintentional injuries	*1,669*	*1,365*	*304*	*3.9*	*6.3*	*1.4*
Cancer (malignant neoplasms)	13,288	5,701	7,587	30.8	26.4	35.3
Heart disease	11,839	8,345	3,494	27.5	38.7	16.2
Suicide	6,722	5,152	1,570	15.6	23.9	7.3
Human immunodeficiency virus infection	3,572	2,506	1,066	8.3	11.6	5.0
Homicide	3,052	2,289	763	7.1	10.6	3.5
Chronic liver disease and cirrhosis	2,570	1,722	848	6.0	8.0	3.9
Stroke (cerebrovascular disease)	2,133	1,143	990	5.0	5.3	4.6
Diabetes mellitus	1,984	1,228	756	4.6	5.7	3.5
Septicemia	910	463	447	2.1	2.1	2.1

See source and footnotes on page 12.

LEADING CAUSES OF DEATH (CONT.)

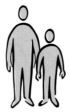

DEATHS AND DEATH RATES BY AGE AND SEX, 2007 (Cont.)

Cause	Number of deaths			Death rates[a]		
	Total	Male	Female	Total	Male	Female
45 to 54 years						
All causes	**184,686**	**114,456**	**70,230**	**421.0**	**530.1**	**315.2**
Cancer (malignant neoplasms)	50,167	25,370	24,797	114.3	117.5	111.3
Heart disease	37,434	26,911	10,523	85.3	124.6	47.2
Unintentional injuries	**20,315**	**14,017**	**6,298**	**46.3**	**64.9**	**28.3**
Poisoning	*9,006*	*5,535*	*3,471*	*20.5*	*25.6*	*15.6*
Motor vehicle	*6,530*	*4,789*	*1,741*	*14.9*	*22.2*	*7.8*
Falls	*1,304*	*982*	*322*	*3.0*	*4.5*	*1.4*
Fires and flames	*488*	*306*	*182*	*1.1*	*1.4*	*0.8*
Drowning	*481*	*385*	*96*	*1.1*	*1.8*	*0.4*
All other unintentional injuries	*2,506*	*2,020*	*486*	*5.7*	*9.4*	*2.2*
Chronic liver disease and cirrhosis	8,212	5,788	2,424	18.7	26.8	10.9
Suicide	7,778	5,824	1,954	17.7	27.0	8.8
Stroke (cerebrovascular disease)	6,385	3,507	2,878	14.6	16.2	12.9
Diabetes mellitus	5,753	3,513	2,240	13.1	16.3	10.1
Human immunodeficiency virus infection	4,156	3,028	1,128	9.5	14.0	5.1
Chronic lower respiratory diseases	4,153	2,125	2,028	9.5	9.8	9.1
Viral hepatitus	2,815	1,997	818	6.4	9.2	3.7
55 to 64 years						
All causes	**287,110**	**173,618**	**113,492**	**877.3**	**1,100.1**	**669.8**
Cancer (malignant neoplasms)	103,171	56,559	46,612	315.3	358.4	275.1
Heart disease	65,527	45,558	19,969	200.2	288.7	117.9
Chronic lower respiratory diseases	12,777	6,733	6,044	39.0	42.7	35.7
Unintentional injuries	**12,193**	**8,357**	**3,836**	**37.3**	**53.0**	**22.6**
Motor vehicle	*4,359*	*3,065*	*1,294*	*13.3*	*19.4*	*7.6*
Poisoning	*3,120*	*1,905*	*1,215*	*9.5*	*12.1*	*7.2*
Falls	*1,739*	*1,183*	*556*	*5.3*	*7.5*	*3.3*
Fires and flames	*492*	*330*	*162*	*1.5*	*2.1*	*1.0*
Choking[c]	*425*	*240*	*185*	*1.3*	*1.5*	*1.1*
All other unintentional injuries	*2,058*	*1,634*	*424*	*6.3*	*10.4*	*2.5*
Diabetes mellitus	11,304	6,644	4,660	34.5	42.1	27.5
Stroke (cerebrovascular disease)	10,500	5,992	4,508	32.1	38.0	26.6
Chronic liver disease and cirrhosis	8,004	5,732	2,272	24.5	36.3	13.4
Suicide	5,069	3,826	1,243	15.5	24.2	7.3
Nephritis and nephrosis	4,440	2,478	1,962	13.6	15.7	11.6
Septicemia	4,231	2,203	2,028	12.9	14.0	12.0
65 to 74 years						
All causes	**389,238**	**218,344**	**170,894**	**2,009.5**	**2,454.3**	**1,631.7**
Cancer (malignant neoplasms)	138,466	75,924	62,542	714.9	853.4	597.1
Heart disease	89,589	55,532	34,057	462.5	624.2	325.2
Chronic lower respiratory diseases	28,664	14,679	13,985	148.0	165.0	133.5
Stroke (cerebrovascular disease)	18,007	9,351	8,656	93.0	105.1	82.6
Diabetes mellitus	15,112	8,279	6,833	78.0	93.1	65.2
Unintentional injuries	**8,753**	**5,593**	**3,160**	**45.2**	**62.9**	**30.2**
Motor vehicle	*2,940*	*1,924*	*1,016*	*15.2*	*21.6*	*9.7*
Falls	*2,594*	*1,582*	*1,012*	*13.4*	*17.8*	*9.7*
Poisoning	*602*	*354*	*248*	*3.1*	*4.0*	*2.4*
Choking[c]	*561*	*323*	*238*	*2.9*	*3.6*	*2.3*
Fires and flames	*421*	*252*	*169*	*2.2*	*2.8*	*1.6*
All other unintentional injuries	*1,635*	*1,158*	*477*	*8.4*	*13.0*	*4.6*
Nephritis and nephrosis	7,752	4,044	3,708	40.0	45.5	35.4
Septicemia	6,345	3,256	3,089	32.8	36.6	29.5
Influenza and pneumonia	5,547	3,044	2,503	28.6	34.2	23.9
Chronic liver disease and cirrhosis	5,167	3,219	1,948	26.7	36.2	18.6
75 years and older[b]						
All causes	**1,366,530**	**569,825**	**796,705**	**7,357.7**	**8,022.4**	**6,946.1**
Heart disease	406,533	170,146	236,387	2,188.9	2,395.5	2,061.0
Cancer (malignant neoplasms)	251,272	125,895	125,377	1,352.9	1,772.4	1,093.1
Stroke (cerebrovascular disease)	97,960	33,619	64,341	527.4	473.3	561.0
Chronic lower respiratory diseases	80,904	36,925	43,979	435.6	519.9	383.4
Alzheimer's disease	69,816	19,730	50,086	375.9	277.8	436.7
Influenza and pneumonia	40,397	17,057	23,340	217.5	240.1	203.5
Diabetes mellitus	36,418	15,338	21,080	196.1	215.9	183.8
Nephritis and nephrosis	30,732	14,121	16,611	165.5	198.8	144.8
Unintentional injuries	**29,573**	**13,501**	**16,072**	**159.2**	**190.1**	**140.1**
Falls	*15,742*	*6,828*	*8,914*	*84.8*	*96.1*	*77.7*
Motor vehicle	*4,131*	*2,411*	*1,720*	*22.2*	*33.9*	*15.0*
Choking[c]	*2,529*	*1,186*	*1,343*	*13.6*	*16.7*	*11.7*
Fires and flames	*712*	*330*	*382*	*3.8*	*4.6*	*3.3*
Poisoning	*550*	*222*	*328*	*3.0*	*3.1*	*2.9*
All other unintentional injuries	*5,909*	*2,524*	*3,385*	*31.8*	*35.5*	*29.5*
Septicemia	20,019	8,133	11,886	107.8	114.5	103.6

Source: National Safety Council analysis of National Center for Health Statistics mortality data and U.S. Census Bureau population data.
[a]Deaths per 100,000 population in each age group.
[b]Includes 201 deaths where the age is unknown.
[c]Inhalation or ingestion of food or other objects.

The rank of unintentional injuries as a cause of death varies with race and Hispanic origin. While ranking fifth overall (following heart disease, cancer, stroke, and chronic lower respiratory diseases), unintentional injuries rank third for Hispanics after heart disease and cancer.

By race, unintentional injuries rank fifth for whites (after heart disease, cancer, stroke, and chronic lower respiratory diseases) and fourth for blacks, Asians, Pacific Islanders, American Indians, and Alaskan Natives.

UNINTENTIONAL INJURY DEATH RATES BY RACE, HISPANIC ORIGIN, AND SEX, UNITED STATES, 2007

| | Total | | | Hispanic origin | | | | | |
| | | | | Non-Hispanic | | | Hispanic | | |
Race and sex	Rank	Number	Rate	Rank	Number	Rate	Rank	Number	Rate
All races	5	123,706	41.1	5	111,641	43.6	3	11,723	25.8
Males	3	79,827	53.8	3	70,739	56.6	3	8,844	37.6
Females	6	43,879	28.7	6	40,902	31.2	5	2,879	13.1
White	5	106,252	44.1	5	94,584	47.5	3	11,414	(b)
Males	3	68,059	57.0	3	59,274	60.6	3	8,604	(b)
Females	6	38,193	31.4	6	35,310	34.8	5	2,810	(b)
Black	4	13,559	35.0	4	13,332	36.1	3	155	(b)
Males	3	9,268	50.1	3	9,093	51.7	3	121	(b)
Females	6	4,291	21.2	6	4,239	21.9	5	34	(b)
Not White or Black[a]	4	3,895	17.8	4	3,725	18.6	3	154	(b)
Males	3	2,500	23.4	3	2,372	24.3	3	119	(b)
Females	4	1,395	12.5	4	1,353	13.2	4	35	(b)

Source: National Safety Council analysis of National Center for Health Statistics mortality data and U.S. Census Bureau population data.
Note: Rates are deaths per 100,000 population in each race/sex/Hispanic origin group. Total column includes 342 deaths for which Hispanic origin was not determined.
[a]Includes American Indian, Alaskan Native, Asian, Native Hawaiian and Pacific Islander.
[b]Race is not well-reported for persons of Hispanic origin. Population death rates are unreliable.

LEADING CAUSES OF UNINTENTIONAL INJURY DEATH BY RACE, HISPANIC ORIGIN, AND SEX, UNITED STATES, 2007

| | All races | | | White | | | Black | | | Not White or Black[a] | | |
Cause of death	Both	Male	Female	Both	Male	Female	Both	Male	Female	Both	Male	Female
Total	123,706	79,827	43,879	106,252	68,059	38,193	13.559	9,268	4,291	3,895	2,500	1,395
Motor vehicle	43,945	31,102	12,843	36,653	25,903	10,750	5,519	4,058	1,461	1,773	1,141	632
Poisoning	29,846	19,644	10,202	25,973	17,135	8,838	3,273	2,150	1,123	600	359	241
Fall	22,631	11,597	11,034	21,020	10,643	10,377	1,015	602	413	596	358	244
Choking[b]	4,344	2,294	2,050	3,712	1,954	1,758	525	276	249	107	64	43
Drowning	3,443	2,681	762	2,714	2,090	624	511	419	92	218	172	46
Fires, flames, smoke	3,286	1,943	1,343	2,420	1,426	994	772	459	313	94	58	36
Population (thousands)	301,290	148,466	152,824	240,947	119,428	121,519	38,742	18,484	20,258	21,891	10,700	11,191

| | Non-Hispanic | | | Hispanic | | | Unknown | | |
Cause of death	Both	Male	Female	Both	Male	Female	Both	Male	Female
Total	111,641	70,739	40,902	11,723	8,844	2,879	342	244	98
Motor vehicle	38,013	26,626	11,387	5,824	4,390	1,434	108	86	22
Poisoning	27,307	17,640	9,667	2,436	1,943	493	103	61	42
Fall	21,374	10,803	10,571	1,212	762	450	45	32	13
Choking[b]	4,114	2,156	1,958	223	133	90	7	5	2
Drowning	2,946	2,256	690	480	410	70	17	15	2
Fires, flames, smoke	3,041	1,786	1,255	230	150	80	15	7	8
Population (thousands)	256,071	125,080	130,991	45,508	23,532	21,977	—	—	—

Source: National Safety Council analysis of National Center for Health Statistics mortality data.
Note: Dashes (—) indicate not applicable.
[a]Includes American Indian, Alaskan Native, Asian, Native Hawaiian and Pacific Islander.
[b]Suffocation by inhalation or ingestion.

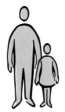

UNINTENTIONAL INJURY DEATHS BY AGE AND EVENT, UNITED STATES, 2007

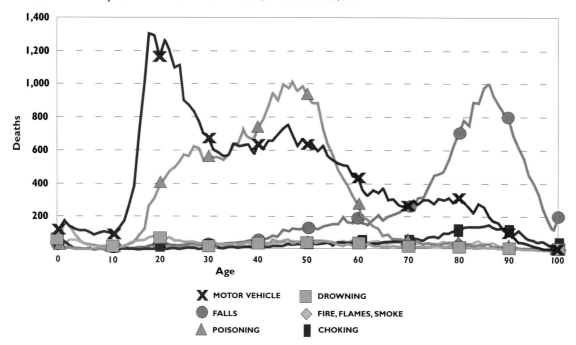

X MOTOR VEHICLE   ◼ DROWNING

● FALLS   ◆ FIRE, FLAMES, SMOKE

▲ POISONING   ◼ CHOKING

Motor vehicle crashes; poisonings; falls; choking (suffocation by inhalation or ingestion of food or other object); drownings; and fires, flames, and smoke were the six leading causes of unintentional injury death in the United States in 2007. The graph above depicts the number of deaths attributed to the top six causes by single years of age through age 99 and an aggregate age group of those 100 and older.

In 2007, motor vehicle crashes were the leading cause of unintentional injury death for all ages combined and the leading cause of unintentional injury death for each single year of age from 1 to 33, for age 35, and from ages 56 to 71. Among infants younger than 1 year old, motor vehicle death was second only to mechanical suffocation, which occurred more than 7 times as often.

The distribution of 2007 motor vehicle fatalities shows a sharp increase during adolescence, rising to 1,303 for 18 year olds from 383 for 15 year olds. The greatest number of motor vehicle fatalities in 2007 occurred to people age 18.

The second leading cause of unintentional injury death overall in 2007 was poisoning. Poisoning fatalities reached a high of 1,013 for 47 year olds and **poisoning was the leading cause of unintentional injury death for people age 34 and for those ages 36 to 55.** For these ages, motor vehicle deaths were the second leading cause of unintentional injury death. Poisonings were the second

most common cause of death for people age 14, for every single year of age from 16 to 33, at age 35, and from ages 56 to 62.

Falls were the third leading cause of unintentional injury death in the United States in 2007. **Falls were the leading cause of unintentional injury death of people age 72 and older** and the second leading cause for ages 63-71 for each year of age; deaths resulting from falls peaked at 997 for individuals age 86.

The fourth leading cause of unintentional injury death in the United States in 2007 was choking.[a] Choking deaths peaked at age 86 with 150 deaths. Choking was the second leading cause of unintentional injury death for people age 89 and older.

Drowning was the fifth leading cause of unintentional injury death in 2007, which peaked at 168 fatalities for 1 year olds. Drownings were the second leading cause of injury death for children ages 1-5, 8, 10, and 13-15 in 2007.

Fires, flames, and smoke were the sixth leading cause of unintentional injury death in 2007. Fatalities due to fires, flames, and smoke were neither the leading nor second leading cause of death for any age group, but peaked at 59 deaths among 3 year olds.

Source: National Safety Council tabulations of National Center for Health Statistics data. See the Technical Appendix for ICD-10 codes for the leading causes and comparability with prior years.
[a]*Inhalation or ingestion of food or other objects.*

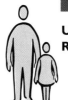

UNINTENTIONAL INJURY DEATH RATES BY AGE, 2007

UNINTENTIONAL INJURY DEATHS PER 100,000 POPULATION BY AGE AND EVENT, UNITED STATES, 2007

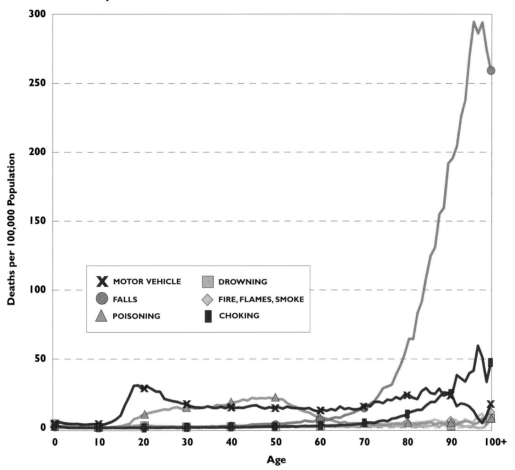

The graph above depicts U.S. death rates per 100,000 population for the six leading causes of unintentional injury deaths in 2007 for single years of age through age 99 and an aggregate age group of people 100 years of age and older.

Unintentional motor vehicle fatalities had the highest overall death rate, with an average of 14.6 deaths per 100,000 population. Motor vehicle death rates in 2007 peaked at 30.9 for people age 19, closely followed by a rate of 30.6 for people age 18. This rate generally declined for those ages 30 to 70, where it began an increase to another peak at 28.9 for people age 85, followed by a secondary peak at 28.5 for those age 88.

Poisoning had the second highest overall death rate from unintentional injury in the United States, with an average rate of 9.9 deaths per 100,000 population. The poisoning death rate remains low until about age 16, where it starts to increase steadily up to its peak rate of 21.9 at 49 years of age and then falls again.

While motor vehicle crashes are a significant problem

for all ages, deaths resulting from falls for certain older ages had even higher death rates. Beginning at about age 70, the death rate from falls increases dramatically. At age 72, the falls death rate surpassed that for motor vehicle, with the death rate continuing to rise steeply with increasing age, peaking at age 98 with a rate of 294.2. Based on 100,000 population, falls have an overall fatality rate of 7.5.

Death rates due to choking on inhaled or ingested food or other objects were quite low for most ages. Rates rise rapidly beginning at about age 70. While relatively stable and low for all ages, the death rates for drownings show peaks in the first few years of life and again at some very old ages. Death rates for fire, flames, and smoke were only slightly elevated at very young ages and began to climb at about age 75. The overall death rates per 100,000 U.S. population for choking; drowning; and fire, flames and smoke do not exceed 1.4.

Source: National Safety Council tabulations of National Center for Health Statistics mortality data and U.S. Census Bureau population data. See the Technical Appendix for ICD-10 codes for the leading causes and comparability with prior years.
[a]Inhalation or ingestion of food or other objects.

UNINTENTIONAL INJURY DEATHS BY SEX AND AGE, 2007

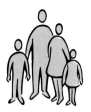

UNINTENTIONAL INJURY DEATHS BY SEX AND AGE, UNITED STATES, 2007

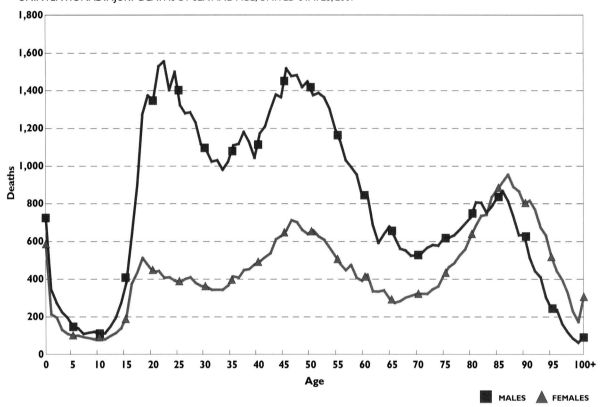

Males incur more deaths due to unintentional injuries than females at all ages from birth to age 82. The difference between the unintentional injury death totals ranges from 10 more male deaths than female deaths at age 82 to 1,164 more deaths at age 22. The excess number of deaths for males compared to females is most evident from the late teenage years to the mid-fifties, where the gap begins to narrow. From age 83 on, deaths of females exceed those of males by as little as 42 at age 84 to as much as 333 deaths nationwide at age 93.

Unintentional injury deaths are at their lowest level for both sexes from about age 4 to about age 13. For males, the highest number of deaths (1,562) occurs at age 22,

with high totals—including another peak of 1,523 deaths for those age 45—occurring from the mid-teens until the late fifties. For females, however, the highest totals occur among the elderly throughout the eighties and into the early nineties. The greatest number of female deaths (952) occurs at age 86.

The graph above shows the number of unintentional injury deaths in the United States during 2007 for each sex by single years of age from younger than 1 to age 99 and an aggregate age group of those 100 years of age and older. It is based on death certificate data from the National Center for Health Statistics.

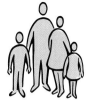

UNINTENTIONAL INJURY DEATHS PER 100,000 POPULATION BY SEX AND AGE, UNITED STATES, 2007

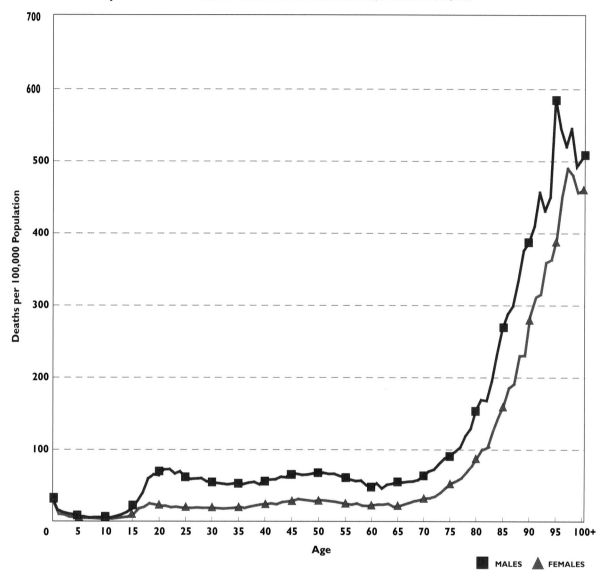

Throughout their lifespan, males have greater unintentional injury death rates for each year of age compared to females. The graph above shows the unintentional injury death rates for males and females by single years of age from younger than 1 to age 99 and an aggregate age group of people 100 years of age and older. It is based on National Center for Health Statistics mortality data and U.S. Census Bureau population data.

Death rates for both sexes were lowest from birth until the mid-teenage years, where rates rise rapidly. Rates then remain fairly constant until the early seventies, where they again rise steadily with increasing age. Across all ages, males had an overall death rate of 53.8 unintentional injury deaths per 100,000 males, while the rate among females in the United States was 28.7. The overall unintentional injury death rate for all ages and both sexes was 41.1 deaths per 100,000 population.

ALL DEATHS DUE TO INJURY

MORTALITY BY SELECTED EXTERNAL CAUSES, UNITED STATES, 2005-2007

Type of accident or manner of injury	2007[a]	2006	2005
All external causes of mortality, V01–Y89, *U01, *U03[b]	185,076	181,586	176,406
Deaths due to unintentional (accidental) injuries, V01–X59, Y85–Y86	123,706	121,599	117,809
Transport accidents, V01–V99, Y85	46,844	48,412	48,441
Motor vehicle accidents, V02–V04, V09.0, V09.2, V12–V14, V19.0–V19.2, V19.4–V19.6, V20–V79, V80.3–V80.5, V81.0–V81.1, V82.0–V82.1, V83–V86, V87.0–V87.8, V88.0–V88.8, V89.0, V89.2	43,945	45,316	45,343
Pedestrian, V01–V09	5,958	6,162	6,074
Pedalcyclist, V10–V19	820	926	927
Motorcycle rider, V20–V29	5,024	4,787	4,387
Occupant of three-wheeled motor vehicle, V30–V39	10	17	5
Car occupant, V40–V49	12,772	14,119	14,584
Occupant of pick-up truck or van, V50–V59	3,100	3,411	3,797
Occupant of heavy transport vehicle, V60–V69	441	432	450
Bus occupant, V70–V79	43	36	59
Animal rider or occupant of animal-drawn vehicle, V80	101	126	120
Occupant of railway train or railway vehicle, V81	17	17	33
Occupant of streetcar, V82	2	2	0
Other and unspecified land transport accidents, V83–V89	16,740	16,462	16,148
Occupant of special industrial vehicle, V83	*14*	*13*	*19*
Occupant of special agricultural vehicle, V84	*148*	*135*	*154*
Occupant of special construction vehicle, V85	*26*	*32*	*33*
Occupant of all-terrain or other off-road motor vehicle, V86	*1,093*	*1,073*	*1,040*
Other and unspecified person, V87–V89	*15,459*	*15,209*	*14,902*
Water transport accidents, V90–V94	486	514	523
Drowning, V90, V92	*349*	*351*	*394*
Other and unspecified injuries, V91, V93–V94	*137*	*163*	*129*
Air and space transport accidents, V95–V97	550	655	590
Other and unspecified transport accidents and sequelae, V98–V99, Y85	780	746	744
Other specified transport accidents, V98	*0*	*0*	*2*
Unspecified transport accident, V99	*3*	*19*	*18*
Nontransport unintentional (accidental) injuries, W00–X59, Y86	**76,862**	**73,187**	**69,368**
Falls, W00–W19	22,631	20,823	19,656
Fall on same level from slipping, tripping and stumbling, W01	*691*	*687*	*698*
Other fall on same level, W00, W02–W03, W18	*6,264*	*5,539*	*5,224*
Fall involving bed, chair or other furniture, W06–W08	*984*	*906*	*899*
Fall on and from stairs and steps, W10	*1,917*	*1,818*	*1,690*
Fall on and from ladder or scaffolding, W11–W12	*434*	*468*	*477*
Fall out of or through building or structure, W13	*587*	*628*	*533*
Other fall from one level to another, W09, W14–W17	*695*	*700*	*694*
Other and unspecified fall, W04–W05, W19	*11,059*	*10,077*	*9,441*
Exposure to inanimate mechanical forces, W20–W49	2,591	2,726	2,845
Struck by or striking against object, W20–W22	*812*	*843*	*854*
Caught between objects, W23	*153*	*119*	*103*
Contact with machinery, W24, W30–W31	*659*	*740*	*755*
Contact with sharp objects, W25–W29	*104*	*119*	*85*
Firearms discharge, W32–W34	*613*	*642*	*789*
Explosion and rupture of pressurized devices, W35–W38	*39*	*44*	*26*
Fireworks discharge, W39	*10*	*8*	*4*
Explosion of other materials, W40	*111*	*140*	*147*
Foreign body entering through skin or natural orifice, W44–W45	*30*	*30*	*37*
Other and unspecified inanimate mechanical forces, W41–W43, W49	*60*	*41*	*45*
Exposure to animate mechanical forces, W50–W64	148	138	161
Struck by or against another person, W50–W52	*20*	*12*	*26*
Bitten or struck by dog, W54	*32*	*32*	*33*
Bitten or struck by other mammals, W53, W55	*76*	*73*	*80*
Bitten or stung by nonvenomous insect and other arthropods, W57	*11*	*7*	*9*
Bitten or crushed by other reptiles, W59	*0*	*1*	*0*
Other and unspecified animate mechanical forces, W56, W58, W60, W64	*9*	*13*	*13*
Accidental drowning and submersion, W65–W74	3,443	3,579	3,582
Drowning and submersion while in or falling into bath tub, W65–W66	*396*	*413*	*344*
Drowning and submersion while in or falling into swimming pool, W67–W68	*705*	*698*	*607*
Drowning and submersion while in or falling into natural water, W69–W70	*1,630*	*1,611*	*1,603*
Other and unspecified drowning and submersion, W73–W74	*712*	*857*	*1,028*
Other accidental threats to breathing, W75–W84	5,997	5,912	5,900
Accidental suffocation and strangulation in bed, W75	*741*	*661*	*573*
Other accidental hanging and strangulation, W76	*244*	*283*	*274*
Threat to breathing due to cave-in, falling earth and other substances, W77	*42*	*44*	*50*
Inhalation of gastric contents, W78	*315*	*351*	*333*
Inhalation and ingestion of food causing obstruction of respiratory tract, W79	*940*	*872*	*864*
Inhalation and ingestion of other objects causing obstruction of respiratory tract, W80	*3,089*	*3,109*	*3,189*
Confined to or trapped in a low-oxygen environment, W81	*25*	*7*	*14*
Other and unspecified threats to breathing, W83–W84	*601*	*585*	*603*

See source and footnotes on page 19.

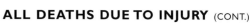

ALL DEATHS DUE TO INJURY (CONT.)

ALL DEATHS DUE TO INJURY (CONT.)

MORTALITY BY SELECTED EXTERNAL CAUSES, UNITED STATES, 2005-2007 (Cont.)

Type of accident or manner of injury	2007[a]	2006	2005
Exposure to electric current, radiation, temperature and pressure, W85–W99	389	408	420
Electric transmission lines, W85	88	93	105
Other and unspecified electric current, W86–W87	281	299	293
Radiation, W88–W91	0	0	0
Excessive heat or cold of man-made origin, W92–W93	8	6	13
High and low air pressure and changes in air pressure, W94	12	10	9
Other and unspecified man-made environmental factors, W99	0	0	0
Exposure to smoke, fire and flames, X00–X09	3,286	3,109	3,197
Uncontrolled fire in building or structure, X00	2,655	2,511	2,617
Uncontrolled fire not in building or structure, X01	65	65	52
Controlled fire in building or structure, X02	42	36	28
Controlled fire not in building or structure, X03	30	37	33
Ignition of highly flammable material, X04	59	65	63
Ignition or melting of nightwear, X05	3	5	6
Ignition or melting of other clothing and apparel, X06	113	99	97
Other and unspecified smoke, fire and flames, X08–X09	319	291	301
Contact with heat and hot substances, X10–X19	89	93	102
Contact with hot tap water, X11	34	32	43
Other and unspecified heat and hot substances, X10, X12–X19	55	61	59
Contact with venomous animals and plants, X20–X29	73	83	105
Contact with venomous snakes and lizards, X20	7	8	7
Contact with venomous spiders, X21	8	4	10
Contact with hornets, wasps and bees, X23	54	61	82
Contact with other and unspecified venomous animal or plant, X22, X24–X29	4	10	6
Exposure to forces of nature, X30–X39	1,217	1,340	2,179
Exposure to excessive natural heat, X30	309	622	466
Exposure to excessive natural cold, X31	711	519	700
Lightning, X33	46	47	48
Earthquake and other earth movements, X34–X36	26	25	37
Cataclysmic storm, X37	84	75	874
Flood, X38	22	10	12
Exposure to other and unspecified forces of nature, X32, X39	19	42	42
Accidental poisoning by and exposure to noxious substances, X40–X49	29,846	27,531	23,618
Nonopioid analgesics, antipyretics and antirheumatics, X40	290	246	226
Antiepileptic, sedative-hypnotic, antiparkinsonism and psychotropic drugs n.e.c., X41	1,545	1,486	1,496
Narcotics and psychodysleptics (hallucinogens) n.e.c., X42	13,030	13,302	11,050
Other and unspecified drugs, medicaments, and biologicals, X43–X44	12,793	11,366	9,676
Alcohol, X45	1,356	352	346
Gases and vapors, X46–X47	680	656	703
Other and unspecified chemicals and noxious substances, X48–X49	152	123	121
Overexertion, travel and privation, X50–X57	20	36	32
Accidental exposure to other and unspecified factors and sequelae, X58–X59, Y86	7,132	7,409	7,571
Intentional self-harm, X60–X84, Y87.0, *U03	**34,598**	**33,300**	**32,637**
Intentional self-poisoning, X60–X69	6,358	6,109	5,744
Intentional self-harm by hanging, strangulation and suffocation, X70	8,161	7,491	7,248
Intentional self-harm by firearm, X72–X74	17,352	16,883	17,002
Other and unspecified means and sequelae, X71, X75–X84, Y87.0	2,727	2,817	2,643
Terrorism, *U03	0	0	0
Assault, X85–Y09, Y87.1, *U01	**18,361**	**18,573**	**18,124**
Assault by firearm, X93–X95	12,632	12,791	12,352
Assault by sharp object, X99	1,981	2,080	2,097
Other and unspecified means and sequelae, X85–X92, X96–X98, Y00–Y09, Y87.1	3,748	3,702	3,675
Terrorism, *U01	0	0	0
Event of undetermined intent, Y10–Y34, Y87.2, Y89.9	**5,381**	**5,131**	**4,742**
Poisoning, Y10–Y19	3,770	3,541	3,240
Hanging, strangulation and suffocation, Y20	135	152	139
Drowning and submersion, Y21	236	255	242
Firearm discharge, Y22–Y24	276	220	221
Exposure to smoke, fire and flames, Y26	98	128	120
Falling, jumping or pushed from a high place, Y30	66	80	69
Other and unspecified means and sequelae, Y25, Y27–Y29, Y31–Y34, Y87.2, Y89.9	800	755	711
Legal intervention, Y35, Y89.0	**412**	**434**	**414**
Legal intervention involving firearm discharge, Y35.0	351	360	330
Legal execution, Y35.5	40	48	54
Other and unspecified means and sequelae, Y35.1–Y35.4, Y35.6–Y35.7, Y89.0	21	26	30
Operations of war and sequelae, Y36, Y89.1	**21**	**28**	**27**
Complications of medical and surgical care and sequelae, Y40–Y84, Y88.0–Y88.3	**2,597**	**2,521**	**2,653**

Source: National Center for Health Statistics. Deaths are classified on the basis of the 10th revision of The International Classification of Diseases (ICD-10), which went into effect in 1999.
Note: "n.e.c." means "not elsewhere classified."
[a]*Latest official figures.*
[b]*Numbers following titles refer to external cause of injury and poisoning classifications in ICD-10.*

DEATHS BY AGE, SEX, AND TYPE

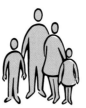

UNINTENTIONAL INJURY DEATHS BY AGE, SEX, AND TYPE, UNITED STATES, 2007[a]

Age & sex	Total[b]	Motor vehicle	Poisoning	Falls	Choking[c]	Drowning[d]	Fires, flames, smoke	Mechanical suffocation	Natural heat/cold	All types	
										Males	Females
Total	123,706	43,945	29,846	22,631	4,344	3,443	3,286	1,653	1,020	79,827	43,879
0-4	2,873	675	53	60	147	515	239	961	30	1,702	1,171
5-14	2,194	1,285	81	32	30	224	211	72	7	1,346	848
15-24	15,897	10,568	3,159	233	42	630	194	91	38	11,905	3,992
25-44	31,908	13,457	13,275	927	262	798	529	220	160	23,406	8,502
45-64	32,508	10,889	12,126	3,043	773	805	980	190	368	22,374	10,134
65-74	8,753	2,940	602	2,594	561	194	421	48	116	5,593	3,160
75+	29,573	4,131	550	15,742	2,529	277	712	71	301	13,501	16,072
Males	79,827	31,102	19,644	11,597	2,294	2,681	1,943	1,069	693		
Females	43,879	12,843	10,202	11,034	2,050	762	1,343	584	327		

Source: National Safety Council analysis of National Center for Health Statistics mortality data.
[a]Latest official figures.
[b]Includes types not shown separately.
[c]Inhalation or ingestion of food or other object obstructing breathing.
[d]Excludes water transport drownings.

Of the 123,706 unintentional injury deaths in 2007, males accounted for 65% of all deaths. Females had the greatest share of deaths only in the 75 and older age group (54% female). For each type of accident listed above, males are disproportionably represented over females. The largest differences in the proportion of fatalities include drowning (78% male) and motor vehicle deaths (71% male). The smallest difference between the proportion of male and female fatalities includes falls (51% male) and choking (53% male).

UNINTENTIONAL INJURY DEATH RATES BY TYPE AND SEX, UNITED STATES, 2007[a]

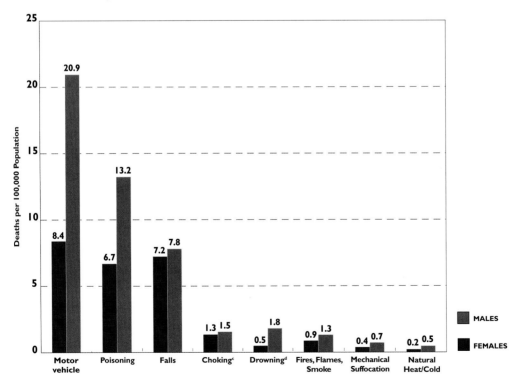

[a]Latest official figures.
[b]Includes types not shown separately.
[c]Inhalation or ingestion of food or other object obstructing breathing.
[d]Excludes water transport drownings.

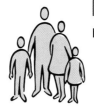
UNINTENTIONAL INJURY DEATHS BY MONTH AND TYPE, UNITED STATES, 2007[a]

Month	All types	Motor vehicle	Poisoning	Falls	Choking[b]	Drowning[c]	Fires, flames, smoke	Mechanical suffocation	Natural heat/cold	Struck by/ against	All other types
Total	**123,706**	**43,945**	**29,846**	**22,631**	**4,344**	**3,443**	**3,286**	**1,653**	**1,020**	**812**	**12,726**
January	10,058	3,227	2,622	1,905	377	127	418	127	152	63	1,040
February	9,526	3,083	2,501	1,746	388	128	388	114	177	64	937
March	10,466	3,688	2,603	1,926	363	222	324	131	66	52	1,091
April	10,046	3,566	2,532	1,819	369	236	274	114	38	57	1,041
May	10,376	3,881	2,400	1,754	339	369	258	179	25	68	1,103
June	10,362	3,860	2,414	1,752	319	523	184	140	41	52	1,077
July	10,998	4,079	2,451	1,895	327	570	203	148	74	88	1,163
August	10,837	3,915	2,443	1,863	349	519	177	158	147	85	1,181
September	10,242	3,790	2,419	1,920	328	292	174	134	48	62	1,075
October	10,288	3,769	2,374	2,011	386	202	213	149	24	88	1,072
November	9,926	3,606	2,399	1,936	368	116	282	123	71	75	950
December	10,581	3,481	2,688	2,104	431	139	391	136	157	58	996
Average	**10,309**	**3,662**	**2,487**	**1,886**	**362**	**287**	**274**	**138**	**85**	**68**	**1,061**

Source: National Safety Council analysis of National Center for Health Statistics mortality data.
[a]*Latest official figures.*
[b]*Inhalation or ingestion of food or other object obstructing breathing.*
[c]*Excludes water transport drownings.*

UNINTENTIONAL INJURY DEATHS BY MONTH AND TYPE, UNITED STATES, 2007[a]

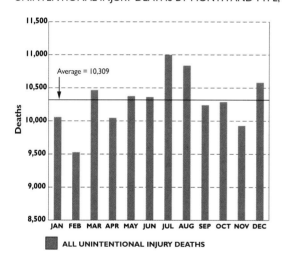

ALL UNINTENTIONAL INJURY DEATHS

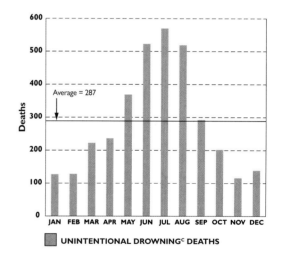

UNINTENTIONAL DROWNING[c] DEATHS

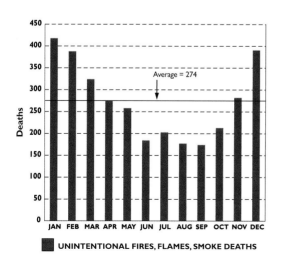

UNINTENTIONAL FIRES, FLAMES, SMOKE DEATHS

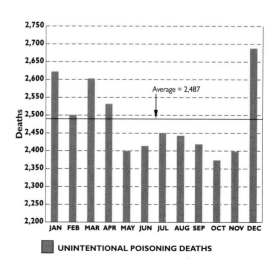

UNINTENTIONAL POISONING DEATHS

See page 117 for motor vehicle deaths by month and page 53 for pedalcycle deaths by month.

THE NATIONAL HEALTH INTERVIEW SURVEY, 2008

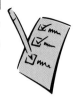

The National Health Interview Survey, conducted by the National Center for Health Statistics, is a continuous, personal interview sampling of households to obtain information about the health status of household members, including injuries experienced during the five weeks prior to the interview.

Responsible family members residing in the household supplied the information found in the survey. In 2008, interviews were completed for 74,236 people living in 28,790 households throughout the United States. See page 23 for definitions.

NUMBER OF LEADING EXTERNAL CAUSES OF INJURY AND POISONING EPISODES BY AGE, UNITED STATES, 2008

| | Population[a] (000) | External cause of injury and poisoning (number in thousands) | | | | | | |
		Falls	Struck by or against person or object	Trans-portation[b]	Overexertion	Cutting-piercing instruments	Other injury causes[b]	Poisoning[b]
All ages	298,688	12,804	3,684	4,223	4,046	2,144	5,741	614[d]
Under 12 years	24,888	2,599	693	(c)	248[d]	(c)	673	(c)
12-17 years	110,154	1,261	576[d]	424[d]	859	310[d]	1,073	(c)
18-44 years	77,518	3,381	1,315	2,468	1,489	1,208	2,547	164[d]
45-64 years	19,879	3,236	758	635	1,080	392[d]	964	305[d]
65-74 years	17,353	853	(c)	403[d]	(c)	(c)	(c)	0
75 years & older	24,888	1,474	234[d]	(c)	(c)	0	295[d]	0

[a]Civilian noninstitutionalized population.
[b]"Transportation" includes motor vehicle, bicycle, motorcycle, pedestrian, train, boat, or airplane. "Poisoning" does not include food poisoning or allergic reaction. "Other injury causes" includes fire/burn/scald-related, animal or insect bites, machinery, and unspecified causes.
[c]Estimate is not shown because it does not meet standard of reliability or precision.
[d]Estimate does not meet standard of reliability or precision and should be used with caution.

LEADING EXTERNAL CAUSES OF INJURY AND POISONING EPISODES BY SEX, UNITED STATES, 2008

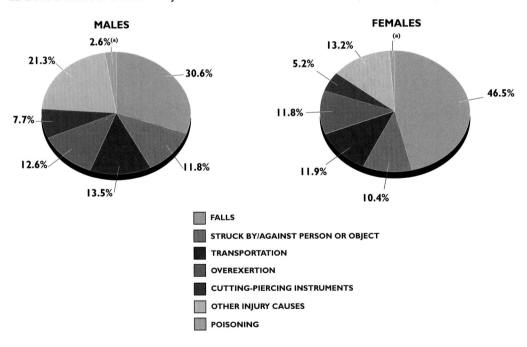

[a]For females, poisoning estimate is not shown because it does not meet standard of reliability or precision. For males, poisoning estimate does not meet standard of reliability or precision and should be used with caution.

Source: Adams, P.F., Barnes, P.M., and Vickerie, J.L. (2009, December). Summary health statistics for the U.S. population: National Health Interview Survey, 2008. National Center for Health Statistics. Vital and Health Statistics, Series 10 (No. 243).

In 2008, an estimated 33.2 million medically consulted injury and poisoning episodes were recorded, of which 50.2% were among males and 49.8% among females. The overall injury rate was 111 episodes per 1,000 population, with males experiencing higher rates (114 per 1,000 males) than females (109 per 1,000 females). Most injuries occurred in or around the home (42.9%), followed by injuries on streets, highways, sidewalks, and parking lots (14.0%), and injuries at recreational and sport facilities (12.5%). Nationwide, injuries in public areas, such as schools, hospitals, streets, recreational facilities, industrial and trade areas, and public buildings, accounted for 47.0% of the total injuries.

Among the 16.7 million injuries reported for males, the single most common place of occurrence was at home, with 17.2% occurring inside the home while injuries occurring outside contributed an additional 19.7%. Nearly half of the injuries among females occurred at home. More than twice as many injuries to females occurred inside the home than outside, consistent with 2007 NHIS findings. Streets, parking lots, sidewalks, and highways, as well as sport facilities and recreational areas, were the next most common locations for injuries among females, accounting for 14.6% and 9.3% of injuries, respectively. For males, sport facilities and recreational areas were the most common non-home places for injuries to occur (15.8%), followed by streets, parking lots, sidewalks, and highways (13.4%).

The 2008 NHIS injury definitions are listed below for comparability with prior years and other injury figures published in *Injury Facts*.

NUMBER AND PERCENT OF INJURY EPISODES BY PLACE OF OCCURRENCE AND SEX, UNITED STATES, 2008

Place of occurrence of injury episode	Both sexes		Male		Female	
	Number of episodes (000)	%	Number of episodes (000)	%	Number of episodes (000)	%
Total episodes[a]	33,255	100.0%	16,692	100.0%	16,563	100.0%
Home (inside)	8,344	25.1	2,877	17.2	5,466	33.0
Home (outside)	5,925	17.8	3,296	19.7	2,628	15.9
School/child care center/preschool	3,361	10.1	1,958	11.7	1,403[c]	8.5
Hospital/residential institution	570[c]	1.7	(b)	—	421[c]	2.5
Street/highway/sidewalk/parking lot	4,665	14.0	2,242	13.4	2,423	14.6
Sport facility/recreation area/lake/river/pool	4,172	12.5	2,639	15.8	1,533	9.3
Industrial/construction/farm	922	2.8	795	4.8	(b)	—
Trade/service area	1,661	5.0	927	5.6	734	4.4
Other public building	449[c]	1.4	(b)	—	302[c]	1.8
Other (unspecified)	3,165	9.5	1,431	8.6	1,733	10.5

Source: Adams, P.F., Barnes, P.M., and Vickerie, J.L. (2009, December). Summary health statistics for the U.S. population: National Health Interview Survey, 2008. National Center for Health Statistics. Vital and Health Statistics, Series 10 (No. 243).
[a]Numbers and percents may not sum to respective totals due to rounding and unknowns.
[b]Estimate is not shown because it does not meet standard of reliability or precision.
[c]Estimate does not meet standard of reliability or precision and should be used with caution.

Injury definitions

National Health Interview Survey definitions. The 2008 National Health Interview Survey figures include medically consulted injury and poisoning episodes (e.g., call to a poison control center; use of an emergency vehicle or emergency department; visit to a doctor's office or other health clinic; phone call to a doctor, nurse, or other health care professional) that reportedly occurred during the three months prior to the date of the interview and resulted in one or more conditions. Beginning in 2004, injury and poisoning estimates were calculated using only those episodes that occurred five weeks or less before the interview date. This reflects a change from 1997-2003, when NHIS data contained injury and poisoning episodes that were reported to occur within four months of the interview, and estimates were calculated using a three-month recall period. Also, an imputation procedure was performed for injury and poisoning episodes to assign a date of occurrence if it was not reported. Therefore, figures for 2004 and subsequent years are not comparable to estimates from prior years.

In the 2008 NHIS Injury and Poisoning file, an injury episode refers to the traumatic event in which the person was injured one or more times from an external cause (e.g., a fall, a motor vehicle traffic accident). An injury condition is the acute condition or the physical harm caused by the traumatic event. Likewise, a poisoning episode refers to the event resulting from ingestion of or contact with harmful substances, as well as overdoses or wrong use of any drug or medication, while a poisoning condition is the acute condition or the physical harm caused by the event. Each episode must have at least one injury condition or poisoning classified according to the nature-of-injury codes 800–909.2, 909.4, 909.9, 910–994.9, 995.5–995.59, and 995.80–995.85 in the 9th revision of the International Classification of Diseases (ICD-9-CM). Poisoning episodes exclude food poisoning, sun poisoning, or poison ivy rashes.

National Safety Council definition of injury. A medically consulted injury is defined as one that is serious enough that a medical professional was consulted, or is a recordable work injury based on OSHA definitions (see Glossary). All injury totals labeled "medically consulted" in *Injury Facts* are based on this definition.

THE NATIONAL HEALTH INTERVIEW SURVEY, 2008 (CONT.)

24

Of the 33.2 million medically consulted injuries in 2008, 41.3% were related to sports and leisure activities. Sports and leisure injuries accounted for 63.1% of all injury episodes among children younger than 12 and 78.6% of injury episodes among teenagers between the ages of 12 and 17.

The rate of injuries occurring during leisure activities was similar for both sexes (25 cases per 1,000 males and 30 cases per 1,000 females). However, the rate of sports injuries among males (26 per 1,000 males) was substantially higher than among females (11 per 1,000 females). The charts on this page illustrate these gender differences in terms of percentages and rates.

NUMBER OF INJURY EPISODES BY AGE AND ACTIVITY AT TIME OF INJURY, UNITED STATES, 2008

	Total episodes[a] (000)	Activity at time of injury[b] (number in thousands)						
		Driving[c]	Working at paid job	Working around house or yard	Attending school	Sports	Leisure activities	Other[d]
All ages	**33,255**	**1,990**	**4,082**	**4,107**	**1,221**	**5,535**	**8,207**	**8,073**
Under 12 years	4,573	(e)	0	0	629	1,020	1,864	1,086
12-17 years	4,578	0	0	(e)	403[f]	2,339	1,259	505[f]
18-44 years	12,572	1,320	2,617	1,845	(e)	1,790	2,076	2,620
45-64 years	7,370	287[f]	1,348	1,298	0	386[f]	1,997	1,995
65-74 years	1,721	279[f]	(e)	422[f]	0	0	498[f]	506[f]
75 years and older	2,440	(e)	(e)	477[f]	0	0	513[f]	1,360

Source: Adams, P.F., Barnes, P.M., and Vickerie, J.L. (2009, December). Summary health statistics for the U.S. population: National Health Interview Survey, 2008. National Center for Health Statistics. Vital and Health Statistics, Series 10 (No. 243).
[a]Numbers may not sum to respective totals due to rounding and unknowns.
[b]Activity at time of injury and poisoning episodes is based on the question, "What was [person] doing when the injury/poisoning happened?" Respondents could indicate up to two activities.
[c]Driving includes both drivers and passengers.
[d]"Other" includes unpaid work such as housework, shopping, volunteer work, sleeping, resting, eating, drinking, cooking, hands-on care from another person, and other unspecified activities.
[e]Estimate is not shown because it does not meet standard of reliability or precision.
[f]Estimate does not meet standard of reliability or precision and should be used with caution.

PERCENT AND RATES OF INJURY EPISODES BY SEX AND ACTIVITY AT TIME OF INJURY, UNITED STATES 2008

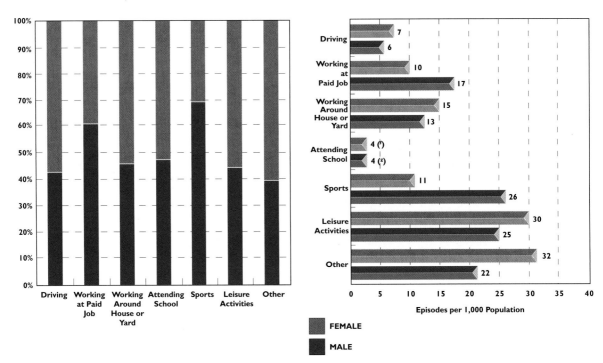

Source: Adams, P.F., Barnes, P.M., and Vickerie, J.L. (2009, December). Summary health statistics for the U.S. population: National Health Interview Survey, 2008. National Center for Health Statistics. Vital and Health Statistics, Series 10 (No. 243).

THE NATIONAL HEALTH INTERVIEW
SURVEY, 2008 (CONT.)

25

There is a wealth of research demonstrating the role of socioeconomic status (SES) in the etiology of medical conditions and disease. In general, people with the highest levels of income and education are healthier than those with median income and education, who, in turn, tend to be in better health than the poor and least educated.[a]

Lower SES is known to contribute to increased rates of fatal injuries. Although research provides some evidence of links between SES and nonfatal injuries, the results of this survey appear to be inconsistent and may depend in part on the survey's design, population, and context. The National Health Interview Survey provides an opportunity to look at the occurrence of unintentional injuries in the U.S. population as a function of socioeconomic position using two SES measures—family income and education.[b]

Although NHIS data indicate that all people are affected by injuries, those with family incomes from $50,000 to $74,999 had the highest injury rate, while those with family incomes of $75,000 to $99,999 had the lowest injury rates (122 compared to 111 injuries per 1,000 population). In contrast, those with less than a high school education had the lowest medically consulted injury rate in 2008 (94 injuries per 1,000 population). This bell-shaped curve, with the highest rate among people with some college education, does not seem to support the typical SES pattern.

[a]Banks, J., Marmot, M., Oldfield, Z., and Smith, J.P. (2006). Disease and disadvantage in the United States and in England. Journal of the American Medical Association, 295 (17); 2037–2045.
[b]Education data are shown for people age 25 years and older.

PERCENTAGES AND RATES OF MEDICALLY CONSULTED INJURIES BY FAMILY INCOME, UNITED STATES, 2008

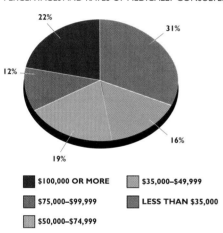

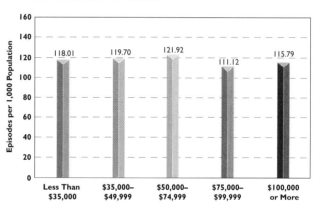

PERCENTAGES AND RATES OF MEDICALLY CONSULTED INJURIES BY LEVEL OF EDUCATION, UNITED STATES, 2008

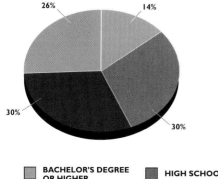

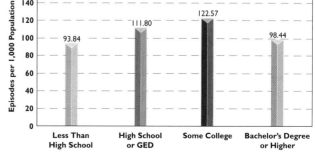

Source: Adams, P.F., Barnes, P.M., and Vickerie, J.L. (2009, December). Summary health statistics for the U.S. population: National Health Interview Survey, 2008. National Center for Health Services. Vital and Health Statistics, Series 10 (No. 243).

ALL UNINTENTIONAL INJURIES

NATIONAL SAFETY COUNCIL® INJURY FACTS® 2011 EDITION

INJURY-RELATED HOSPITAL EMERGENCY DEPARTMENT VISITS, 2007

About 39.4 million visits to hospital emergency departments in 2007 were due to injuries.

About 34% of all hospital emergency department visits in the United States were injury-related in 2007, according to information from the 2007 National Hospital Ambulatory Medical Care Survey conducted for the National Center for Health Statistics. There were approximately 116.8 million visits made to emergency departments, of which about 39.4 million were injury-related. This resulted in an annual rate of about 39.4 emergency department visits per 100 people, of which about 13.3 visits per 100 people were injury-related.

Males had a higher overall rate of injury-related visits than females. For males, about 14.4 visits per 100 people were recorded; for females, the rate was 12.2 per 100 people. Males also had higher rates of injury-related visits than females for age groups from younger than 15 through age 64, while females had higher rates for age groups beginning at age 75. Males and females in the 65- to 74-year-old age group had identical rates of 10.3 visits per 100 people. Those ages 15 to 24 had the highest rate of

injury-related visits for males, while those age 75 and older had the highest rate for females.

Falls and motor vehicle accidents were the leading causes of injury-related emergency department visits, accounting for 23% and 11% of the total, respectively. In total, about 8.9 million visits to emergency departments were made in 2007 due to accidental falls, and about 4.3 million were made due to motor vehicle accidents. The next leading types were struck against or struck accidentally by objects or people with more than 3.0 million visits (8% of the total), and accidents caused by overexertion and strenuous movements, which accounted for about 2.1 million visits (5% of the total).

The upper extremities were the most frequent body site of injuries treated in hospital emergency rooms, followed by injuries to the lower extremities and to the head and neck. These three body sites accounted for about 45% of all injury-related visits. The most commonly mentioned body sites for injuries were wrist, hand and fingers, followed by the vertebral column.

NUMBER AND PERCENT DISTRIBUTION OF EMERGENCY DEPARTMENT VISITS BY CAUSE OF INJURY, UNITED STATES, 2007

Cause of injury and E-code[a]	Number of visits (000)	%
All injury-related visits	**39,395**	**100.0**
Unintentional Injuries, E800–E869, E880–E929	**26,036**	**66.1**
Accidental Falls, E880.0–E886.9, E888	8,898	22.6
Total Motor Vehicle Accidents, E810–E825 (.0–.5, .7–.9)	4,287	10.9
Motor vehicle traffic, E810–E819	*3,836*	*9.7*
Motor vehicle, nontraffic, E820–E825 (.0–.5, .7–.9)	*451*	*1.1*
Striking Against or Struck Accidentally by Objects or Persons, E916–E917	3,044	7.7
Overexertion and Strenuous Movements, E927	2,116	5.4
Accidents Caused by Cutting or Piercing Instruments or Objects, E920	2,089	5.3
Accidents Due to Natural and Environmental Factors, E900–E909, E928.0–E928.2	1,522	3.9
Foreign Body, E914–E915	638	1.6
Accidental Poisoning by Drugs, Medicinal Substances, Biologicals, Other Solid and Liquid Substances, Gases and Vapors, E850–E869	486	1.2
Accidents Caused by Fire and Flames, Hot Substances or Object, Caustic or Corrosive Material, and Steam, E890–E899, E924	416	1.1
Caught Accidentally In or Between Objects, E918	359	0.9
Pedalcycle, Nontraffic and Other, E800–E807(.3), E820–E825(.6), E826.1, E826.9	330	0.8
Machinery, E919	280	0.7
Other Transportation, E800-807(.0–.2, .8–.9), E826(.0, .2–.8), E827–E829, E831, E833–E845	209	0.5

Cause of injury and E-code[a]	Number of visits (000)	%
Other Mechanism[b], E830, E832, E846–E848, E910, E921–E923, E925–E926, E928.3, E928.8, E929.0–E929.5	1,182	3.0
Mechanism Unspecified, E887, E928.9, E929.8, E929.9	179	0.4
Intentional injuries, E950–E959, E960–E969, E970–E978, E990–E999	**1,998**	**5.1**
Assault, E960–E969	1,447	3.7
Unarmed Fight or Brawl and Striking by Blunt or Thrown Object, E960.0, E968.2	*784*	*2.0*
Assault by Cutting and Piercing Instrument, E966	*76*	*0.2*
Assault by Other and Unspecified Mechanism,[c] E960.1, E961–E964, E965.0–E965.9, E967–E968.1, E968.3–E969	*587*	*1.5*
Self-Inflicted Injury, E950–E959	472	1.2
Poisoning by Solid or Liquid Substances, Gases or Vapors, E950–E952	*294*	*0.7*
Other and Unspecified Mechanism,[d] E954–E959	*178*	*0.4*
Other Causes of Violence, E970–E979, E990–E999	79	0.2
Injuries of undetermined intent, E980–E989	**293**	**0.7**
Adverse effects of medical treatment, E870–E879, E930–E949	**1,684**	**4.3**
Medical and Surgical Complications, E870–E879	968	2.5
Adverse Drug Effects, E930–E949	716	1.8
Alcohol and/or drug abuse[e]	**1,766**	**4.5**
Other and unknown[f]	**7,618**	**19.3**

Source: Niska, R., Bhuiya, F., and Jianmin, X. (2010). National Hospital Ambulatory Medical Care Survey: 2007 Emergency Department Summary (National Health Statistics Reports, No. 26, Aug. 6, 2010). Hyattsville, MD: National Center for Health Statistics

Note: Sum of parts may not add to total due to rounding.

[a]*Based on the International Classification of Diseases, 9th revision, Clinical Modification (ICD-9-CM).*
[b]*Includes drowning, firearms, and other and not elsewhere classified mechanism.*
[c]*Includes assault by firearms and explosives, and other mechanism.*
[d]*Includes injury by cutting and piercing instrument, and other and unspecified mechanism.*
[e]*Alcohol and drug abuse are not contained in the "Supplementary Classification of External Causes of Injury and Poisoning," but frequently are recorded as a cause of injury or poisoning.*
[f]*Includes illegible and blank E-codes.*

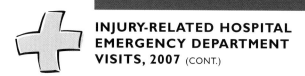

RATE[a] OF INJURY-RELATED VISITS TO EMERGENCY DEPARTMENTS BY PATIENT AGE AND SEX, 2007

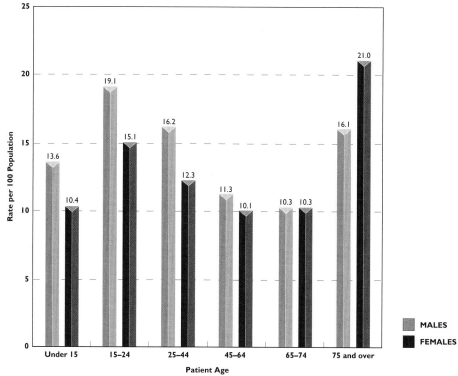

[a]Number of visits per 100 population in each age group.

PERCENT OF INJURY-RELATED[a] EMERGENCY DEPARTMENT VISITS BY BODY SITE OF PRIMARY DIAGNOSIS, UNITED STATES, 2007

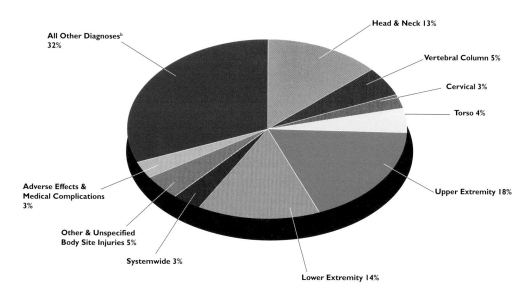

[a]Injury-related includes injuries, poisoning, and adverse effects.

[b]"All other diagnoses" includes musculoskeletal system, symptoms and ill-defined conditions, skin and subcutaneous tissue, mental disorders, nervous system and sense organs, other illnesses, supplementary classification, and unknown diagnoses.

LEADING CAUSES OF FATAL UNINTENTIONAL INJURIES

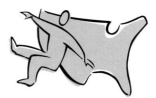

Motor vehicle (MV) traffic fatalities are the leading cause of fatal unintentional injuries in the United States, according to the latest data from the National Center for Health Statistics. There were a total of 42,031 MV traffic fatalities in 2007, which accounted for about 34% of all unintentional injury-related deaths. MV traffic fatalities were the leading cause of unintentional injury deaths in age groups from 5-9 through 25-34, and again for the 55-64 age group.

Suffocation was the leading cause of unintentional injury deaths for people younger than 1, while drowning was the leading cause for those ages 1-4. The leading cause of unintentional injury deaths among the 35-44 and 45-54 age groups was poisoning, and the leading cause for those age 65 and older was falls. In addition to MV traffic, poisoning and falls, drowning also was a leading cause of unintentional injury deaths for most age groups.

LEADING CAUSES OF FATAL UNINTENTIONAL INJURIES BY AGE GROUP, UNITED STATES, 2007

Rank	All ages	Age group									
		<1	1–4	5–9	10–14	15–24	25–34	35–44	45–54	55–64	65+
1	MV traffic 42,031	Suffocation 959	Drowning 458	MV traffic 456	MV traffic 696	MV traffic 10,272	MV traffic 6,842	Poisoning 7,575	Poisoning 9,006	MV traffic 4,177	Falls 18,334
2	Poisoning 29,846	MV traffic 122	MV traffic 428	Fire, flames, smoke 136	Drowning 102	Poisoning 3,159	Poisoning 5,700	MV traffic 6,135	MV traffic 6,262	Poisoning 3,120	MV traffic 6,632
3	Falls 22,631	Drowning 57	Fire, flames, smoke 204	Drowning 122	Other land transport 80	Drowning 630	Drowning 381	Falls 593	Falls 1,304	Falls 1,739	Unspecified 4,855
4	Unspecified 6,019	Fire, flames, smoke 39	Suffocation 149	Suffocation 42	Fire, flames, smoke 78	Other land transport 310	Falls 334	Drowning 417	Fire, flames, smoke 496	Fire, flames, smoke 505	Suffocation 3,209
5	Suffocation 5,997	Falls 24	Pedestrian, other 124	Other land transport 40	Poisoning 69	Falls 233	Other specified 244	Fire, flames, smoke 313	Drowning 481	Suffocation 484	Fire, flames, smoke 1,179
6	Drowning 3,443	Other specified 20	Struck by/against 44	Pedestrian, other 32	Suffocation 60	Fire, flames smoke 196	Other land transport 233	Suffocation 289	Suffocation 479	Unspecified 392	Poisoning 1,149
7	Fire, flames, smoke 3,375	Poisoning 19	Falls 36	Firearms 20	Firearms 26	Other specified 156	Fire, flames, smoke 225	Other specified 251	Other specified 370	Drowning 324	Natural/ environment 539
8	Other land transport 1,617	Natural/ environment 18	Poisoning 34	Struck by/against 20	Falls 21	Firearms 155	Suffocation 193	Other land transport 227	Unspecified 318	Other specified 229	Other specified, n.e.c.[a] 515
9	Other specified 1,542	Unspecified 14	Natural/ environment 27	Other specified 17	Pedestrian, other 17	Pedestrian, other 139	Other transport 138	Unspecified 195	Natural/ environment 282	Natural/ environment 220	Drowning 466
10	Natural/ environment 1,449	Struck by/against 6	Firearms 18	Unspecified 16	Other transport 16	Other transport 135	Pedestrian, other 120	Other transport 162	Other land transport 256	Other transport 209	Other land transport 304
All causes of injury											
Number	123,706	1,285	1,588	965	1,229	15,897	14,977	16,931	20,315	12,193	38,326[b]
Per 100,00 population	41.1	30.1	9.6	4.9	6.1	37.5	37.1	39.3	46.3	37.3	101.0[b]

Source: Centers for Disease Control and Prevention, National Center for Injury Prevention and Control. Web-based Injury Statistics Query and Reporting System (WISQARS), data accessed June 8, 2010, at www.cdc.gov/injury/wisqars/index.html.
[a]"n.e.c." means not elsewhere classified.
[b]Includes 34 cases with age unknown.

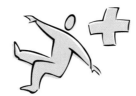

LEADING CAUSES OF NONFATAL UNINTENTIONAL INJURIES

LEADING CAUSES OF NONFATAL UNINTENTIONAL INJURIES

Falls are the leading cause of nonfatal unintentional injuries that are treated in hospital emergency departments, according to data from the All Injury Program, a cooperative program involving the National Center for Injury Prevention and Control, the Centers for Disease Control and Prevention and the Consumer Product Safety Commission. More than 8.5 million people were treated in an emergency department for fall-related injuries in 2008. Falls were the leading cause of nonfatal injuries for all age groups except for the 15-24 year old age group, for which struck by or against an object or person was the leading cause. Struck by or against, overexertion, and motor vehicle crashes involving vehicle occupants were also leading causes for most age groups.

LEADING CAUSES OF NONFATAL UNINTENTIONAL INJURIES TREATED IN HOSPITAL EMERGENCY DEPARTMENTS BY AGE GROUP, UNITED STATES, 2008

Rank	All ages	Age group									
		<1	1–4	5–9	10–14	15–24	25–34	35–44	45–54	55–64	65+
1	Falls 8,551,037	Falls 125,097	Falls 878,612	Falls 639,091	Falls 607,365	Struck by/against 1,031,192	Falls 813,125	Falls 798,775	Falls 913,341	Falls 742,735	Falls 2,114,113
2	Struck by/against 4,492,287	Struck by/against 37,010	Struck by/against 371,404	Struck by/against 399,995	Struck by/against 583,948	Falls 918,574	Overexertion 675,349	Overexertion 584,738	Overexertion 448,656	Struck by/against 230,874	Struck by/against 229,304
3	Overexertion 3,278,300	Other bite/sting[a] 13,092	Other bite/sting[a] 134,920	Cut/pierce 106,907	Overexertion 283,813	MV occupant 743,738	Struck by/against 654,918	Struck by/against 529,223	Struck by/against 424,305	Overexertion 213,174	Overexertion 178,344
4	MV occupant 2,581,605	Foreign body 11,035	Foreign body 123,369	Other bite/sting[a] 83,107	Cut/pierce 135,610	Overexertion 735,400	MV occupant 528,571	MV occupant 412,047	MV occupant 350,291	MV occupant 197,380	MV occupant 176,571
5	Cut/pierce 2,072,604	Fire, flames, smoke 9,101	Cut/pierce 81,571	Pedalcyclist 80,743	Pedalcyclist 108,016	Cut/pierce 452,297	Cut/pierce 411,514	Cut/pierce 320,785	Cut/pierce 289,857	Cut/pierce 156,046	Cut/pierce 112,015
6	Other specified[b] 1,109,782	Other specified[b] 8,271	Overexertion 78,018	Overexertion 75,796	Unknown/ unspecified 100,842	Other specified[b] 203,484	Other specified[b] 196,247	Other specified[b] 228,808	Other specified[b] 225,469	Other specified[b] 95,934	Poisoning 74,623
7	Other bite/sting[a] 993,923	Unknown/ unspecified 6,722	Other specified[b] 69,043	MV occupant 57,236	MV occupant 75,969	Unknown/ unspecified 191,276	Other bite/sting[a] 146,982	Poisoning 132,444	Poisoning 169,088	Poisoning 84,040	Other bite/sting[a] 73,062
8	Unknown/ unspecified 806,819	Cut/pierce 5,916	Fire, flames, smoke 50,708	Foreign body 56,624	Other transport[c] 57,597	Other bite/sting[a] 167,310	Unknown/ unspecified 126,719	Other bite/sting[a] 128,813	Other bite/sting[a] 122,059	Other bite/sting[a] 72,088	Unknown/ unspecified 65,524
9	Poisoning 732,316	Inhalation/ suffocation 4,975	Unknown/ unspecified 45,017	Other transport[c] 45,158	Other bite/sting[a] 52,489	Other transport[c] 125,828	Poisoning 103,881	Unknown/ unspecified 101,767	Unknown/ unspecified 81,359	Unknown/ unspecified 45,563	Other transport[c] 60,997
10	Other transport[c] 620,386	MV occupant 4,818	Dog bite 38,214	Unknown/ unspecified 41,967	Dog bite 32,733	Poisoning 110,601	Other transport[c] 98,565	Other transport[c] 89,849	Other transport[c] 72,507	Other transport[c] 44,176	Other specified[b] 44,520
All causes of injury											
Number	27,877,748	237,485	2,008,655	1,693,564	2,151,639	5,170,713	4,143,130	3,680,896	3,433,363	2,070,337	3,287,968[d]
Per 100,000 population	9,219.2	5,506.1	12,033.1	8,440.3	10,728.9	12,145.4	10,122.1	8,660.7	7,737.7	6,145.9	8,458.9[d]

Source: NEISS All Injury Program, Office of Statistics and Programming, National Center for Injury Prevention and Control, the Centers for Disease Control and Prevention, and Consumer Product Safety Commission.
[a] Other than dog bite.
[b] Includes electric current, explosions, fireworks, radiation, animal scratch, etc. Excludes all causes listed in the table and bb/pellet gunshot, drowning and near drowning, firearm gunshot, suffocation, machinery, natural and environmental conditions, pedestrians, and motorcyclists.
[c] Includes occupant of any transport vehicle other than a motor vehicle or motor cycle (e.g., airplane, rail car, boat, all-terrain vehicle, animal rider).
[d] Includes 3,297 cases with age unknown.

ALL UNINTENTIONAL INJURIES   NATIONAL SAFETY COUNCIL® INJURY FACTS® 2011 EDITION

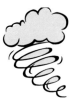

Disasters are front-page news stories even though the lives lost in the United States are relatively few when compared with the day-to-day life losses from unintentional injuries (see "While You Speak!" page 31). Listed below are the U.S. disasters, of which the National Safety Council is aware, that occurred in 2009 and took five or more lives.

There also were 31 motor vehicle traffic crashes in 2009 that resulted in five or six deaths each.

DISASTER DEATHS, UNITED STATES, 2009

Type and location	No. of deaths	Date of disaster
Major disasters (25 or more deaths)		
Passenger airline crash; Buffalo, NY	50	Feb. 12
Other Disasters (5–24 deaths)		
Snow and ice storm; Arkansas, Kentucky, Missouri, Ohio, Oklahoma, Texas	23	Jan. 27-28
Motor vehicle traffic crash; Arizona	11	June 6
Motor vehicle traffic crash; Oklahoma	10	June 26
Residential fire; Mississippi	9	December
Subway train crash; Washington, D.C.	9	June 22
Helicopter and plane collision; New York	9	Aug. 8
Residential fire; New York	8	January
Tornado; Oklahoma	8	Feb. 10
Motor vehicle traffic crash; New York	8	July 26
Motor vehicle traffic crash; California	8	Aug. 8
Motor vehicle traffic crash; Arizona	7	Jan. 30
Extreme heat; Tennessee	7	June 17
Residential fire; Washington, D.C.	6	January
Residential fire; Kentucky	6	July
Residential fire; South Carolina	5	January
Homeless shelter fire; Texas	5	January
Residential fire; West Virginia	5	January
Residential fire; Alabama	5	March
Residential fire; Michigan	5	April
Flash flood; Texas	5	April 18
Residential fire; Missouri	5	May
Residential fire; Florida	5	November

Source: National Climatic Data Center, www.infoplease.com/world/disasters/2009.html, retrieved on Aug. 2, 2010, National Fire Protection Association, and National Highway Traffic Safety Administration.
Note: Some death totals are estimates and may differ among sources.

WHILE YOU SPEAK!

While you make a 10-minute safety speech, 2 people in the United States will be killed and about 740 will suffer an injury severe enough to require consultation with a medical professional.[a] Costs will amount to $13,190,000. On average, 15 unintentional injury deaths and about 4,440 medically consulted injuries occur every hour during the year.

Deaths and medically consulted injuries by class occurred in the nation at the following rates in 2009:

DEATHS AND DISABLING INJURIES BY CLASS, 2009

Class	Severity	One every—	Number per ...			2009 total
			Hour	Day	Week	
All	Deaths	4 minutes	15	351	2,470	128,000
	Injuries[a]	<1 second	4,440	106,600	748,100	38,900,000
Motor vehicle	Deaths	15 minutes	4	98	690	35,900
	Injuries	9 seconds	400	9,600	67,300	3,500,000
Work	Deaths	147 minutes	<1	10	70	3,582
	Injuries	6 seconds	580	14,000	98,100	5,100,000
Workers off the job	Deaths	9 minutes	6	153	1,070	55,800
	Injuries	2 seconds	1,640	39,500	276,900	14,400,000
Home	Deaths	8 minutes	7	179	1,250	65,200
	Injuries	1 second	2,410	57,800	405,800	21,100,000
Public non-motor vehicle	Deaths	21 minutes	3	69	480	25,100
	Injuries	3 seconds	1,070	25,800	180,000	9,400,000

Source: National Safety Council estimates.
[a]Starting with the 2011 Edition of Injury Facts, the National Safety Council adopted the definition of medically consulted injuries to replace disabling injuries. For a full description of medically consulted injuries, please see the Technical Appendix.

DEATHS EVERY HOUR ...

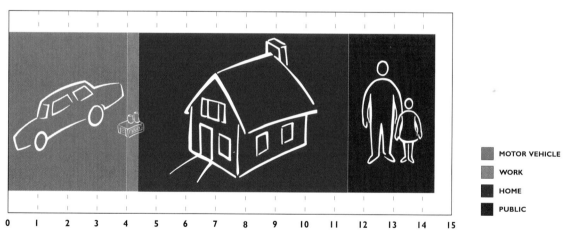

MOTOR VEHICLE
WORK
HOME
PUBLIC

| 0 | 1 | 2 | 3 | 4 | 5 | 6 | 7 | 8 | 9 | 10 | 11 | 12 | 13 | 14 | 15 |

AN UNINTENTIONAL INJURY DEATH EVERY FOUR MINUTES ...

Four Minutes

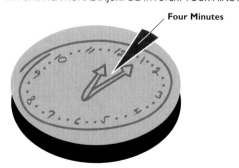

CHILDREN AND YOUTHS

Motor vehicle crashes are the leading cause of injury deaths among children.

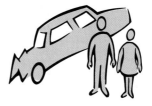

Unintentional injuries are a major public health concern affecting children and adolescents in the United States. They are the underlying cause of death in nearly 3 out of every 7 childhood mortality cases for people ages 1-19 years, and 15- to 19-year-olds account for more than 60% of the total.

Fatal injuries in the first year of life numbered 1,285 in 2007, or approximately 30 deaths per 100,000 population. Mechanical suffocation constituted the majority (69%) of all injury-related mortality cases for infants. Motor vehicle crashes were the second leading cause of injury mortality. In addition, 352 infant deaths that year were attributed to homicide (for more information on intentional injuries, see pages 160-165).

In the second year of life, the risk of fatal injury is reduced by more than half. In 2007, 532 fatal injury cases, or about 13 deaths per 100,000 population, were recorded among 1-year-old children. Motor vehicle crashes were the leading cause of injury death in this age group, followed by drowning.

In the following three-year period (ages 2-4), the injury mortality rate drops even lower, averaging about 9

deaths per 100,000 population in 2007. Motor vehicle crashes were the number one cause of injury mortality, followed by drowning and flames, fire, and smoke.

From age 5 to early adolescence (ages 12-14), the injury mortality rate shows a general U-shaped pattern, reaching its lowest level at around age 11. Motor vehicle crashes, unintentional drowning, and incidents related to fire, flames, and smoke were the leading causes of injury mortality for children ages 5-14 in 2007.

Teenagers (15-19 years) make up 27% of the U.S. population between the ages of 1 and 19 and 63% of all injury mortality cases in that age group. Most importantly, nearly 3 out of every 4 teenage injury deaths are attributed to motor vehicle crashes. Of the 6,493 injury deaths among teens in 2007, more than 4,700 occurred in crashes. That same year, the injury mortality rate for 19 year olds was 44 deaths per 100,000 population.

For all children and adolescents younger than 19, the injury mortality rate by age can be described as a J-shaped relationship, peaking during infancy and again in the late teenage years.

UNINTENTIONAL INJURY DEATHS BY EVENT, AGES 0-19, UNITED STATES, 2007

Age	Population (000)	Unintentional injury deaths										
		Total	Rates[a]	Motor vehicle	Falls	Poisoning	Drowning	Fire, flames smoke	Choking[b]	Mechanical suffocation	Firearms	All other
<1 year	4,274	1,285	30.1	124	24	19	57	38	70	889	1	63
1-19 years	78,031	10,275	13.2	6,559	154	953	999	498	118	186	137	671
1 year	4,165	532	12.8	173	9	15	168	35	45	47	0	40
2 years	4,114	444	10.8	140	10	13	139	58	24	14	3	43
3 years	4,114	331	8.0	123	8	4	89	59	4	6	8	30
4 years	4,064	281	6.9	115	9	2	62	49	4	5	7	28
5 years	4,031	225	5.6	115	2	2	36	35	3	4	6	22
6 years	4,087	213	5.2	103	2	3	31	32	7	6	3	26
7 years	3,933	176	4.5	89	4	2	23	27	0	4	4	23
8 years	3,888	177	4.6	101	2	5	19	18	2	7	4	19
9 years	3,897	174	4.5	107	1	0	13	22	5	4	3	19
10 years	3,923	169	4.3	102	5	5	19	17	0	9	1	11
11 years	4,006	166	4.1	93	4	4	17	19	1	7	7	14
12 years	4,070	220	5.4	133	4	12	14	17	2	13	4	21
13 years	4,105	285	6.9	179	4	15	19	14	7	13	4	30
14 years	4,189	389	9.3	263	4	33	33	10	3	5	10	28
15 years	4,261	562	13.2	383	7	48	49	9	2	5	14	45
16 years	4,330	982	22.7	724	11	90	55	14	1	10	12	65
17 years	4,410	1,320	29.9	1,017	13	126	58	16	3	8	21	58
18 years	4,251	1,784	42.0	1,303	23	266	74	19	3	12	10	74
19 years	4,194	1,845	44.0	1,296	32	308	81	28	2	7	16	75
0-4 years	20,731	2,873	13.9	675	60	53	515	239	147	961	19	204
5-9 years	19,836	965	4.9	515	11	12	122	134	17	25	20	109
10-14 years	20,293	1,229	6.1	770	21	69	102	77	13	47	26	104
15-19 years	21,446	6,493	30.3	4,723	86	838	317	86	11	42	73	317

Source: National Safety Council tabulations of National Center for Health Statistics mortality data.
Note: Data does not include "age unknown" cases, which totaled 34 in 2007.
[a]Deaths per 100,000 population in each age group.
[b]Suffocation by inhalation or ingestion of food or other object.

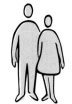

ADULTS

Injury mortality and fall-related mortality rates increase with age.

Unintentional injuries cause significant mortality among adults in the United States. In 2007 alone, injuries were responsible for more than 112,000 deaths among Americans age 20 and older.

The leading causes of injury mortality include motor vehicle crashes; poisoning; falls; choking; fire, flames, and smoke; and drowning. Motor vehicle crashes (33.2%), poisoning (25.8%), and falls (20.0%), the three leading causes of injury mortality, combined to account for nearly four-fifths of all fatal injuries sustained by adults older than 20 in 2007.

Age plays an important role in the occurrence of injuries. Motor vehicle crashes are the leading cause of injury mortality up to the fourth decade of life, when the incidence of poisoning cases reaches its peak. Beginning at age 55, motor vehicle crashes once again take over as the leading cause of injury mortality until superseded by falls beginning in the early seventies.

The increase in the incidence of fatal falls appears to be the driving force behind a surge in the overall injury mortality rate in later life. The highest fall mortality rates occur among adults in age groups beginning at age 70 and older. As the table below illustrates, the number of injury-related deaths per 100,000 population in 2007 increased to 349 for 90-94 year olds from 53 for 70-74 year olds – a nearly sevenfold increase.

A recent study compared two different methods of expressing the risk of falls among community-dwelling older people: the commonly used population incidence (fallers per 1,000 person-years) and the new FAlls Risk by Exposure (FARE), expressed as the number of fallers per 1,000 physically active person-days.[a] A total of 771 people (42% men) between the ages of 71 and 96 completed a baseline questionnaire that contained questions about their age, gender, specific disabilities, and level of physical activity. They then participated in a follow-up at 10 months that asked about their involvement in falls. Individuals who reported no difficulty controlling their balance were about 5 times more active than those who reported severe difficulty controlling their balance. Whether expressed as population incidence or FARE, the falls risk rose with increasing difficulty controlling balance. However, with FARE, the risk of falling increased exponentially compared to the linear increase of the population incidence. Thus, FARE was more indicitive of the real risk people face and recommended for use in public health policy and research on falls prevention because it takes into account reduced physical activity of older people who experience increased difficulty controlling their balance.

[a]Wijlhuizen, G.J., Chorus, A.M.J., and Hopman-Rock, M. (2010). The FARE: A new way to express FAlls Risk among older persons including physical activity as a measure of exposure. Preventive Medicine, 50 (3); 143-147.

UNINTENTIONAL INJURY DEATHS BY EVENT, AGE 20 AND OLDER, UNITED STATES, 2007

Age	Population (000)	Unintentional injury deaths											
		Total	Rates[a]	Motor vehicle	Falls	Poisoning	Drowning	Fire, flames smoke	Choking[b]	Mechanical suffocation	Natural heat/cold	Firearms	All other
20-24	20,962	9,404	44.9	5,845	147	2,321	313	108	31	49	22	82	486
25-29	20,956	8,134	38.8	4,086	168	2,919	210	122	44	49	24	64	448
30-34	19,445	6,843	35.2	3,001	166	2,781	171	100	53	47	32	30	462
35-39	21,123	7,737	36.6	3,115	247	3,344	179	118	73	52	32	52	525
40-44	21,959	9,194	41.9	3,255	346	4,231	238	189	92	72	72	39	660
45-49	22,855	10,717	46.9	3,472	612	4,931	244	235	162	66	92	41	862
50-54	21,016	9,598	45.7	3,058	692	4,075	237	253	186	65	115	41	876
55-59	18,244	7,100	38.9	2,525	832	2,198	162	245	207	38	102	30	761
60-64	14,481	5,093	35.2	1,834	907	922	162	247	218	21	59	27	696
65-69	10,758	4,187	38.9	1,508	1,059	371	101	217	233	27	59	21	591
70-74	8,611	4,566	53.0	1,432	1,535	231	93	204	328	21	57	10	655
75-79	7,343	5,922	80.6	1,486	2,543	191	103	201	468	15	56	16	843
80-84	5,715	7,814	136.7	1,359	4,009	164	81	235	671	19	89	15	1,172
85-89	3,479	8,064	231.8	916	4,597	120	59	168	688	21	91	4	1,400
90-94	1,505	5,249	348.8	307	3,111	52	24	73	462	14	41	2	1,163
95-99	451	2,115	469.0	49	1,275	18	4	26	202	2	20	1	518
100 and older	80	375	468.8	5	205	2	1	5	38	0	1	0	118
20 and older	218,983	112,112	51.2	37,253	22,451	28,871	2,382	2,746	4,156	578	964	475	12,236
25 and older	198,021	102,708	51.9	31,408	22,304	26,550	2,069	2,638	4,125	529	942	393	11,750
35 and older	157,620	87,731	55.7	24,321	21,970	20,850	1,688	2,416	4,028	433	886	299	10,840
45 and older	114,538	70,800	61.8	17,951	21,377	13,275	1,271	2,109	3,863	309	782	208	9,655
55 and older	70,667	50,485	71.4	11,421	20,073	4,269	790	1,621	3,515	178	575	126	7,917
65 and older	37,942	38,292	100.9	7,062	18,334	1,149	466	1,129	3,090	119	414	69	6,460
75 and older	18,573	29,539	159.0	4,122	15,740	547	272	708	2,529	71	298	38	5,214

Source: National Safety Council tabulations of National Center for Health Statistics mortality data.
Note: Data does not include "age unknown" cases, which totaled 34 in 2007.
[a]Deaths per 100,000 population in each age group.
[b]Suffocation by inhalation or ingestion of food or other object.

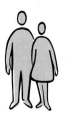

The table on the following pages was prepared in response to frequent inquiries such as, "What are the odds of being killed by lightning?" or "What are the chances of dying in a plane crash?"

The odds given in the table are statistical averages over the whole U.S. population and do not necessarily reflect the chances of death for a particular person from a particular external cause. Any individual's odds of dying from various external causes are affected by the activities in which they participate, where they live and drive, what kind of work they do, and other factors.

The table has four columns. The first column gives the manner of injury, such as motor vehicle crash, fall, fire, etc. The second column gives the total number of deaths nationwide due to the manner of injury in 2007 (the latest year for which data are available). The third column gives the odds of dying in one year due to the manner of injury. The fourth column gives the lifetime odds of dying from the manner of injury. Statements about the odds or chances of dying from a given cause of death may be made as follows:

• The odds of dying from (manner of injury) in 2007 were 1 in (value given in the one-year odds column).

• The lifetime odds of dying from (manner of injury) for a person born in 2007 were 1 in (value given in the lifetime odds column).

For example, referring to the first line of the table:

• The odds of dying from an injury in 2007 were 1 in 1,628.

• The lifetime odds of dying from an injury for a person born in 2007 were 1 in 21.

The one-year odds are approximated by dividing the 2007 population (301,290,332) by the number of deaths. The lifetime odds are approximated by dividing the one-year odds by the life expectancy of a person born in 2007 (77.9 years). Please note that odds based on less than 20 deaths are likely to be unstable from year to year and should be used with caution.

The figure on page 37 represents the lifetime odds of death for selected causes from the odds table. The total lifetime odds of death from any cause are 1 in 1, or 100%, and thus the largest rectangle representing the total odds actually extends off the page in all directions to infinity. The rectangles for selected causes are sized according to their relative lifetime probabilities, with the least probable event—death from earthquakes and other earth movements—depicted using the smallest box.

Source: National Safety Council estimates based on data from National Center for Health Statistics and U.S. Census Bureau. Deaths are classified on the basis of the 10th revision of the World Health Organization's "The International Classification of Diseases" (ICD). Numbers following titles refer to External Cause of Morbidity and Mortality classifications in ICD-10.

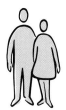

ODDS OF DEATH DUE TO INJURY, UNITED STATES, 2007[a]

Type of accident or manner of injury	Deaths	One-year odds	Lifetime odds
All external causes of mortality, V01–Y89, *U01, *U03[b]	**185,076**	**1,628**	**21**
Deaths due to unintentional (accidental) injuries, V01–X59, Y85–Y86	**123,706**	**2,436**	**31**
Transport accidents, V01–V99, Y85	**48,844**	**6,432**	**83**
Motor vehicle accidents, V02–V04, V09.0, V09.2, V12–V14, V19.0–V19.2, V19.4–V19.6, V20–V79, V80.3–V80.5, V81.0–V81.1, V82.0–V82.1, V83–V86, V87.0–V87.8, V88.0–V88.8, V89.0, V89.2	**43,945**	**6,856**	**88**
Pedestrian, V01–V09	5,958	50,569	649
Pedalcyclist, V10–V19	820	367,427	4,717
Motorcycle rider, V20–V29	5,024	59,970	770
Occupant of three-wheeled motor vehicle, V30–V39	10	30,129,033	386,766
Car occupant, V40–V49	12,772	23,590	303
Occupant of pick-up truck or van, V50–V59	3,100	97,190	1,248
Occupant of heavy transport vehicle, V60–V69	441	683,198	8,770
Bus occupant, V70–V79	43	7,006,752	89,945
Animal rider or occupant of animal-drawn vehicle, V80	101	2,983,073	38,294
Occupant of railway train or railway vehicle, V81	17	17,722,961	227,509
Occupant of streetcar, V82	2	150,645,166	1,933,828
Other and unspecified land transport accidents, V83–V89	16,740	17,998	231
Occupant of special industrial vehicle, V83	*14*	*21,520,738*	*276,261*
Occupant of special agricultural vehicle, V84	*148*	*2,035,745*	*26,133*
Occupant of special construction vehicle, V85	*26*	*11,588,090*	*148,756*
Occupant of all-terrain or other off-road motor vehicle, V86	*1,093*	*275,654*	*3,539*
Other and unspecified person, V87–V89	*15,459*	*19,490*	*250*
Water transport accidents, V90–V94	486	619,939	7,958
Drowning, V90, V92	*349*	*854,908*	*10,974*
Other and unspecified injuries, V91, V93–V94	*137*	*2,177,832*	*27,957*
Air and space transport accidents, V95–V97	550	547,801	7,032
Other and unspecified transport accidents and sequelae, V98–V99, Y85	780	386,270	4,959
Other specified transport accidents, V98	*0*	*0*	*0*
Unspecified transport accident, V99	*3*	*100,430,111*	*1,289,218*
Nontransport unintentional (accidental) injuries, W00–X59, Y86	**76,862**	**3,920**	**50**
Falls, W00–W19	22,631	13,313	171
Fall on same level from slipping, tripping and stumbling, W01	*691*	*436,021*	*5,597*
Other fall on same level, W00, W02–W03, W18	*6,264*	*48,099*	*617*
Fall involving bed, chair, other furniture, W06–W08	*984*	*306,189*	*3,931*
Fall on and from stairs and steps, W10	*1,917*	*157,168*	*2,018*
Fall on and from ladder or scaffolding, W11–W12	*434*	*694,217*	*8,912*
Fall from out of or through building or structure, W13	*587*	*513,271*	*6,589*
Other fall from one level to another, W09, W14–W17	*695*	*433,511*	*5,565*
Other and unspecified fall, W04–W05, W19	*11,059*	*27,244*	*350*
Exposure to inanimate mechanical forces, W20–W49	2,591	116,283	1,493
Struck by or striking against object, W20–W22	*812*	*371,047*	*4,763*
Caught between objects, W23	*153*	*1,969,218*	*25,279*
Contact with machinery, W24, W30–W31	*659*	*457,193*	*5,869*
Contact with sharp objects, W25–W29	*104*	*2,897,022*	*37,189*
Firearms discharge, W32–W34	*613*	*491,501*	*6,309*
Explosion and rupture of pressurized devices, W35–W38	*39*	*7,725,393*	*99,171*
Fireworks discharge, W39	*10*	*30,129,033*	*386,766*
Explosion of other materials, W40	*111*	*2,714,327*	*34,844*
Foreign body entering through skin or natural orifice, W44–W45	*30*	*10,043,011*	*128,922*
Other and unspecified inanimate mechanical forces, W41–W43, W49	*60*	*5,021,506*	*64,461*
Exposure to animate mechanical forces, W50–W64	148	2,035,745	26,133
Struck by or against another person, W50–W52	*20*	*15,064,517*	*193,383*
Bitten or struck by dog, W54	*32*	*9,415,323*	*120,864*
Bitten or struck by other mammals, W53, W55	*76*	*3,964,346*	*50,890*
Bitten or stung by nonvenomous insect and other arthropods, W57	*11*	*27,390,030*	*351,605*
Bitten or crushed by other reptiles, W59	*0*	*0*	*0*
Other and unspecified animate mechanical forces, W56, W58, W60, W64	*9*	*33,476,704*	*429,739*
Accidental drowning and submersion, W65–W74	3,443	87,508	1,123
Drowning and submersion while in or falling into bath tub, W65–W66	*396*	*760,834*	*9,767*
Drowning and submersion while in or falling into swimming pool, W67–W68	*705*	*427,362*	*5,486*
Drowning and submersion while in or falling into natural water, W69–W70	*1,630*	*184,841*	*2,373*
Other and unspecified drowning and submersion, W73–W74	*712*	*423,161*	*5,432*
Other accidental threats to breathing, W75–W84	5,997	50,240	645
Accidental suffocation and strangulation in bed, W75	*741*	*406,600*	*5,220*
Other accidental hanging and strangulation, W76	*244*	*1,234,796*	*15,851*
Threat to breathing due to cave-in, falling earth and other substances, W77	*42*	*7,173,579*	*92,087*
Inhalation of gastric contents, W78	*315*	*956,477*	*12,278*
Inhalation and ingestion of food causing obstruction of respiratory tract, W79	*940*	*320,522*	*4,115*
Inhalation and ingestion of other objects causing obstruction of respiratory tract, W80	*3,089*	*97,537*	*1,252*
Confined to or trapped in a low-oxygen environment, W81	*25*	*12,051,613*	*154,706*
Other and unspecified threats to breathing, W83–W84	*601*	*501,315*	*6,435*

See source and footnotes on page 36.

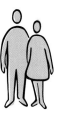

ODDS OF DEATH DUE TO INJURY, UNITED STATES, 2007[a] (Cont.)

Type of accident or manner of injury	Deaths	One-year odds	Lifetime odds
Exposure to electric current, radiation, temperature and pressure, W85–W99	389	774,525	9,943
Electric transmission lines, W85	88	3,423,754	43,951
Other and unspecified electric current, W86–W87	281	1,072,208	13,764
Radiation, W88–W91	0	0	0
Excessive heat or cold of man-made origin, W92–W93	8	37,661,292	483,457
High and low air pressure and changes in air pressure, W94	12	25,107,528	322,305
Other and unspecified man-made environmental factors, W99	0	0	0
Exposure to smoke, fire and flames, X00–X09	3,286	91,689	1,177
Uncontrolled fire in building or structure, X00	2,655	113,480	1,457
Uncontrolled fire not in building or structure, X01	65	4,635,236	59,502
Controlled fire in building or structure, X02	42	7,173,579	92,087
Controlled fire not in building or structure, X03	30	10,043,011	128,922
Ignition of highly flammable material, X04	59	5,106,616	65,553
Ignition or melting of nightwear, X05	3	100,430,111	1,289,218
Ignition or melting of other clothing and apparel, X06	113	2,666,286	34,227
Other and unspecified smoke, fire and flames, X08–X09	319	944,484	12,124
Contact with heat and hot substances, X10–X19	89	3,385,285	43,457
Contact with hot tap water, X11	34	8,861,480	113,755
Other and unspecified heat and hot substances, X10, X12–X19	55	5,478,006	70,321
Contact with venomous animals and plants, X20–X29	73	4,127,265	52,982
Contact with venomous snakes and lizards, X20	7	43,041,476	552,522
Contact with venomous spiders, X21	8	37,661,292	483,457
Contact with hornets, wasps and bees, X23	54	5,579,451	71,623
Contact with other and unspecified venomous animal or plant, X22, X24–X29	4	75,322,583	966,914
Exposure to forces of nature, X30–X39	1,217	247,568	3,178
Exposure to excessive natural heat, X30	309	975,050	12,517
Exposure to excessive natural cold, X31	711	423,756	5,440
Lightning, X33	46	6,549,790	84,079
Earthquake and other earth movements, X34–X36	26	11,588,090	148,756
Cataclysmic storm, X37	84	3,586,790	46,044
Flood, X38	22	13,695,015	175,803
Exposure to other and unspecified forces of nature, X32, X39	19	15,857,386	203,561
Accidental poisoning by and exposure to noxious substances, X40–X49	29,846	10,095	130
Nonopioid analgesics, antipyretics, and antirheumatics, X40	290	1,038,932	13,337
Antiepileptic, sedative-hypnotic, antiparkinsonism, and psychotropic drugs n.e.c., X41	1,545	195,010	2,503
Narcotics and psychodysleptics (hallucinogens) n.e.c., X42	13,030	23,123	297
Other and unspecified drugs, medicaments, and biologicals, X43–X44	12,793	23,551	302
Alcohol, X45	1,356	222,191	2,852
Gases and vapors, X46–X47	680	443,074	5,688
Other and unspecified chemicals and noxious substances, X48–X49	152	1,982,173	25,445
Overexertion, travel and privation, X50–X57	20	15,064,517	193,383
Accidental exposure to other and unspecified factors and sequelae, X58–X59, Y86	7,132	42,245	542
Intentional self-harm, X60–X84, Y87.0, *U03	**34,598**	**8,708**	**112**
Intentional self-poisoning, X60–X69	6,358	47,388	608
Intentional self-harm by hanging, strangulation and suffocation, X70	8,161	36,918	474
Intentional self-harm by firearm, X72-X74	17,352	17,363	223
Other and unspecified means and sequelae, X71, X75–X84, Y87.0	2,727	110,484	1,418
Terrorism, *U03	0	0	0
Assault, X85–Y09, Y87.1, *U01	**18,361**	**16,409**	**211**
Assault by firearm, X93–X95	12,632	23,851	306
Assault by sharp object, X99	1,981	152,090	1,952
Other and unspecified means and sequelae, X85–X92, X96–X98, Y00–Y09, Y87.1	3,748	80,387	1,032
Terrorism, *U01	0	0	0
Event of undetermined intent, Y10–Y34, Y87.2, Y89.9	**5,381**	**55,992**	**719**
Poisoning, Y10–Y19	3,770	79,918	1,026
Hanging, strangulation and suffocation, Y20	135	2,231,780	28,649
Drowning and submersion, Y21	236	1,276,654	16,388
Firearm discharge, Y22–Y24	276	1,091,632	14,013
Exposure to smoke, fire and flames, Y26	98	3,074,991	39,466
Falling, jumping or pushed from a high place, Y30	66	4,565,005	58,601
Other and unspecified means and sequelae, Y25, Y27–Y29, Y31–Y34, Y87.2, Y89.9	800	376,613	4,835
Legal intervention, Y35, Y89.0	**412**	**731,287**	**9,388**
Legal intervention involving firearm discharge, Y35.0	351	858,377	11,019
Legal execution, Y35.5	40	7,532,258	96,691
Other and unspecified means and sequelae, Y35.1–Y35.4, Y35.6–Y35.7, Y89.0	21	14,347,159	184,174
Operations of war and sequelae, Y36, Y89.1	**21**	**14,347,159**	**184,174**
Complications of medical and surgical care and sequelae, Y40–Y84, Y88.0–Y88.3	**2,597**	**116,015**	**1,489**

Source: National Center for Health Statistics. Deaths are classified on the basis of the 10th revision of "The International Classification of Diseases" (ICD-10), which went into effect in 1999.
Note: "n.e.c." means not elsewhere classified.
[a]*Latest official figures.*
[b]*Numbers following titles refer to external cause of injury and poisoning classifications in ICD-10.*

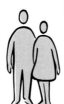

LIFETIME ODDS OF DEATH FOR SELECTED CAUSES, UNITED STATES, 2007[a]

Total, any cause
1 in 1

Heart disease 1 in 6

Cancer 1 in 7

Stroke 1 in 28

Motor vehicle accidents 1 in 88

Intentional self-harm 1 in 112

Accidental poisoning by and exposure to noxious substances 1 in 130

Falls 1 in 171

Car occupant 1 in 303

Assault by firearm 1 in 306

Pedestrian 1 in 649

Motorcycle rider 1 in 770

Accidental drowning and submersion 1 in 1,123

Exposure to smoke, fire and flames 1 in 1,177

Pedalcyclist 1 in 4,717

Firearms discharge 1 in 6,309

Air and space transport accidents 1 in 7,032

Exposure to electric current, radiation, temperature, and pressure 1 in 9,943

Exposure to excessive natural heat 1 in 12,517

Cataclysmic storm 1 in 46,044

Contact with hornets, wasps, and bees 1 in 71,623

Lightning 1 in 84,079

Legal execution 1 in 96,691

Bitten or struck by dog 1 in 120,864

Earthquake and other earth movements 1 in 148,756

Flood 1 in 175,803

Fireworks discharge 1 in 386,766

TRENDS IN UNINTENTIONAL INJURY DEATH RATES

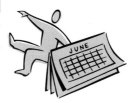

Age-adjusted rates, which eliminate the effect of shifts in the age distribution of the population, have decreased 59% from 1912 to 2009—from 100.4 to 40.9 deaths per 100,000 population. The adjusted rates, which are shown in the graph on the opposite page, are standardized to the year 2000 standard U.S. population. The break in the lines at 1948 shows the estimated effect of changes in the International Classification of Diseases (ICD). The break in the lines at 1992 resulted from the adoption of the Bureau of Labor Statistics Census of Fatal Occupational Injuries for work-related deaths. Another change in the ICD in 1999 also affects the trends. See the Technical Appendix for comparability.

The table below shows the change in the age distribution of the population since 1910.

The age-adjusted death rate for all unintentional injuries increased and decreased significantly several times during the period from 1910 to 1940. Since 1940, some setbacks occurred, such as in the early 1960s, but the overall trend through the early 1990s was positive. The age-adjusted death rates for unintentional injury deaths in the work and home classes declined fairly steadily since they became available in the late 1920s, the home class rates have increased since the early 1990s. The rates in the public class declined for three decades, rose in the 1960s and then continued declining until leveling in the 1990s to the present. The age-adjusted motor vehicle death rate rose steadily from 1910 to the late 1930s as the automobile became more widely used. A sharp drop in use occurred during World War II and a sharp rise in rates occurred in the 1960s, with death rates reflecting economic cycles and a long-term downward trend since then.

UNITED STATES POPULATION, SELECTED YEARS

Year	All ages	0–14	15–24	25–44	45–64	65 and older
Number (in thousands)						
1910	91,973[a]	29,499	18,121	26,810	13,424	3,950
2000[b]	274,634	58,964	38,077	81,892	60,991	34,710
2009	306,803	61,512	42,709	83,322	79,632	39,628
Percent						
1910	100.0%	32.1%	19.7%	29.2%	14.6%	4.3%
2000[b]	100.0%	21.5%	13.9%	29.8%	22.2%	12.6%
2009	100.0%	20.0%	13.9%	27.2%	26.0%	12.9%

Source: For 1910: U.S. Census Bureau. (1960). Historical Statistics of the United States, Colonial Times to 1957. Series A 71-85. Washington, DC: U.S. Government Printing Office. For 2000: Anderson, R.N., and Rosenberg, H.M. (1998). Age standardization of death rates: Implementation of the year 2000 standard. National Vital Statistics Reports, 47(3), 13. For 2008: U.S. Census Bureau, Monthly Postcensal Resident Population, by Single Year of Age, Sex, Race, and Hispanic Origin. Retrieved June 2010 from: www.census.gov/popest/national/asrh/2008-nat-ni.html.
[a]Includes 169,000 persons with age unknown.
[b]This is the population used for standardization (age-adjustment) and differs slightly from the actual 2000 population, which totaled 275,306,000.

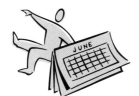

AGE-ADJUSTED DEATH RATES BY CLASS OF INJURY, UNITED STATES, 1910–2009

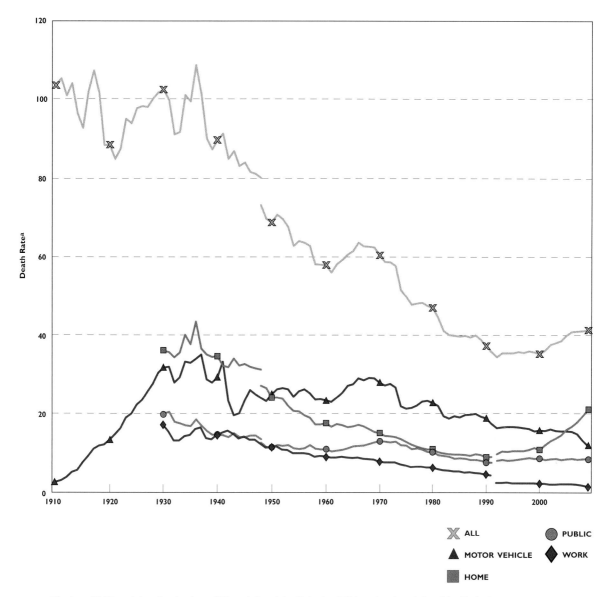

ᵃDeaths per 100,000 population, adjusted to the year 2000 standard population. The break at 1948 shows the estimated effect of classification changes.
The break at 1992 is due to the adoption of the Bureau of Labor Statistics' Census of Fatal Occupational Injuries for work-related deaths.

PRINCIPAL CLASSES OF
UNINTENTIONAL INJURY DEATHS

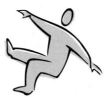

PRINCIPAL CLASSES OF UNINTENTIONAL INJURY DEATHS, UNITED STATES, 1903-2009

Year	Total[a] Deaths	Total[a] Rate[b]	Motor vehicle Deaths	Motor vehicle Rate[b]	Work Deaths	Work Rate[b]	Home Deaths	Home Rate[b]	Public non-motor vehicle Deaths	Public non-motor vehicle Rate[b]
1903	70,600	87.2	(c)	—	(c)	—	(c)	—	(c)	—
1904	71,500	86.6	(c)	—	(c)	—	(c)	—	(c)	—
1905	70,900	84.2	(c)	—	(c)	—	(c)	—	(c)	—
1906	80,000	93.2	400	0.5	(c)	—	(c)	—	(c)	—
1907	81,900	93.6	700	0.8	(c)	—	(c)	—	(c)	—
1908	72,300	81.2	800	0.9	(c)	—	(c)	—	(c)	—
1909	72,700	80.1	1,300	1.4	(c)	—	(c)	—	(c)	—
1910	77,900	84.4	1,900	2.0	(c)	—	(c)	—	(c)	—
1911	79,300	84.7	2,300	2.5	(c)	—	(c)	—	(c)	—
1912	78,400	82.5	3,100	3.3	(c)	—	(c)	—	(c)	—
1913	82,500	85.5	4,200	4.4	(c)	—	(c)	—	(c)	—
1914	77,000	78.6	4,700	4.8	(c)	—	(c)	—	(c)	—
1915	76,200	76.7	6,600	6.6	(c)	—	(c)	—	(c)	—
1916	84,800	84.1	8,200	8.1	(c)	—	(c)	—	(c)	—
1917	90,100	88.2	10,200	10.0	(c)	—	(c)	—	(c)	—
1918	85,100	82.1	10,700	10.3	(c)	—	(c)	—	(c)	—
1919	75,500	71.9	11,200	10.7	(c)	—	(c)	—	(c)	—
1920	75,900	71.2	12,500	11.7	(c)	—	(c)	—	(c)	—
1921	74,000	68.4	13,900	12.9	(c)	—	(c)	—	(c)	—
1922	76,300	69.4	15,300	13.9	(c)	—	(c)	—	(c)	—
1923	84,400	75.7	18,400	16.5	(c)	—	(c)	—	(c)	—
1924	85,600	75.6	19,400	17.1	(c)	—	(c)	—	(c)	—
1925	90,000	78.4	21,900	19.1	(c)	—	(c)	—	(c)	—
1926	91,700	78.7	23,400	20.1	(c)	—	(c)	—	(c)	—
1927	92,700	78.4	25,800	21.8	(c)	—	(c)	—	(c)	—
1928	95,000	79.3	28,000	23.4	19,000	15.8	30,000	24.9	21,000	17.4
1929	98,200	80.8	31,200	25.7	20,000	16.4	30,000	24.6	20,000	16.4
1930	99,100	80.5	32,900	26.7	19,000	15.4	30,000	24.4	20,000	16.3
1931	97,300	78.5	33,700	27.2	17,500	14.1	29,000	23.4	20,000	16.1
1932	89,000	71.3	29,500	23.6	15,000	12.0	29,000	23.2	18,000	14.4
1933	90,932	72.4	31,363	25.0	14,500	11.6	29,500	23.6	18,500	14.7
1934	100,977	79.9	36,101	28.6	16,000	12.7	34,000	26.9	18,000	14.2
1935	99,773	78.4	36,369	28.6	16,500	13.0	32,000	25.2	18,000	14.2
1936	110,052	85.9	38,089	29.7	18,500	14.5	37,000	28.9	19,500	15.2
1937	105,205	81.7	39,643	30.8	19,000	14.8	32,000	24.8	18,000	14.0
1938	93,805	72.3	32,582	25.1	16,000	12.3	31,000	23.9	17,000	13.1
1939	92,623	70.8	32,386	24.7	15,500	11.8	31,000	23.7	16,000	12.2
1940	96,885	73.4	34,501	26.1	17,000	12.9	31,500	23.9	16,500	12.5
1941	101,513	76.3	39,969	30.0	18,000	13.5	30,000	22.5	16,500	12.4
1942	95,889	71.6	28,309	21.1	18,000	13.4	30,500	22.8	16,000	12.0
1943	99,038	73.8	23,823	17.8	17,500	13.0	33,500	25.0	17,000	12.7
1944	95,237	71.7	24,282	18.3	16,000	12.0	32,500	24.5	16,000	12.0
1945	95,918	72.4	28,076	21.2	16,500	12.5	33,500	25.3	16,000	12.1
1946	98,033	70.0	33,411	23.9	16,500	11.8	33,000	23.6	17,500	12.5
1947	99,579	69.4	32,697	22.8	17,000	11.9	34,500	24.1	18,000	12.6
1948 (5th Rev.)[d]	98,001	67.1	32,259	22.1	16,000	11.0	35,000	24.0	17,000	11.6
1948 (6th Rev.)[d]	93,000	63.7	32,259	22.1	16,000	11.0	31,000	21.2	16,000	11.0
1949	90,106	60.6	31,701	21.3	15,000	10.1	31,000	20.9	15,000	10.1
1950	91,249	60.3	34,763	23.0	15,500	10.2	29,000	19.2	15,000	9.9
1951	95,871	62.5	36,996	24.1	16,000	10.4	30,000	19.6	16,000	10.4
1952	96,172	61.8	37,794	24.3	15,000	9.6	30,500	19.6	16,000	10.3
1953	95,032	60.1	37,955	24.0	15,000	9.5	29,000	18.3	16,500	10.4
1954	90,032	55.9	35,586	22.1	14,000	8.7	28,000	17.4	15,500	9.6
1955	93,443	56.9	38,426	23.4	14,200	8.6	28,500	17.3	15,500	9.4
1956	94,780	56.6	39,628	23.7	14,300	8.5	28,000	16.7	16,000	9.6
1957	95,307	55.9	38,702	22.7	14,200	8.3	28,000	16.4	17,500	10.3
1958	90,604	52.3	36,981	21.3	13,300	7.7	26,500	15.3	16,500	9.5
1959	92,080	52.2	37,910	21.5	13,800	7.8	27,000	15.3	16,500	9.3
1960	93,806	52.1	38,137	21.2	13,800	7.7	28,000	15.6	17,000	9.4
1961	92,249	50.4	38,091	20.8	13,500	7.4	27,000	14.8	16,500	9.0
1962	97,139	52.3	40,804	22.0	13,700	7.4	28,500	15.3	17,000	9.2
1963	100,669	53.4	43,564	23.1	14,200	7.5	28,500	15.1	17,500	9.3
1964	105,000	54.9	47,700	25.0	14,200	7.4	28,000	14.6	18,500	9.7
1965	108,004	55.8	49,163	25.4	14,100	7.3	28,500	14.7	19,500	10.1
1966	113,563	58.1	53,041	27.1	14,500	7.4	29,500	15.1	20,000	10.2
1967	113,169	57.3	52,924	26.8	14,200	7.2	29,000	14.7	20,500	10.4
1968	114,864	57.6	54,862	27.5	14,300	7.2	28,000	14.0	21,500	10.8
1969	116,385	57.8	55,791	27.7	14,300	7.1	27,500	13.7	22,500	11.2
1970	114,638	56.2	54,633	26.8	13,800	6.8	27,000	13.2	23,500	11.5
1971	113,439	54.8	54,381	26.3	13,700	6.6	26,500	12.8	23,500	11.4
1972	115,448	55.2	56,278	26.9	14,000	6.7	26,500	12.7	23,500	11.2
1973	115,821	54.8	55,511	26.3	14,300	6.8	26,500	12.5	24,500	11.6

See source and footnotes on page 41.

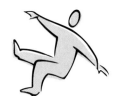

PRINCIPAL CLASSES OF UNINTENTIONAL INJURY DEATHS, UNITED STATES, 1903-2009 (Cont.)

Year	Total[a] Deaths	Total[a] Rate[b]	Motor vehicle Deaths	Motor vehicle Rate[b]	Work Deaths	Work Rate[b]	Home Deaths	Home Rate[b]	Public non-motor vehicle Deaths	Public non-motor vehicle Rate[b]
1974	104,622	49.0	46,402	21.8	13,500	6.3	26,000	12.2	23,000	10.8
1975	103,030	47.8	45,853	21.3	13,000	6.0	25,000	11.6	23,000	10.6
1976	100,761	46.3	47,038	21.6	12,500	5.7	24,000	11.0	21,500	10.0
1977	103,202	47.0	49,510	22.5	12,900	5.9	23,200	10.6	22,200	10.1
1978	105,561	47.5	52,411	23.6	13,100	5.9	22,800	10.3	22,000	9.9
1979	105,312	46.9	53,524	23.8	13,000	5.8	22,500	10.0	21,000	9.4
1980	105,718	46.5	53,172	23.4	13,200	5.8	22,800	10.0	21,300	9.4
1981	100,704	43.9	51,385	22.4	12,500	5.4	21,700	9.5	19,800	8.6
1982	94,082	40.6	45,779	19.8	11,900	5.1	21,200	9.2	19,500	8.4
1983	92,488	39.6	44,452	19.0	11,700	5.0	21,200	9.1	19,400	8.3
1984	92,911	39.4	46,263	19.6	11,500	4.9	21,200	9.0	18,300	7.8
1985	93,457	39.3	45,901	19.3	11,500	4.8	21,600	9.1	18,800	7.9
1986	95,277	39.7	47,865	19.9	11,100	4.6	21,700	9.0	18,700	7.8
1987	95,020	39.2	48,290	19.9	11,300	4.7	21,400	8.8	18,400	7.6
1988	97,100	39.7	49,078	20.1	11,000	4.5	22,700	9.3	18,400	7.5
1989	95,028	38.5	47,575	19.3	10,900	4.4	22,500	9.1	18,200	7.4
1990	91,983	36.9	46,814	18.8	10,100	4.0	21,500	8.6	17,400	7.0
1991	89,347	35.4	43,536	17.3	9,800	3.9	22,100	8.8	17,600	7.0
1992	86,777	34.0	40,982	16.1	4,968[e]	1.9[e]	24,000[e]	9.4[e]	19,000[e]	7.4[e]
1993	90,523	35.1	41,893	16.3	5,035	2.0	26,100	10.1	19,700	7.6
1994	91,437	35.1	42,524	16.3	5,338	2.1	26,300	10.1	19,600	7.5
1995	93,320	35.5	43,363	16.5	5,018	1.9	27,200	10.3	20,100	7.6
1996	94,948	35.8	43,649	16.5	5,058	1.9	27,500	10.4	21,000	7.9
1997	95,644	35.7	43,458	16.2	5,162	1.9	27,700	10.3	21,700	8.1
1998	97,835	36.2	43,501	16.1	5,120	1.9	29,000	10.7	22,600	8.4
1999[f]	97,860	35.9	42,401	15.5	5,185	1.9	30,500	11.2	22,200	8.1
2000	97,900	35.6	43,354	15.7	5,022	1.8	29,200	10.6	22,700	8.2
2001	101,537	35.6	43,788	15.4	5,042	1.8	33,200	11.6	21,800	7.6
2002	106,742	37.1	45,380	15.8	4,726	1.6	36,400	12.6	22,500	7.8
2003	109,277	37.6	44,757	15.4	4,725	1.6	38,800	13.3	23,200	8.0
2004	112,012	38.1	44,933	15.3	5,000	1.7	41,700	14.2	22,700	7.7
2005	117,809	39.7	45,343	15.3	4,987	1.7	46,400	15.6	23,400	7.9
2006	121,599	40.8	45,316	15.2	5,092	1.7	49,600	16.6	23,900	8.0
2007[g]	123,706	41.1	43,945	14.6	4,833	1.6	53,500	17.8	23,700	7.9
2008[g]	125,800	41.4	39,700	13.1	4,425	1.5	59,300	19.5	24,400	8.0
2009[h]	128,200	41.8	35,900	11.7	3,582	1.2	65,200	21.3	25,100	8.2
Changes										
1999 to 2009	+31%	+16%	−15%	−25%	−31%	−37%	+114%	+90%	+13%	+1%
2008 to 2009	+2%	+1%	−10%	−11%	−19%	−20%	+10%	+9%	+3	+3%

Source: Total and motor vehicle deaths, 1903-1932 based on National Center for Health Statistics death registration states; 1933-1948 (5th Rev.), 1949-1963, 1965-2007 are NCHS totals for the United States. Work deaths for 1992-2007 are from the U.S. Bureau of Labor Statistics, Census of Fatal Occupational Injuries. All other figures are National Safety Council estimates.
[a]*Duplications between Motor Vehicle, Work, and Home are eliminated in the Total column.*
[b]*Rates are deaths per 100,000 population.*
[c]*Data insufficient to estimate yearly totals.*
[d]*In 1948, a revision was made in the International Classification of Diseases. The first figures for 1948 are comparable with those for earlier years, the second with those for later years.*
[e]*Adoption of the Census of Fatal Occupational Injuries figure for the Work class necessitated adjustments to the Home and Public classes. See the Technical Appendix for details.*
[f]*In 1999, a revision was made in the International Classification of Diseases. See the Technical Appendix for comparability with earlier years.*
[g]*Revised.*
[h]*Preliminary.*

UNINTENTIONAL INJURY DEATHS BY AGE

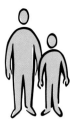

UNINTENTIONAL INJURY DEATHS BY AGE, UNITED STATES, 1903-2009

Year	All ages	Under 5 years	5-14 years	15-24 years	25-44 years	45-64 years	65-74 years	75 years & older[a]
1903	70,600	9,400	8,200	10,300	20,100	12,600	10,000	
1904	71,500	9,700	9,000	10,500	19,900	12,500	9,900	
1905	70,900	9,800	8,400	10,600	19,600	12,600	9,900	
1906	80,000	10,000	8,400	13,000	24,000	13,600	11,000	
1907	81,900	10,500	8,300	13,400	24,900	14,700	10,100	
1908	72,300	10,100	7,600	11,300	20,500	13,100	9,700	
1909	72,700	9,900	7,400	10,700	21,000	13,300	10,400	
1910	77,900	9,900	7,400	11,900	23,600	14,100	11,000	
1911	79,300	11,000	7,500	11,400	22,400	15,100	11,900	
1912	78,400	10,600	7,900	11,500	22,200	14,700	11,500	
1913	82,500	9,800	7,400	12,200	24,500	16,500	12,100	
1914	77,000	10,600	7,900	11,000	21,400	14,300	11,800	
1915	76,200	10,300	8,200	10,800	20,500	14,300	12,100	
1916	84,800	11,600	9,100	7,700	24,900	17,800	13,700	
1917	90,100	11,600	9,700	11,700	24,400	18,500	14,200	
1918	85,100	10,600	10,100	10,600	21,900	17,700	14,200	
1919	75,500	10,100	10,000	10,200	18,600	13,800	12,800	
1920	75,900	10,200	9,900	10,400	18,100	13,900	13,400	
1921	74,000	9,600	9,500	9,800	18,000	13,900	13,200	
1922	76,300	9,700	9,500	10,000	18,700	14,500	13,900	
1923	84,400	9,900	9,800	11,000	21,500	16,900	15,300	
1924	85,600	10,200	9,900	11,900	20,900	16,800	15,900	
1925	90,000	9,700	10,000	12,400	22,200	18,700	17,000	
1926	91,700	9,500	9,900	12,600	22,700	19,200	17,800	
1927	92,700	9,200	9,900	12,900	22,900	19,700	18,100	
1928	95,000	8,900	9,800	13,100	23,300	20,600	19,300	
1929	98,200	8,600	9,800	14,000	24,300	21,500	20,000	
1930	99,100	8,200	9,100	14,000	24,300	22,200	21,300	
1931	97,300	7,800	8,700	13,500	23,100	22,500	21,700	
1932	89,000	7,100	8,100	12,000	20,500	20,100	21,200	
1933	90,932	6,948	8,195	12,225	21,005	20,819	21,740	
1934	100,977	7,034	8,272	13,274	23,288	24,197	24,912	
1935	99,773	6,971	7,808	13,168	23,411	23,457	24,958	
1936	110,052	7,471	7,866	13,701	24,990	26,535	29,489	
1937	105,205	6,969	7,704	14,302	23,955	24,743	27,532	
1938	93,805	6,646	6,593	12,129	20,464	21,689	26,284	
1939	92,628	6,668	6,378	12,066	20,164	20,842	26,505	
1940	96,885	6,851	6,466	12,763	21,166	21,840	27,799	
1941	101,513	7,052	6,702	14,346	22,983	22,509	27,921	
1942	95,889	7,220	6,340	13,732	21,141	20,764	26,692	
1943	99,038	8,039	6,636	15,278	20,212	20,109	28,764	
1944	95,237	7,912	6,704	14,750	19,115	19,097	27,659	
1945	95,918	7,741	6,836	12,446	19,393	20,097	29,405	
1946	98,033	7,949	6,545	13,366	20,705	20,249	29,219	
1947	99,579	8,219	6,069	13,166	21,155	20,513	30,457	
1948 (5th Rev.)[b]	98,001	8,387	5,859	12,595	20,274	19,809	31,077	
1948 (6th Rev.)[b]	93,000	8,350	5,850	12,600	20,300	19,300	9,800	16,800
1949	90,106	8,469	5,539	11,522	19,432	18,302	9,924	16,918
1950	91,249	8,389	5,519	12,119	20,663	18,665	9,750	16,144
1951	95,871	8,769	5,892	12,366	22,363	19,610	10,218	16,653
1952	96,172	8,871	5,980	12,787	21,950	19,892	10,026	16,667
1953	95,032	8,678	6,136	12,837	21,422	19,479	9,927	16,553
1954	90,032	8,380	5,939	11,801	20,023	18,299	9,652	15,938
1955	93,443	8,099	6,099	12,742	29,911	19,199	9,929	16,464
1956	94,780	8,173	6,319	13,545	20,986	19,207	10,160	16,393
1957	95,307	8,423	6,454	12,973	20,949	19,495	10,076	16,937
1958	90,604	8,789	6,514	12,744	19,658	18,095	9,431	15,373
1959	92,080	8,748	6,511	13,269	19,666	18,937	9,475	15,474
1960	93,806	8,950	6,836	13,457	19,600	19,385	9,689	15,829
1961	92,249	8,622	6,717	13,431	19,273	19,134	9,452	15,620
1962	97,139	8,705	6,751	14,557	19,955	20,335	10,149	16,687
1963	100,669	8,688	6,962	15,889	20,529	21,262	10,194	17,145
1964	100,500	8,670	7,400	17,420	22,080	22,100	10,400	16,930
1965	108,004	8,586	7,391	18,688	22,228	22,900	10,430	17,781
1966	113,563	8,507	7,958	21,030	23,134	24,022	10,706	18,206
1967	113,169	7,825	7,874	21,645	23,255	23,826	10,645	18,099
1968	114,864	7,263	8,369	23,012	23,684	23,896	10,961	17,679
1969	116,385	6,973	8,186	24,668	24,410	24,192	10,643	17,313
1970	114,638	6,594	8,203	24,336	23,979	24,164	10,644	16,718
1971	113,439	6,496	8,143	24,733	23,535	23,240	10,494	16,798
1972	115,448	6,142	8,242	25,762	23,852	23,658	10,446	17,346
1973	115,821	6,037	8,102	26,550	24,750	23,059	10,243	17,080

See source and footnotes on page 43.

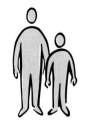

UNINTENTIONAL INJURY DEATHS
BY AGE (CONT.)

43

UNINTENTIONAL INJURY DEATHS BY AGE, UNITED STATES, 1903-2009 (Cont.)

Year	All ages	Under 5 years	5-14 years	15-24 years	25-44 years	45-64 years	65-74 years	75 years & older[a]
1974	104,622	5,335	7,037	24,200	22,547	20,334	9,323	15,846
1975	103,030	4,948	6,818	24,121	22,877	19,643	9,220	15,403
1976	100,761	4,692	6,308	24,316	22,399	19,000	8,823	15,223
1977	103,202	4,470	6,305	25,619	23,460	19,167	9,006	15,175
1978	105,561	4,766	6,118	26,622	25,024	18,774	9,072	15,185
1979	105,312	4,429	5,689	26,574	26,097	18,346	9,013	15,164
1980	105,718	4,479	5,224	26,206	26,722	18,140	8,997	15,950
1981	100,704	4,130	4,866	23,582	26,928	17,339	8,639	15,220
1982	94,082	4,108	4,504	21,306	25,135	15,907	8,224	14,898
1983	92,488	3,999	4,321	19,756	24,996	15,444	8,336	15,636
1984	92,911	3,652	4,198	19,801	25,498	15,273	8,424	16,065
1985	93,457	3,746	4,252	19,161	25,940	15,251	8,583	16,524
1986	95,277	3,843	4,226	19,975	27,201	14,733	8,499	16,800
1987	95,020	3,871	4,198	18,695	27,484	14,807	8,686	17,279
1988	97,100	3,794	4,215	18,507	28,279	15,177	8,971	18,157
1989	95,028	3,770	4,090	16,738	28,429	15,046	8,812	18,143
1990	91,983	3,496	3,650	16,241	27,663	14,607	8,405	17,921
1991	89,347	3,626	3,660	15,278	26,526	13,693	8,137	18,427
1992	86,777	3,286	3,388	13,662	25,808	13,882	8,165	18,586
1993	90,523	3,488	3,466	13,966	27,277	14,434	8,125	19,767
1994	91,437	3,406	3,508	13,898	27,012	15,200	8,279	20,134
1995	93,320	3,067	3,544	13,842	27,660	16,004	8,400	20,803
1996	94,948	2,951	3,433	13,809	27,092	16,717	8,780	22,166
1997	95,644	2,770	3,371	13,367	27,129	17,521	8,578	22,908
1998	97,835	2,689	3,254	13,349	27,172	18,286	8,892	24,193
1999[c]	97,860	2,743	3,091	13,656	27,121	18,924	8,208	24,117
2000	97,900	2,707	2,979	14,113	27,182	19,783	7,698	23,438
2001	101,537	2,690	2,836	14,411	27,784	21,002	7,835	24,979
2002	106,742	2,587	2,718	15,412	29,279	23,020	8,086	25,640
2003	109,277	2,662	2,618	15,272	29,307	25,007	8,081	26,330
2004	112,012	2,693	2,666	15,449	29,503	26,593	8,116	26,992
2005	117,809	2,747	2,415	15,753	30,916	29,192	8,632	28,154
2006	121,599	2,757	2,258	16,229	32,488	31,121	8,420	28,326
2007[d]	123,706	2,873	2,194	15,897	31,908	32,508	8,753	29,573
2008[d]	125,800	2,700	1,900	14,800	32,200	35,000	9,000	30,200
2009[e]	128,200	2,800	1,800	14,100	32,100	37,100	9.300	31,000
Changes								
1999 to 2009	+31%	+2%	−42%	+3%	+18%	+96%	+13%	+29%
2008 to 2009	+2%	+4%	−5%	−5%	− <1%	+6%	+3%	+3%

Source: 1903-1932 based on National Center for Health Statistics data for registration states; 1933-1948 (5th Rev.), 1949-1963, 1965-2007 are NCHS totals. All other figures are National Safety Council estimates. See Technical Appendix for comparability.
[a]Includes age unknown. In 2007, these deaths numbered 34.
[b]In 1948, a revision was made in the International Classification of Diseases. The first figures for 1948 are comparable with those for earlier years, the second with those for later years.
[c]In 1999, a revision was made in the International Classification of Diseases. See the Technical Appendix for comparability with earlier years.
[d]Revised.
[e]Preliminary.

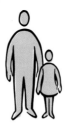

UNINTENTIONAL INJURY DEATH RATES BY AGE

UNINTENTIONAL INJURY DEATH RATES[a] BY AGE, UNITED STATES, 1903-2009

Year	Standardized rate[b]	All ages	Under 5 years	5-14 years	15-24 years	25-44 years	45-64 years	65-74 years	75 years & older[c]
1903	99.4	87.2	98.7	46.8	65.0	87.4	111.7		299.8
1904	103.4	86.6	99.1	50.9	64.9	84.6	108.1		290.0
1905	98.4	84.2	98.6	47.0	64.1	81.4	106.2		282.5
1906	114.2	93.2	99.1	46.5	77.1	97.3	111.7		306.0
1907	112.4	93.6	102.7	45.5	78.0	98.8	117.8		274.2
1908	99.7	81.2	97.5	41.2	64.4	79.5	102.2		256.7
1909	97.4	80.1	94.2	39.6	59.9	79.6	101.0		268.2
1910	103.0	84.4	92.8	39.1	65.3	87.3	104.0		276.0
1911	104.7	84.7	101.9	39.3	62.1	81.4	108.7		292.1
1912	100.4	82.5	97.1	40.5	62.3	79.2	103.2		275.8
1913	103.5	85.5	88.4	37.4	65.2	85.6	112.5		281.7
1914	95.9	78.6	94.3	38.9	58.5	73.2	94.6		268.1
1915	92.1	76.7	90.8	39.7	57.3	69.0	92.1		268.8
1916	101.4	84.1	101.4	43.3	40.8	82.5	112.1		297.6
1917	106.7	88.2	108.4	45.3	62.1	79.8	113.8		301.2
1918	101.2	82.1	91.0	46.5	58.7	72.2	106.3		294.2
1919	87.7	71.9	87.2	45.9	55.3	60.1	81.8		262.0
1920	87.8	71.2	87.4	44.9	55.5	56.9	85.6		289.5
1921	84.3	68.4	80.8	42.4	51.4	55.5	79.4		259.8
1922	86.9	69.4	80.6	41.5	51.4	57.1	81.4		265.1
1923	94.5	75.7	82.0	42.4	55.6	64.5	92.6		282.8
1924	93.3	75.6	82.9	42.4	58.6	61.7	90.2		283.5
1925	97.2	78.4	78.6	42.3	59.7	64.7	97.8		293.9
1926	97.7	78.7	77.9	41.4	59.9	65.4	98.2		298.7
1927	97.5	78.4	75.9	41.0	60.2	65.2	98.0		295.4
1928	99.6	79.3	74.4	40.4	59.9	65.6	99.9		306.2
1929	101.2	80.8	73.3	40.0	63.1	67.7	102.1		308.9
1930	101.8	80.5	71.8	36.9	62.3	67.0	102.9		317.9
1931	99.2	78.5	69.9	35.2	59.7	63.0	102.1		313.3
1932	90.5	71.3	65.1	32.8	52.7	55.6	89.3		296.9
1933	91.1	72.4	65.5	33.4	53.6	56.3	90.8		295.3
1934	100.5	79.9	68.1	33.9	57.8	61.8	103.3		328.5
1935	97.9	78.4	68.5	32.2	56.9	61.6	98.0		319.8
1936	108.1	85.9	74.4	32.9	58.8	65.3	108.6		367.4
1937	100.7	81.7	69.6	32.7	60.9	62.1	99.3		333.4
1938	89.4	72.3	65.3	28.5	51.3	52.5	85.4		308.9
1939	86.7	70.8	62.9	28.2	50.7	51.2	81.0		300.0
1940	89.1	73.4	64.8	28.8	53.5	53.2	83.4		305.7
1941	90.7	76.3	65.0	29.7	60.9	57.2	84.8		297.4
1942	84.3	71.6	63.9	27.9	59.8	52.4	77.1		275.5
1943	86.3	73.8	66.9	29.0	69.7	50.3	73.6		287.8
1944	82.5	71.7	63.2	29.1	72.9	48.9	68.9		268.6
1945	83.4	72.4	59.8	29.5	64.5	50.5	71.6		277.6
1946	81.0	70.0	60.2	28.1	61.7	48.8	70.9		267.9
1947	80.5	69.4	57.4	25.8	59.6	49.0	70.6		270.7
1948 (5th Rev.)[d]	79.5	67.1	56.3	24.6	56.8	46.2	66.8		267.4
1948 (6th Rev.)[d]	72.5	63.7	56.0	24.5	56.8	46.2	65.1	122.4	464.3
1949	69.0	60.6	54.4	23.0	52.2	43.5	60.6	120.4	450.7
1950	68.1	60.3	51.4	22.6	55.0	45.6	60.5	115.8	414.7
1951	70.1	62.5	50.8	23.6	57.7	49.0	62.7	117.1	413.6
1952	69.0	61.8	51.5	22.5	60.9	47.7	62.7	111.1	399.8
1953	67.0	60.1	49.5	22.1	61.4	46.4	60.5	106.7	383.6
1954	62.2	55.9	46.7	20.5	56.4	43.0	55.9	100.7	354.4
1955	63.4	56.9	43.9	20.7	60.1	44.7	57.7	100.8	350.2
1956	63.0	56.6	43.3	20.2	63.3	44.7	56.7	100.6	335.6
1957	62.2	55.9	43.5	19.9	59.5	44.6	56.6	97.5	333.3
1958	57.5	52.3	44.5	19.6	56.2	42.0	51.7	89.3	292.6
1959	57.4	52.2	43.6	18.9	56.5	42.1	53.2	87.7	284.7
1960	57.3	52.1	44.0	19.1	55.6	42.0	53.6	87.6	281.4
1961	55.4	50.4	42.0	18.1	54.0	41.2	52.1	83.8	267.9
1962	57.5	52.3	42.6	18.0	55.0	42.7	54.6	88.5	277.7
1963	58.6	53.4	42.8	18.2	57.2	44.0	56.3	87.9	277.0
1964	60.0	54.9	43.1	19.1	59.9	47.3	57.6	88.9	263.9
1965	61.9	55.8	43.4	18.7	61.6	47.7	58.8	88.5	268.7
1966	63.0	58.1	44.4	19.9	66.9	49.6	60.7	89.8	267.4
1967	62.1	57.3	42.2	19.4	66.9	49.7	59.2	88.5	257.4
1968	62.0	57.6	40.6	20.5	69.2	50.1	58.5	90.2	244.0
1969	61.8	57.8	40.2	20.0	71.8	51.2	58.4	86.6	232.0
1970	59.8	56.2	38.4	20.1	68.0	49.8	57.6	85.2	219.6
1971	58.1	54.8	37.7	20.1	66.1	48.4	54.7	82.7	213.2
1972	58.0	55.2	35.9	20.6	67.6	47.5	55.2	80.8	214.2
1973	57.1	54.8	35.8	20.6	68.2	48.0	53.3	77.3	206.3

See source and footnotes on page 45.

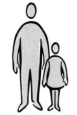
UNINTENTIONAL INJURY DEATH RATES[a] BY AGE, UNITED STATES, 1903-2009 (Cont.)

Year	Standardized rate[b]	All ages	Under 5 years	5-14 years	15-24 years	25-44 years	45-64 years	65-74 years	75 years & older[c]
1974	50.9	49.0	32.4	18.2	60.9	42.7	46.7	68.7	186.7
1975	49.3	47.8	30.7	17.8	59.5	42.3	44.9	66.2	175.5
1976	47.3	46.3	30.0	16.7	58.9	40.3	43.2	62.0	168.4
1977	47.6	47.0	28.7	17.0	61.3	40.9	43.4	61.5	164.0
1978	47.8	47.5	30.3	16.9	63.1	42.3	42.4	60.5	159.7
1979	47.0	46.9	27.6	16.1	62.6	42.7	41.3	58.8	154.8
1980	46.5	46.5	27.2	15.0	61.7	42.3	40.8	57.5	158.6
1981	44.0	43.9	24.4	14.2	55.9	41.2	39.0	54.4	147.4
1982	40.6	40.6	23.8	13.2	51.2	37.3	35.8	50.9	140.0
1983	39.6	39.6	22.8	12.7	48.2	36.0	34.7	50.8	142.8
1984	39.4	39.4	20.6	12.4	48.9	35.7	34.3	50.7	142.8
1985	39.2	39.3	21.0	12.6	47.9	35.3	34.2	50.9	143.0
1986	39.4	39.7	21.4	12.6	50.5	36.1	33.0	49.6	141.5
1987	39.0	39.2	21.4	12.4	48.1	35.7	33.0	49.8	141.6
1988	39.5	39.7	20.9	12.3	48.5	36.1	33.4	50.9	145.3
1989	38.4	38.5	20.4	11.8	44.8	35.7	32.8	49.3	141.5
1990	36.8	36.9	18.5	10.4	44.0	34.2	31.6	46.4	136.5
1991	35.3	35.4	18.9	10.2	42.0	32.3	29.3	44.5	136.7
1992	34.0	34.0	16.8	9.3	37.8	31.3	28.7	44.2	134.5
1993	35.0	35.1	17.7	9.4	38.8	33.0	29.1	43.6	139.9
1994	35.0	35.1	17.3	9.4	38.4	32.5	29.9	44.3	139.2
1995	35.0	35.5	15.7	9.3	38.2	33.2	30.6	44.8	140.6
1996	35.3	35.8	15.3	8.9	38.1	32.3	31.1	47.0	145.9
1997	35.1	35.7	14.5	8.7	36.5	32.5	31.6	46.3	146.2
1998	35.5	36.2	14.2	8.3	35.9	32.6	31.9	48.3	151.1
1999[e]	35.2	35.9	14.5	7.8	36.1	32.7	32.0	45.0	147.7
2000	34.8	35.6	14.3	7.5	36.7	33.0	32.3	42.3	140.8
2001	35.7	35.6	13.9	6.9	36.1	32.7	32.6	42.8	146.8
2002	37.1	37.1	13.2	6.6	37.9	34.7	34.6	44.2	148.2
2003	37.6	37.6	13.5	6.4	37.0	34.8	36.4	44.0	149.6
2004	38.1	38.1	13.4	6.5	37.1	35.1	37.6	43.9	151.4
2005	39.5	39.7	13.5	6.0	37.4	36.8	40.1	46.3	155.2
2006	40.4	40.8	13.5	5.6	38.5	38.9	41.6	44.5	154.4
2007[f]	40.5	41.1	13.9	5.5	37.5	38.2	42.4	45.2	159.2
2008[f]	40.6	41.4	12.9	4.7	34.8	38.6	44.8	46.5	161.1
2009[g]	40.8	41.8	13.2	4.5	33.0	38.5	46.6	44.8	164.5
Changes									
1999 to 2009	+16%	–9%	–42%	–9%	+18%	+46%	– <1%	+11%	
2008 to 2009	+1%	+2%	–4%	–5%	– <1%	+4%	–4%	+2%	
2008 population (millions)									
Total[h]	306,803	21,268	40,244	42,709	83,322	79,632	20,781	18,847	
Male	151,367	10,883	20,583	21,930	42,233	38,889	9,583	7,265	
Female	155,436	10,385	19,662	20,779	41,089	40,742	11,198	11,582	

Source: All figures are National Safety Council estimates. See Technical Appendix for comparability.
[a]Rates are deaths per 100,000 resident population in each age group.
[b]Adjusted to the year 2000 standard population to remove the influence of changes in age distribution between 1903 and 2007.
[c]Includes age unknown.
[d]In 1948, a revision was made in the International Classification of Diseases. The first figures for 1948 are comparable with those for earlier years, the second with those for later years.
[e]In 1999, a revision was made in the International Classification of Diseases. See the Technical Appendix for comparability.
[f]Revised.
[g]Preliminary.
[h]Sum of parts may not equal total due to rounding.

PRINCIPAL TYPES OF UNINTENTIONAL INJURY DEATHS

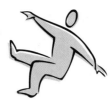

PRINCIPAL TYPES OF UNINTENTIONAL INJURY DEATHS, UNITED STATES, 1903-1998

Year	Total	Motor vehicle	Falls	Drowning[a]	Fire, flames, smoke[b]	Choking[b]	Firearms	Poison (solid, liquid)	Poison (gas, vapor)	All other
1903	70,600	(c)	(c)	9,200	(c)	(c)	2,500	(c)	(c)	58,900
1904	71,500	(c)	(c)	9,300	(c)	(c)	2,800	(c)	(c)	59,400
1905	70,900	(c)	(c)	9,300	(c)	(c)	2,000	(c)	(c)	59,600
1906	80,000	400	(c)	9,400	(c)	(c)	2,100	(c)	(c)	68,100
1907	81,900	700	(c)	9,000	(c)	(c)	1,700	(c)	(c)	70,500
1908	72,300	800	(c)	9,300	(c)	(c)	1,900	(c)	(c)	60,300
1909	72,700	1,300	(c)	8,500	(c)	(c)	1,600	(c)	(c)	61,300
1910	77,900	1,900	(c)	8,700	(c)	(c)	1,900	(c)	(c)	65,400
1911	79,300	2,300	(c)	9,000	(c)	(c)	2,100	(c)	(c)	65,900
1912	78,400	3,100	(c)	8,600	(c)	(c)	2,100	(c)	(c)	64,600
1913	82,500	4,200	15,100	10,300	8,900	(c)	2,400	3,200	(c)	38,400
1914	77,000	4,700	15,000	8,700	9,100	(c)	2,300	3,300	(c)	33,900
1915	76,200	6,600	15,000	8,600	8,400	(c)	2,100	2,800	(c)	32,700
1916	84,800	8,200	15,200	8,900	9,500	(c)	2,200	2,900	(c)	37,900
1917	90,100	10,200	15,200	7,600	10,800	(c)	2,300	2,800	(c)	41,200
1918	85,100	10,700	13,200	7,000	10,200	(c)	2,500	2,700	(c)	38,800
1919	75,500	11,200	11,900	9,100	9,100	(c)	2,800	3,100	(c)	28,300
1920	75,900	12,500	12,600	6,100	9,300	(c)	2,700	3,300	(c)	29,400
1921	74,000	13,900	12,300	7,800	7,500	(c)	2,800	2,900	(c)	26,800
1922	76,300	15,300	13,200	7,000	8,300	(c)	2,900	2,800	(c)	26,800
1923	84,400	18,400	14,100	6,800	9,100	(c)	2,900	2,800	2,700	27,600
1924	85,600	19,400	14,700	7,400	7,400	(c)	2,900	2,700	2,900	28,200
1925	90,000	21,900	15,500	7,300	8,600	(c)	2,800	2,700	2,800	28,400
1926	91,700	23,400	16,300	7,500	8,800	(c)	2,800	2,600	3,200	27,100
1927	92,700	25,800	16,500	8,100	8,200	(c)	3,000	2,600	2,700	25,800
1928	95,000	28,000	17,000	8,600	8,400	(c)	2,900	2,800	2,800	24,500
1929	98,200	31,200	17,700	7,600	8,200	(c)	3,200	2,600	2,800	24,900
1930	99,100	32,900	18,100	7,500	8,100	(c)	3,200	2,600	2,500	24,200
1931	97,300	33,700	18,100	7,600	7,100	(c)	3,100	2,600	2,100	23,000
1932	89,000	29,500	18,600	7,500	7,100	(c)	3,000	2,200	2,100	19,000
1933	90,932	31,363	18,962	7,158	6,781	(c)	3,014	2,135	1,633	19,886
1934	100,977	36,101	20,725	7,077	7,456	(c)	3,033	2,148	1,643	22,794
1935	99,773	36,369	21,378	6,744	7,253	(c)	2,799	2,163	1,654	21,413
1936	110,052	38,089	23,562	6,659	7,939	(c)	2,817	2,177	1,665	27,144
1937	105,205	39,643	22,544	7,085	7,214	(c)	2,576	2,190	1,675	22,278
1938	93,805	32,582	23,239	6,881	6,491	(c)	2,726	2,077	1,428	18,381
1939	92,623	32,386	23,427	6,413	6,675	(c)	2,618	1,963	1,440	17,701
1940	96,885	34,501	23,356	6,202	7,521	(c)	2,375	1,847	1,583	19,500
1941	101,513	39,969	22,764	6,389	6,922	(c)	2,396	1,731	1,464	19,878
1942	95,889	28,309	22,632	6,696	7,901	(c)	2,678	1,607	1,741	24,325
1943	99,038	23,823	24,701	7,115	8,726	921	2,282	1,745	2,014	27,711
1944	95,237	24,282	22,989	6,511	8,372	896	2,392	1,993	1,860	25,942
1945	95,918	28,076	23,847	6,624	7,949	897	2,385	1,987	2,120	22,033
1946	98,033	33,411	23,109	6,442	7,843	1,076	2,801	1,961	1,821	19,569
1947	99,579	32,697	24,529	6,885	8,033	1,206	2,439	1,865	1,865	14,060
1948 (5th Rev.)[d]	98,001	32,259	24,836	6,428	7,743	1,315	2,191	1,753	2,045	19,611
1948 (6th Rev.)[d]	93,000	32,259	22,000	6,500	6,800	1,299	2,330	1,600	2,020	17,192
1949	90,106	31,701	22,308	6,684	5,982	1,341	2,326	1,634	1,617	16,513
1950	91,249	34,763	20,783	6,131	6,405	1,350	2,174	1,584	1,769	16,290
1951	95,871	36,996	21,376	6,489	6,788	1,456	2,247	1,497	1,627	17,395
1952	96,172	37,794	20,945	6,601	6,922	1,434	2,210	1,440	1,397	17,429
1953	95,032	37,955	20,631	6,770	6,579	1,603	2,277	1,391	1,223	16,603
1954	90,032	35,586	19,771	6,334	6,083	1,627	2,271	1,339	1,223	15,798
1955	93,443	38,426	20,192	6,344	6,352	1,608	2,120	1,431	1,163	15,807
1956	94,780	39,628	20,282	6,263	6,405	1,760	2,202	1,422	1,213	15,605
1957	95,307	38,702	20,545	6,613	6,269	2,043	2,369	1,390	1,143	16,233
1958	90,604	36,981	18,248	6,582e	7,291e	2,191e	2,172	1,429	1,187	14,523
1959	92,080	37,910	18,774	6,434	6,898	2,189	2,258	1,661	1,141	14,815
1960	93,806	38,137	19,023	6,529	7,645	2,397	2,334	1,679	1,253	14,809
1961	92,249	38,091	18,691	6,525	7,102	2,499	2,204	1,804	1,192	14,141
1962	97,139	40,804	19,589	6,439	7,534	1,813	2,092	1,833	1,376	15,659
1963	100,669	43,564	19,335	6,347	8,172	1,949	2,263	2,061	1,489	15,489
1964	105,000	47,700	18,941	6,709	7,379	1,865	2,275	2,100	1,360	16,571
1965	108,004	49,163	19,984	6,799	7,347	1,836	2,344	2,110	1,526	16,895
1966	113,563	53,041	20,066	7,084	8,084	1,831	2,558	2,283	1,648	16,968
1967	113,169	52,924	20,120	7,076	7,423	1,980	2,896	2,506	1,574	16,670
1968	114,864	54,862	18,651	7,372e	7,335	3,100e	2,394e	2,583	1,526	17,041
1969	116,385	55,791	17,827	7,699	7,163	3,712	2,309	2,967	1,549	16,368
1970	114,638	54,633	16,926	7,860	6,718	2,753	2,406	3,679	1,620	18,043
1971	113,439	54,381	16,755	7,396	6,776	2,877	2,360	3,710	1,646	17,538
1972	115,448	56,278	16,744	7,586	6,714	2,830	2,442	3,728	1,690	17,436
1973	115,821	55,511	16,506	8,725	6,503	3,013	2,618	3,683	1,652	17,610

See source and footnotes on page 47.

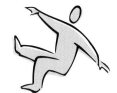

PRINCIPAL TYPES OF UNINTENTIONAL INJURY DEATHS, UNITED STATES, 1903-1998 (Cont.)

Year	Total	Motor vehicle	Falls	Drowning[a]	Fire, flames, smoke[b]	Choking[b]	Firearms	Poison (solid, liquid)	Poison (gas, vapor)	All other
1974	104,622	46,402	16,339	7,876	6,236	2,991	2,513	4,016	1,518	16,731
1975	103,030	45,853	14,896	8,000	6,071	3,106	2,380	4,694	1,577	16,453
1976	100,761	47,038	14,136	6,827	6,338	3,033	2,059	4,161	1,569	15,600
1977	103,202	49,510	13,773	7,126	6,357	3,037	1,982	3,374	1,596	16,447
1978	105,561	52,411	13,690	7,026	6,163	3,063	1,806	3,035	1,737	16,630
1979	105,312	53,524	13,216	6,872	5,991	3,243	2,004	3,165	1,472	15,825
1980	105,718	53,172	13,294	7,257	5,822	3,249	1,955	3,089	1,242	16,638
1981	100,704	51,385	12,628	6,277	5,697	3,331	1,871	3,243	1,280	14,992
1982	94,082	45,779	12,077	6,351	5,210	3,254	1,756	3,474	1,259	14,922
1983	92,488	44,452	12,024	6,353	5,028	3,387	1,695	3,382	1,251	14,916
1984	92,911	46,263	11,937	5,388	5,010	3,541	1,668	3,808	1,103	14,193
1985	93,457	45,901	12,001	5,316	4,938	3,551	1,649	4,091	1,079	14,931
1986	95,277	47,865	11,444	5,700	4,835	3,692	1,452	4,731	1,009	14,549
1987	95,020	48,290	11,733	5,100	4,710	3,688	1,440	4,415	900	14,744
1988	97,100	49,078	12,096	4,966	4,965	3,805	1,501	5,353	873	14,463
1989	95,028	47,575	12,151	4,015	4,716	3,578	1,489	5,603	921	14,980
1990	91,983	46,814	12,313	4,685	4,175	3,303	1,416	5,055	748	13,474
1991	89,347	43,536	12,662	4,818	4,120	3,240	1,441	5,698	736	13,096
1992	86,777	40,982	12,646	3,542	3,958	3,182	1,409	6,449	633	13,976
1993	90,523	41,893	13,141	3,807	3,900	3,160	1,521	7,877	660	14,564
1994	91,437	42,524	13,450	3,942	3,986	3,065	1,356	8,309	685	14,120
1995	93,320	43,363	13,986	4,350	3,761	3,185	1,225	8,461	611	14,378
1996	94,948	43,649	14,986	3,959	3,741	3,206	1,134	8,872	638	14,763
1997	95,644	43,458	15,447	4,051	3,490	3,275	981	9,587	576	14,779
1998	97,835	43,501	16,274	4,406	3,255	3,515	866	10,255	546	15,217

PRINCIPAL TYPES OF UNINTENTIONAL INJURY DEATHS, UNITED STATES, 1999-2009

Year	Total	Motor vehicle	Falls	Poisoning	Choking[b]	Drowning[f]	Fire, flames, smoke[b]	Mechanical suffocation	Firearms	All other
1999[g]	97,860	42,401	13,162	12,186	3,885	3,529	3,348	1,618	824	16,907
2000	97,900	43,354	13,322	12,757	4,313	3,482	3,377	1,335	776	15,184
2001	101,537	43,788	15,019	14,078	4,185	3,281	3,309	1,370	802	15,705
2002	106,742	45,380	16,257	17,550	4,128	3,447	3,159	1,389	762	13,670
2003	109,277	44,757	17,229	19,457	4,272	3,306	3,369	1,309	730	14,850
2004	112,012	44,933	18,807	20,950	4,470	3,308	3,229	1,421	649	14,245
2005	117,809	45,343	19,656	23,617	4,386	3,582	3,197	1,514	789	15,725
2006	121,599	45,316	20,823	27,531	4,332	3,579	3,109	1,580	642	14,687
2007[h]	123,706	43,945	22,631	29,846	4,344	3,443	3,286	1,653	613	14,558
2008[h]	125,800	39,700	24,300	34,400	4,600	3,500	3,200	1,700	610	14,400
2009[i]	128,200	35,900	26,100	39,000	4,600	3,700	3,200	1,800	600	13,900
Changes										
1999 to 2009	+31%	−15%	+98%	+220%	+18%	+5%	−4%	+11%	−27%	−18%
2008 to 2009	+2%	−10%	+7%	+13%	0%	+6%	0%	+6%	−2%	−3%

Source: National Center for Health Statistics and National Safety Council. See Technical Appendix for comparability.
[a]Includes drowning in water transport accidents.
[b]Fires, Flames, Smoke includes burns by fire and deaths resulting from conflagration regardless of nature of injury. Choking is the inhalation of food or other object obstructing breathing.
[c]Comparable data not available.
[d]In 1948, a revision was made in the International Classification of Diseases. The first figures for 1948 are comparable with those for earlier years, the second with those for later years.
[e]Data are not comparable to previous years shown due to classification changes in 1958 and 1968.
[f]Excludes water transport drownings.
[g]In 1999, a revision was made in the International Classification of Diseases. See the Technical Appendix for comparability.
[h]Revised.
[i]Preliminary.

UNINTENTIONAL INJURY DEATH RATES FOR PRINCIPAL TYPES

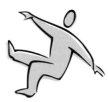

UNINTENTIONAL INJURY DEATH RATES[a] FOR PRINCIPAL TYPES, UNITED STATES, 1903-1998

Year	Total	Motor vehicle	Falls	Drowning[b]	Fire, flames, smoke[c]	Choking[c]	Firearms	Poison (solid, liquid)	Poison (gas, vapor)	All other
1903	87.2	(d)	(d)	11.4	(d)	(d)	3.1	(d)	(d)	72.7
1904	86.6	(d)	(d)	11.3	(d)	(d)	3.4	(d)	(d)	71.9
1905	84.2	(d)	(d)	11.1	(d)	(d)	2.4	(d)	(d)	70.7
1906	93.2	0.5	(d)	11.0	(d)	(d)	2.4	(d)	(d)	79.3
1907	93.6	0.8	(d)	10.4	(d)	(d)	2.0	(d)	(d)	80.4
1908	81.2	0.9	(d)	10.5	(d)	(d)	2.1	(d)	(d)	67.7
1909	80.1	1.4	(d)	9.4	(d)	(d)	1.8	(d)	(d)	67.5
1910	84.4	2.0	(d)	9.4	(d)	(d)	2.1	(d)	(d)	70.9
1911	84.7	2.5	(d)	9.6	(d)	(d)	2.2	(d)	(d)	70.4
1912	82.5	3.3	(d)	9.0	(d)	(d)	2.2	(d)	(d)	68.0
1913	85.5	4.4	15.5	10.6	9.1	(d)	2.5	3.3	(d)	40.1
1914	78.6	4.8	15.1	8.8	9.1	(d)	2.3	3.3	(d)	35.2
1915	76.7	6.6	14.9	8.6	8.4	(d)	2.1	2.8	(d)	33.3
1916	84.1	8.1	14.9	8.7	9.3	(d)	2.2	2.8	(d)	38.1
1917	88.2	10.0	14.7	7.4	10.5	(d)	2.2	2.7	(d)	40.7
1918	82.1	10.3	12.8	6.8	9.9	(d)	2.4	2.6	(d)	37.3
1919	71.9	10.7	11.4	6.9	8.7	(d)	2.7	3.0	(d)	28.5
1920	71.2	11.7	11.8	5.7	8.7	(d)	2.5	3.1	(d)	27.7
1921	68.4	12.9	11.3	7.2	6.9	(d)	2.6	2.7	(d)	24.8
1922	69.4	13.9	12.0	6.4	7.5	(d)	2.6	2.5	(d)	24.5
1923	75.7	16.5	12.6	6.1	8.1	(d)	2.6	2.5	2.4	24.9
1924	75.6	17.1	12.9	6.5	8.4	(d)	2.5	2.4	2.5	23.3
1925	78.4	19.1	13.4	6.3	7.4	(d)	2.4	2.3	2.4	25.1
1926	78.7	20.1	13.9	6.4	7.5	(d)	2.4	2.2	2.7	23.5
1927	78.4	21.8	13.9	6.8	6.9	(d)	2.5	2.2	2.3	22.0
1928	79.3	23.4	14.1	7.1	7.0	(d)	2.4	2.3	2.3	20.7
1929	80.8	25.7	14.5	6.2	6.7	(d)	2.6	2.1	2.3	20.7
1930	80.5	26.7	14.7	6.1	6.6	(d)	2.6	2.1	2.0	19.7
1931	78.5	27.2	14.6	6.1	5.7	(d)	2.5	2.1	1.7	18.6
1932	71.3	23.6	14.9	6.0	5.7	(d)	2.4	1.8	1.7	15.2
1933	72.4	25.0	15.1	5.7	5.4	(d)	2.4	1.7	1.3	15.8
1934	79.9	28.6	16.4	5.6	5.9	(d)	2.4	1.7	1.3	18.0
1935	78.4	28.6	16.8	5.3	5.7	(d)	2.2	1.7	1.3	16.8
1936	85.9	29.7	18.4	5.2	6.2	(d)	2.2	1.7	1.3	21.2
1937	81.7	30.8	17.5	5.5	5.6	(d)	2.0	1.7	1.3	17.3
1938	72.3	25.1	17.9	5.3	5.0	(d)	2.1	1.6	1.1	14.2
1939	70.8	24.7	17.9	4.9	5.1	(d)	2.0	1.5	1.1	13.6
1940	73.4	26.1	17.7	4.7	5.7	(d)	1.8	1.4	1.2	14.8
1941	76.3	30.0	17.1	4.8	5.2	(d)	1.8	1.3	1.1	15.0
1942	71.6	21.1	16.9	5.0	5.9	(d)	2.0	1.2	1.3	18.2
1943	73.8	17.8	18.4	5.3	6.5	0.7	1.7	1.3	1.5	20.6
1944	71.7	18.3	17.3	4.9	6.3	0.7	1.8	1.5	1.4	19.5
1945	72.4	21.2	18.0	5.0	6.0	0.7	1.8	1.5	1.6	16.6
1946	70.0	23.9	16.5	4.6	5.6	0.8	2.0	1.4	1.3	13.9
1947	69.4	22.8	17.1	4.8	5.6	0.8	1.7	1.3	1.3	14.0
1948 (5th Rev.)[e]	67.1	22.1	17.0	4.4	5.3	0.9	1.5	1.2	1.4	13.3
1948 (6th Rev.)[e]	63.7	22.1	15.1	4.5	4.7	0.9	1.6	1.1	1.4	12.3
1949	60.6	21.3	15.0	4.5	4.0	0.9	1.6	1.1	1.1	11.1
1950	60.3	23.0	13.7	4.1	4.2	0.9	1.4	1.1	1.2	10.7
1951	62.5	24.1	13.9	4.2	4.4	1.0	1.5	1.0	1.1	11.3
1952	61.8	24.3	13.5	4.2	4.5	0.9	1.4	0.9	0.9	11.2
1953	60.1	24.0	13.0	4.3	4.2	1.0	1.4	0.9	0.8	10.2
1954	55.9	22.1	12.3	3.9	3.8	1.0	1.4	0.8	0.8	9.8
1955	56.9	23.4	12.3	3.9	3.9	1.0	1.3	0.9	0.7	9.5
1956	56.6	23.7	12.1	3.7	3.8	1.1	1.3	0.8	0.7	9.4
1957	55.9	22.7	12.1	3.9	3.7	1.2	1.4	0.8	0.7	9.4
1958	52.3	21.3	10.5	3.8[f]	4.2[f]	1.3[f]	1.3	0.8	0.7	8.4
1959	52.2	21.5	10.6	3.7	3.9	1.2	1.3	0.9	0.7	8.4
1960	52.1	21.2	10.6	3.6	4.3	1.3	1.3	0.9	0.7	8.2
1961	50.4	20.8	10.2	3.6	3.9	1.4	1.2	1.0	0.7	7.6
1962	52.3	22.0	10.5	3.5	4.1	1.0	1.1	1.0	0.7	8.4
1963	53.4	23.1	10.3	3.4	4.3	1.0	1.2	1.1	0.8	8.2
1964	54.9	25.0	9.9	3.5	3.9	1.0	1.2	1.1	0.7	8.4
1965	55.8	25.4	10.3	3.5	3.8	1.0	1.2	1.1	0.8	8.7
1966	58.1	27.1	10.3	3.6	4.8	0.9	1.3	1.2	0.8	8.1
1967	57.3	26.8	10.2	3.6	3.8	1.0	1.5	1.3	0.8	8.3
1968	57.6	27.5	9.4	3.7[f]	3.7[f]	1.6[f]	1.2[f]	1.3	0.8	8.4
1969	57.8	27.7	8.9	3.8	3.6	1.8	1.2	1.5	0.8	8.5
1970	56.2	26.8	8.3	3.9	3.3	1.4	1.2	1.8	0.8	8.7
1971	54.8	26.3	8.1	3.6	3.3	1.4	1.1	1.8	0.8	8.4
1972	55.2	26.9	8.0	3.6	3.2	1.4	1.2	1.8	0.8	8.3
1973	54.8	26.3	7.8	4.1	3.1	1.4	1.2	1.7	0.8	8.4

See source and footnotes on page 49.

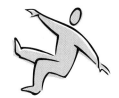

UNINTENTIONAL INJURY DEATH RATES[a] FOR PRINCIPAL TYPES, UNITED STATES, 1903-1998 (Cont.)

Year	Total	Motor vehicle	Falls	Drowning[b]	Fire, flames, smoke[c]	Choking[c]	Firearms	Poison (solid, liquid)	Poison (gas, vapor)	All other
1974	49.0	21.8	7.7	3.7	2.9	1.4	1.2	1.8	0.7	7.8
1975	47.8	21.3	6.9	3.7	2.8	1.4	1.1	2.2	0.7	7.7
1976	46.3	21.6	6.5	3.1	2.9	1.4	0.9	1.9	0.7	7.3
1977	47.0	22.5	6.3	3.2	2.9	1.4	0.9	1.5	0.7	7.6
1978	47.5	23.6	6.2	3.2	2.8	1.4	0.8	1.4	0.8	7.3
1979	46.9	23.8	5.9	3.1	2.7	1.4	0.9	1.4	0.7	7.0
1980	46.5	23.4	5.9	3.2	2.6	1.4	0.9	1.4	0.5	7.2
1981	43.9	22.4	5.5	2.7	2.5	1.5	0.8	1.4	0.6	6.5
1982	40.6	19.8	5.2	2.7	2.2	1.4	0.8	1.5	0.5	6.5
1983	39.6	19.0	5.1	2.7	2.2	1.4	0.7	1.4	0.5	6.6
1984	39.4	19.6	5.1	2.3	2.1	1.5	0.7	1.6	0.5	6.0
1985	39.3	19.3	5.0	2.2	2.1	1.5	0.7	1.7	0.5	6.3
1986	39.7	19.9	4.8	2.4	2.0	1.5	0.6	2.0	0.4	6.1
1987	39.2	19.9	4.8	2.1	1.9	1.5	0.6	1.8	0.4	6.2
1988	39.7	20.1	4.9	2.0	2.0	1.6	0.6	2.2	0.4	5.9
1989	38.5	19.3	4.9	1.9	1.9	1.4	0.6	2.3	0.4	5.8
1990	36.9	18.8	4.9	1.9	1.7	1.3	0.6	2.0	0.3	5.4
1991	35.4	17.3	5.0	1.8	1.6	1.3	0.6	2.3	0.3	5.2
1992	34.0	16.1	5.0	1.4	1.6	1.2	0.6	2.5	0.2	5.4
1993	35.1	16.3	5.1	1.5	1.5	1.2	0.6	3.1	0.3	5.5
1994	35.1	16.3	5.2	1.5	1.5	1.2	0.5	3.2	0.3	5.4
1995	35.5	16.5	5.3	1.7	1.4	1.2	0.5	3.2	0.2	5.5
1996	35.8	16.5	5.6	1.5	1.4	1.2	0.4	3.3	0.2	5.7
1997	35.7	16.2	5.8	1.5	1.3	1.2	0.4	3.6	0.2	5.5
1998	36.2	16.1	6.0	1.6	1.2	1.3	0.3	3.8	0.2	5.7

UNINTENTIONAL INJURY DEATH RATES[a] FOR PRINCIPAL TYPES, UNITED STATES, 1999-2009

Year	Total	Motor vehicle	Falls	Poisoning	Choking[c]	Drowning[g]	Fire, flames, and smoke[c]	Mechanical suffocation	Firearms	All other
1999[h]	35.9	15.5	4.8	4.5	1.4	1.3	1.2	0.6	0.3	6.3
2000	35.6	15.7	4.8	4.6	1.6	1.3	1.2	0.5	0.3	5.5
2001	35.6	15.4	5.3	4.9	1.5	1.2	1.2	0.5	0.3	5.5
2002	37.1	15.8	5.6	6.4	1.4	1.2	1.1	0.5	0.3	4.7
2003	37.6	15.4	5.9	6.7	1.5	1.1	1.2	0.4	0.3	5.1
2004	38.1	15.3	6.4	7.1	1.5	1.1	1.1	0.5	0.2	4.9
2005	39.7	15.3	6.6	8.0	1.5	1.2	1.1	0.5	0.3	5.3
2006	40.8	15.2	7.0	9.2	1.5	1.2	1.0	0.5	0.2	4.9
2007[i]	41.1	14.6	7.5	9.9	1.4	1.1	1.1	0.5	0.2	4.8
2008[i]	41.4	13.1	8.0	11.3	1.5	1.2	1.1	0.6	0.2	4.7
2009[i]	41.8	11.7	8.5	12.7	1.5	1.2	1.0	0.6	0.2	4.5
Changes										
1999 to 2009	+16%	−24%	+77%	+182%	+7%	−8%	−17%	0%	−33%	−29%
2008 to 2009	+1%	−11%	−6%	+12%	0%	0%	−9%	0%	0%	−4%

Source: National Safety Council estimates. See Technical Appendix for comparability.
[a]*Deaths per 100,000 population.*
[b]*Includes drowning in water transport accidents.*
[c]*Flames, fire, smoke includes burns by fire and deaths resulting from conflagration regardless of nature of injury. Choking is the inhalation of food or other object obstructing breathing.*
[d]*Comparable data not available.*
[e]*In 1948, a revision was made in the International Classification of Diseases. The first figures for 1948 are comparable with those for earlier years, the second with those for later years.*
[f]*Data are not comparable to previous years shown due to classification changes in 1958 and 1968.*
[g]*Excludes water transport drownings.*
[h]*In 1999, a revision was made in the International Classification of Diseases. See the Technical Appendix for comparability.*
[i]*Revised.*
[j]*Preliminary.*

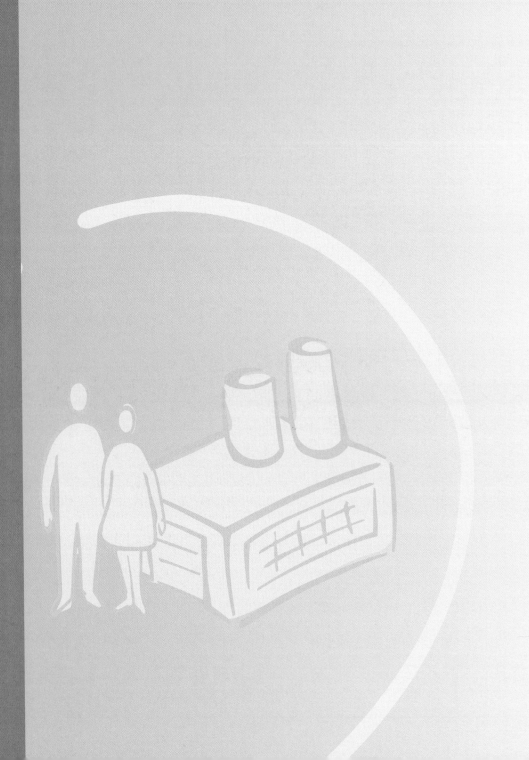

OVERVIEW OF WORK-RELATED UNINTENTIONAL INJURY DEATHS, 2009

128,200
Unintentional Injury Deaths

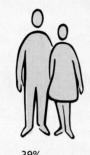

39%
All Others

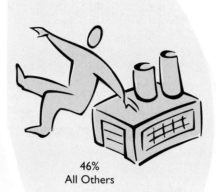

46%
All Others

15%
Workers' Spouses
and Children

59,400
Worker Deaths from
Unintentional Injuries

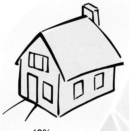

48%
Off-the-Job
Home

31%
Off-the-Job
Motor Vehicle

15%
Off-the-Job
Public

6%
On-the-Job

3,582
On-The-Job Deaths from
Unintentional Injuries

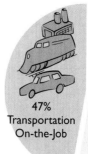

47%
Transportation
On-the-Job

53%
All Other
On-the-Job

WORK, 2009

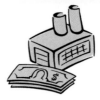

The 2009 data presented in this section is preliminary. All Census of Fatal Occupational Injuries fatal injury rates published by the Bureau of Labor Statistics for 1992-2007 were employment-based and measured the risk of fatal injury for people employed during a given period of time, regardless of hours worked. Starting in 2008, BLS moved to hours-based rates to measure fatal injury risk per standardized length of exposure, which generally are considered more accurate than employment-based rates. Caution should be used when comparing rates prior to 2008.

In addition to unintentional (accidental) fatal work injuries, 758 homicides and suicides occurred in the workplace in 2009. These intentional injuries are not included in the unintentional injury data shown here.

The State Data section, which begins on page 168, shows fatal occupational injuries and nonfatal injury and illness incidence rates by state.

Unintentional injury deaths **3,582**

Unintentional injury deaths per 100,000 full-time equivalent workers[a] **2.8**

Medically consulted injuries **5,100,000**

Workers **141,102,000**

Costs . . . . **$168.9 billion**

UNINTENTIONAL INJURIES AT WORK BY INDUSTRY (PRELIMINARY), UNITED STATES, 2009

Industry division	Hours worked[a] (millions)	Deaths[a]		Deaths per 100,000 full-time equivalent workers[a]		Medically Consulted Injuries
		2009	Change from 2008	2009	Change from 2008	
All industries	254,771	3,582	—19%	2.8	—15%	5,100,000
Agriculture[b]	4,147	527	–18%	25.4	–14%	110,000
Mining[b]	1,580	101	–42%	12.8	–28%	20,000
Construction	16,685	776	–17%	9.3	–1%	360,000
Manufacturing	28,049	280	–23%	2.0	–13%	600,000
Wholesale trade	7,665	165	5%	4.3	13%	130,000
Retail trade	27,469	133	–16%	1.0	–9%	580,000
Transportation & warehousing	9,527	526	–27%	11.0	–19%	250,000
Utilities	1,849	17	–54%	1.8	–55%	30,000
Information	5,874	28	–22%	1.0	–9%	60,000
Financial activities	18,075	53	–18%	0.6	–14%	140,000
Professional & business services	27,221	341	–3%	2.5	4%	240,000
Educational & health services	36,879	92	–16%	0.5	–17%	920,000
Leisure & hospitality	19,857	110	–7%	1.1	0%	390,000
Other services[b]	11,927	103	–21%	1.7	–19%	170,000
Government	37,822	336	–19%	1.8	–14%	1,100,000

Source: Deaths are preliminary data from the U.S. Bureau of Labor Statistics, Census of Fatal Occupational Injuries. All other figures are National Safety Council estimates based on data from BLS.
[a]Deaths include persons of all ages. Workers and death rates include persons 16 years and older. The rate is calculated as: (number of fatal work injuries x 200,000,000/total hours worked). The base for 100,000 full-time equivalent worker is 200,000,000 hours. Prior to 2008, rates were based on estimated employment, not hours worked.
[b]Agriculture includes forestry, fishing, and hunting. Mining includes oil and gas extraction. Other services excludes public administration.
[c]See Technical Appendix for definition of medically consulted injury.

OCCUPATIONAL UNINTENTIONAL INJURY DEATHS AND DEATH RATES BY INDUSTRY, UNITED STATES, 2009

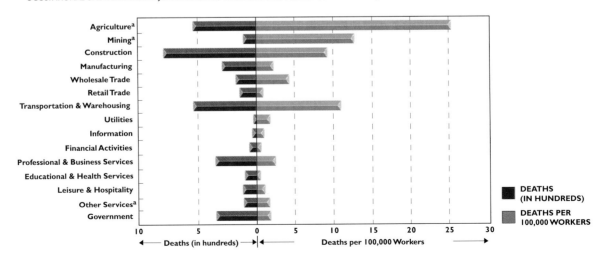

[a]Agriculture includes forestry, fishing, and hunting. Mining includes oil and gas extraction. Other services excludes public administration.

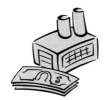

UNINTENTIONAL WORK INJURY DEATHS AND DEATH RATES, UNITED STATES, 1992-2009

Year	Deaths	Workers (in thousands)	Hours worked[a] (in millions)	Deaths per 100,000 workers[a]
1992	4,965	119,168	—	4.2
1993	5,034	120,778	—	4.2
1994	5,338	124,470	—	4.3
1995	5,015	126,248	—	4.0
1996	5,069	127,997	—	4.0
1997	5,160	130,810	—	3.9
1998	5,117	132,772	—	3.9
1999	5,184	134,688	—	3.8
2000	5,022	136,402	—	3.7
2001	5,042	136,246	—	3.7
2002	4,726	137,731	—	3.4
2003	4,725	138,988	—	3.4
2004	4,995	140,504	—	3.6
2005	4,984	142,946	—	3.5
2006	5,088	145,607	—	3.5
2007	4,829	147,203		3.3
2008[a,b]	4,423	146,535	271,958	3.3[a]
2009[c]	3,582	141,102	254,771	2.8

Source: Deaths and hours worked are from the Bureau of Labor Statistics, Census of Fatal Occupational Injuries. Employment is from BLS and is based on the Current Population Survey. All other data are National Safety Council estimates.
Note: Deaths include persons of all ages. Workers and death rates include persons 16 years and older. Workers are persons ages 16 and older gainfully employed, including owners, managers, other paid employees, the self-employed, unpaid family workers, and active duty resident military personnel. Because of adoption of CFOI, deaths and rates from 1992 to the present are not comparable to prior years. See the Technical Appendix for additional information.
[a]Starting in 2008, BLS moved from employment-based rates to hours-based rates to measure fatal injury risk per standardized length of exposure, which are generally considered more accurate than employment-based rates. Caution should be used when comparing to rates prior to 2008.
[b]Revised.
[c]Preliminary. BLS urges caution when using preliminary estimates.

WORKERS, UNINTENTIONAL INJURY DEATHS, AND DEATH RATES, UNITED STATES, 1992–2009

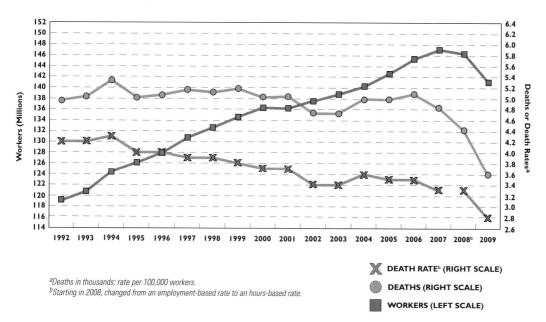

[a]Deaths in thousands; rate per 100,000 workers.
[b]Starting in 2008, changed from an employment-based rate to an hours-based rate.

✕ **DEATH RATE[b] (RIGHT SCALE)**

⬤ **DEATHS (RIGHT SCALE)**

■ **WORKERS (LEFT SCALE)**

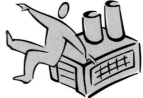

OCCUPATIONAL INJURY DEATHS AND DEATH RATES, UNITED STATES, 1992-2002

Year	Total	Homicide & suicide	Unintentional								
			All industries[a]	Agriculture[b]	Mining, quarrying[c]	Construction	Manufacturing	Transportation & public utilities	Trade[d]	Services[e]	Government
Deaths											
1992	6,217	1,252	4,965	779	175	889	707	767	415	601	586
1993	6,331	1,297	5,034	842	169	895	698	753	450	631	527
1994	6,632	1,294	5,338	814	177	1,000	734	819	492	676	534
1995	6,275	1,260	5,015	769	155	1,021	640	784	461	608	528
1996	6,202	1,133	5,069	762	151	1,025	660	883	451	615	321
1997	6,238	1,078	5,160	799	156	1,075	678	882	451	593	504
1998	6,055	938	5,117	808	143	1,136	631	830	443	634	465
1999	6,054	870	5,184	776	122	1,168	671	918	425	623	451
2000	5,920	898	5,022	693	153	1,114	624	872	447	643	460
2001	5,915	873[f]	5,042	714	169	1,183	546	844	431	636	507
2002	5,534	808	4,726	758	120	1,092	523	843	381	569	437
Deaths per 100,000 workers											
1992	5.2	1.0	4.2	23.1	26.4	13.7	3.6	11.5	1.7	1.6	3.0
1993	5.2	1.0	4.2	26.0	25.3	13.3	3.6	11.0	1.8	1.6	2.6
1994	5.3	1.0	4.3	22.8	26.5	14.4	3.7	11.6	1.9	1.7	2.7
1995	4.9	1.0	4.0	21.4	24.8	14.3	3.1	11.0	1.8	1.5	2.7
1996	4.8	0.9	4.0	21.2	26.6	13.7	3.2	12.2	1.7	1.4	1.6
1997	4.8	0.8	3.9	22.5	24.7	13.7	3.3	11.6	1.7	1.3	2.6
1998	4.5	0.7	3.9	22.7	23.1	14.1	3.1	10.8	1.6	1.4	2.4
1999	4.5	0.6	3.8	22.6	21.7	13.8	3.4	11.5	1.5	1.3	2.2
2000	4.3	0.7	3.7	20.1	29.4	12.4	3.1	10.8	1.6	1.4	2.3
2001	4.3	0.6[f]	3.7	22.0	29.9	13.0	2.9	10.4	1.6	1.3	2.5
2002	4.0	0.6	3.4	21.8	23.3	11.9	2.9	10.5	1.4	1.1	2.1

Source: Deaths are from Bureau of Labor Statistics, Census of Fatal Occupational Injuries. Rates are National Safety Council estimates based on BLS employment data. Deaths include persons of all ages. Death rates include persons 16 years and older. Industry divisions based on the Standard Industrial Classification Manual.
[a]*Includes deaths with industry unknown.*
[b]*Agriculture includes forestry, fishing, and agricultural services.*
[c]*Mining includes oil and gas extraction.*
[d]*Trade includes wholesale and retail trade.*
[e]*Services includes finance, insurance, and real estate.*
[f]*Excludes 2,886 homicides of workers on Sept. 11, 2001.*

OCCUPATIONAL INJURY DEATHS AND DEATH RATES, UNITED STATES, 2003-2009

Year	Total	Homicide & suicide	Unintentional															
			All industries[a]	Agriculture, forestry, Fishing & hunting	Mining	Construction	Manufacturing	Wholesale trade	Retail trade	Transportation & warehousing	Utilities	Information	Financial activities	Professional & business services	Educational & health services	Leisure & hospitality	Other services	Government
Deaths																		
2003	5,575	850	4,725	676	141	1,094	379	169	148	735	29	57	82	396	116	142	123	434
2004	5,764	769	4,995	651	151	1,203	421	187	189	779	49	49	68	401	123	144	144	432
2005	5,734	750	4,984	697	154	1,161	357	197	198	831	28	56	66	442	122	114	149	404
2006	5,840	752	5,088	635	190	1,199	423	210	190	803	52	61	82	407	142	136	142	409
2007	5,657	828	4,829	564	180	1,163	364	193	160	819	33	70	69	415	121	138	116	421
2008[b]	5,214	791	4,423	640	173	937	364	157	158	724	37	36	65	351	110	118	130	414
2009[c]	4,340	758	3,582	527	101	776	280	165	133	526	17	28	53	341	92	110	103	336
Deaths per 100,000 workers[d]																		
2003	4.0	0.6	3.4	30.0	26.9	11.4	2.3	3.8	0.9	16.0	3.3	1.6	0.9	2.9	0.6	1.3	1.8	2.1
2004	4.1	0.5	3.6	29.7	28.1	11.7	2.6	4.1	1.2	16.7	5.9	1.5	0.7	2.9	0.7	1.3	2.1	2.0
2005	4.0	0.5	3.5	31.7	24.8	10.8	2.2	4.3	1.2	16.7	3.4	1.7	0.7	3.2	0.6	1.0	2.1	1.9
2006	4.0	0.5	3.5	29.1	27.8	10.6	2.6	4.6	1.1	15.7	6.2	1.8	0.8	2.8	0.7	1.2	2.0	1.9
2007	3.8	0.5	3.3	26.9	24.7	10.2	2.2	4.4	1.0	15.6	3.9	2.1	0.7	2.7	0.6	1.2	1.7	1.9
2008[b,d]	3.8	0.6	3.3	29.4	17.8	9.4	2.3	3.8	1.1	13.6	4.0	1.1	0.7	2.4	0.6	1.1	2.1	2.1
2009[c]	3.4	0.6	2.8	25.4	12.8	9.3	2.0	4.3	1.0	11.0	1.8	1.0	0.6	2.5	0.5	1.1	1.7	1.8

Source: Deaths are from Bureau of Labor Statistics, Census of Fatal Occupational Injuries. Rates are National Safety Council estimates based on BLS employment data. Deaths include persons of all ages. Death rates include persons 16 years and older. Industry sectors based on the North American Industry Classification System.
[a]*Includes deaths with industry unknown.*
[b]*Revised.*
[c]*Preliminary. BLS urges particular caution when using preliminary estimates.*
[d]*Starting in 2008, BLS moved from employment-based rates to hours-based rates to measure fatal injury risk per standardized length of exposure. Caution should be used when comparing rates prior to 2008.*

WORK INJURY COSTS

The true cost to the nation, employers, and individuals of work-related deaths and injuries is much greater than the cost of workers' compensation insurance alone. The figures presented below show the National Safety Council's estimates of the total economic costs of occupational deaths and injuries. Cost estimating procedures were revised for the 1993 edition of *Accident Facts®* and additional revisions were made for the 2005-2006 edition. For this reason, *costs should not be compared to prior years.*

TOTAL COST IN 2009 . . . . **$168.9 billion**

Includes wage and productivity losses of $82.4 billion, medical costs of $38.3 billion, and administrative expenses of $33.1 billion. Includes employers' uninsured costs of $10.3 billion, such as the money value of time lost by workers other than those with

disabling injuries, who are directly or indirectly involved in injuries, and the cost of time required to investigate injuries, write up injury reports, etc. Also includes damage to motor vehicles in work injuries of $2.0 billion and fire losses of $2.8 billion.

Cost per worker **$1,200**
Includes the value of goods or services each worker must produce to offset the cost of work injuries. It is *not* the average cost of a work injury.

Cost per death **$1,330,000**
Cost per medically consulted injury **$36,000**

Includes estimates of wage losses, medical expenses, administrative expenses, and employer costs, but excludes property damage costs except to motor vehicles.

TIME LOST DUE TO WORK INJURIES

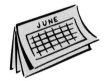

DAYS LOST

TOTAL TIME LOST IN 2009 . . . . **95,000,000**
Due to injuries in 2009 . . . . **55,000,000**
Includes primarily the actual time lost during the year from disabling injuries, except that it does not include time lost on the day of the injury or time required for further medical treatment or check-up following the injured person's return to work.

Fatalities are included at an average loss of 150 days per case and permanent impairments are included at actual days lost plus an allowance for lost efficiency resulting from the impairment.

Not included is time lost by people with nondisabling injuries or other people directly or indirectly involved in the incidents.

DAYS LOST

Due to injuries in prior years **40,000,000**
Represents productive time lost in 2009 due to permanently disabling injuries that occurred in prior years.

DAYS LOST

TIME LOSS IN FUTURE YEARS
FROM 2009 INJURIES **45,000,000**
Includes time lost in future years due to on-the-job deaths and permanently disabling injuries that occurred in 2009.

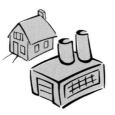

WORKER DEATHS AND INJURIES
ON AND OFF THE JOB

56

Nine out of every 10 deaths and nearly three-fourths of medically consulted injurie[a] suffered by workers in 2009 occurred off the job. While more than 15 times the number of deaths occur off the job compared with on the job (15.8 to 1), nearly three times as many medically consulted injuries[a] occur off the job (2.8 to 1).

Production time lost due to off-the-job injuries totaled about 255,000,000 days in 2009, compared with 55,000,000 days lost by workers injured on the job.

Production time lost in future years due to off-the-job injuries in 2009 will total an estimated 545,000,000 days, more than 12 times the 45,000,000 days lost in future years from 2009's on-the-job injuries.

Off-the-job injuries to workers cost the nation at least $246.8 billion in 2009 compared with $168.9 billion for on-the-job injuries.

WORKERS' ON- AND OFF-THE-JOB INJURIES, UNITED STATES, 2009

Place	Deaths		Medically consulted injuries[a]	
	Number	Rate[b]	Number	Rate[b]
On and off the job	59,382	0.014	19,500,000	4.7
On the job	3,582	0.002	5,100,000	3.4
Off the job	55,800	0.021	14,400,000	5.3
Motor vehicle	*18,200*	*0.064*	*1,800,000*	*6.4*
Public non-motor vehicle	*8,700*	*0.020*	*3,300,000*	*7.5*
Home	*28,900*	*0.015*	*9,300,000*	*4.7*

Source: National Safety Council estimates. Procedures for allocating time spent on and off the job were revised for the 1990 edition. Rate basis changed to 200,000 hours for the 1998 edition. Death and injury rates are not comparable to rate estimates prior to the 1998 edition.
[a]Medically consulted injuries are not comparable to estimates provided in earlier editions that used the definition of disabling injury. Please see the Technical Appendix for more information regarding medically consulted injuries.
[b]Per 200,000 hours exposure by place.

WORKERS' ON- AND OFF-THE-JOB INJURIES, 2009

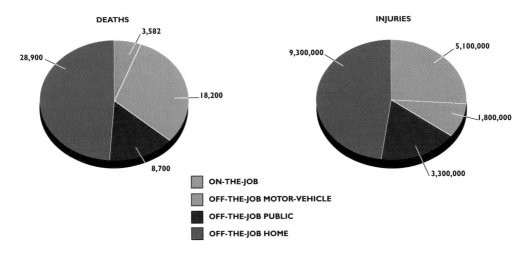

WORKERS' OFF-THE-JOB FATALITIES BY EVENT, 2009

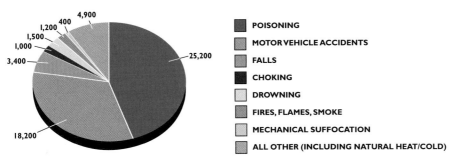

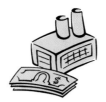

WORKERS COMPENSATION CASES

57

According to the National Academy of Social Insurance, an estimated $57.6 billion, including benefits under deductible provisions, was paid out under workers' compensation in 2008 (the latest year for which data were available), an increase of about 4.4% from 2007. Of this total, $28.6 billion was for income benefits and $29.1 billion was for medical and hospitalization costs. Private carriers paid about $30.1 billion of the total workers' compensation benefits in 2008. In 2008,

approximately 130.6 million workers were covered by workers' compensation—a decrease of 0.8% from the 131.7 million in 2007.

The table below shows the trend in the number of compensated or reported cases in each reporting state. Due to the differences in population, industries, and coverage of compensation laws, comparisons across states should not be made.

WORKERS' COMPENSATION CASES, 2007-2009

State	Deaths[a]			Cases[a]			2008 compensation paid ($000)
	2009	2008	2007	2009	2008	2007	
Alabama[b]	58	64	70	14,386	15,574	16,607	648,094
Alaska	17	21	27	20,099	22,927	22,718	205,263
Arizona	—	100	97	102,870	122,101	121,699	648,664
Arkansas[b]	95	71	80	8,903	9,622	10,024	215,404
California[c]	421	578	685	537,887	635,649	695,700	9,426,019
Colorado	—	126	125	—	29,096	30,293	875,440
District of Columbia	4	5	12	10,034	9,979	10,091	81,263
Hawaii	—	26	27	—	24,542	26,105	245,763
Idaho[d]	22	31	36	36,211	42,425	44,400	280,276
Iowa[b]	53	63	72	16,051	19,617	19,965	575,072
Kansas[e]	41	32	56	59,045	68,268	72,464	417,517
Kentucky	—	38	42	—	29,836	32,446	696,185
Louisiana[e]	80	52	59	12,960[f]	14,550[g]	16,150	733,650
Massachusetts	—	61	75	31,216	32,794	33,476	842,705
Minnesota[e]	30	42	50	—	112,600	119,000	1,007,193
Mississippi[e]	48	67	81	11,138	11,787	12,450	361,015
Missouri	120	109	123	109,123	122,700	131,574	937,299
Montana	70	22	32	26,393	31,061	31,861	252,648
Nebraska	61	46	55	45,761	48,530	49,345	345,108
Nevada[e]	—	42	86	—	65,077	65,842	392,663
New Hampshire	14	13	23	42,189	45,208	46,171	239,290
New Mexico	34	38	37	21,761	20,937	24,072	271,573
North Carolina	—	—	—	64,405	62,462	64,405	1,526,320
North Dakota	16	19	24	20,544	21,061	21,309	105,837
Ohio	197	236	176	132,549	159,611	171,692	2,490,080
Oregon[e]	31	45	35	18,948	21,659	23,431	601,849
Pennsylvania[c]	—	154	148	—	104,275	115,845	2,902,243
Rhode Island	3	3	2	20,723	22,583	25,544	158,006
South Dakota	6	13	14	22,018	25,455	24,604	113,555
Tennessee	65	74	97	105,413	106,276	124,359	827,757
Utah	44	73	73	51,851	62,272	68,105	301,116
West Virginia	39	59	55	44,802	45,944	46,540	603,073
Wisconsin[b]	—	77	103	—	38,857	41,390	1,011,334

Source: Deaths and Cases data from National Safety Council survey of state workers' compensation authorities for calendar or fiscal year. States not listed did not respond to the survey. Compensation Paid data from Sengupta, I., Reno, V., and Burton, J. F., Jr. (September 2010). Workers' compensation: benefits, coverage, and costs, 2008. Washington, DC: National Academy of Social Insurance.
Note: Dash (—) indicates data not available.

Definitions:
Reported case—a reported case may or may not be work-related and may not receive compensation.
Compensated case—a case determined to be work-related and for which compensation was paid.

[a]Reported cases involving medical and indemnity benefits, unless otherwise noted.
[b]Reported cases involving indemnity benefits only.
[c]Reported and closed or compensated cases.
[d]Reported cases involving medical benefits only.
[e]Closed or compensated cases only.
[f]Preliminary.
[g]Updated.

WORKERS COMPENSATION CLAIMS COSTS, 2007-2008

Head injuries are the most costly workers' compensation claims.

Data in the graphs on this and the next page are from the National Council on Compensation Insurance's (NCCI) Workers Compensation Statistical Plan (WCSP) database. The WCSP database includes details on virtually all lost-time claims for 36 states, while NCCI provides ratemaking services. Total incurred costs consist of medical and indemnity payments plus case reserves on open claims, and are calculated as of the second report (30 months after the inception date of the policy). Injuries that result in medical payments only, without lost time, are not included. For open claims, costs include all payments as of the second report plus case reserves for future payments. The average cost for all claims combined in 2007-2008 was $34,377.

NCCI data that previously appeared in *Injury Facts* was sourced to its Detailed Claim Information (DCI) file, which was a stratified random sample of lost-time claims in 42 states. Data from the current WCSP database are not comparble to those provided in previous years from the DCI file.

Cause of injury. The most costly lost-time workers'

compensation claims by cause of injury, according to the NCCI data, are for those resulting from motor vehicle crashes. These injuries averaged $65,875 per workers' compensation claim filed in 2007 and 2008. The only other causes with above average costs were falls or slips ($40,043) and burns ($36,974).

Nature of injury. The most costly lost-time workers' compensation claims by nature of the injury are for those resulting from amputation. These injuries averaged $63,494 per workers' compensation claim filed in 2007 and 2008. The next highest costs were for injuries resulting in fracture, crush, or dislocation ($47,947), other trauma ($41,104), and burns ($41,092).

Part of body. The most costly lost-time workers' compensation claims are for those involving the head or central nervous system. These injuries averaged $84,362 per workers' compensation claim filed in 2007 and 2008. The next highest costs were for injuries involving multiple body parts ($54,117) and neck ($52,654). Injuries to the arm or shoulder; hip, thigh, and pelvis; leg; and lower back also had above-average costs.

AVERAGE TOTAL INCURRED COSTS PER CLAIM BY CAUSE OF INJURY, 2007–2008

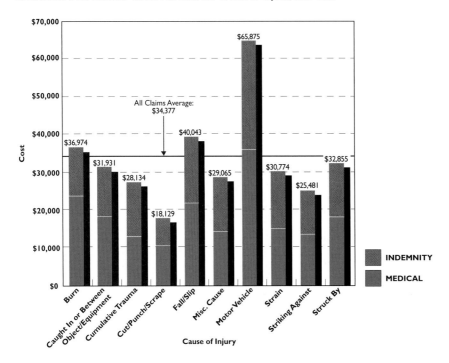

AVERAGE TOTAL INCURRED COSTS PER CLAIM BY NATURE OF INJURY, 2007–2008

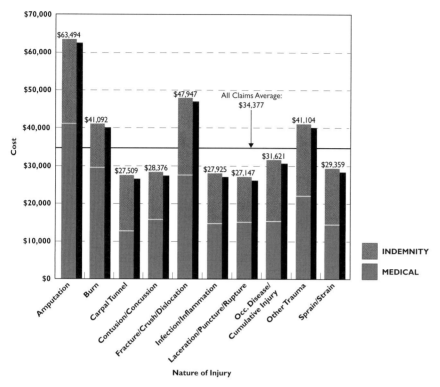

AVERAGE TOTAL INCURRED COSTS PER CLAIM BY PART OF BODY, 2007–2008

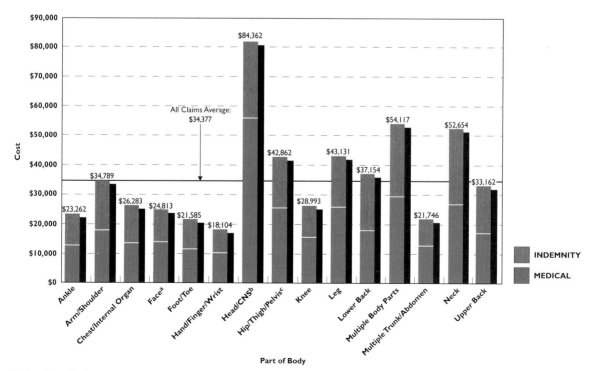

[a]Includes teeth, mouth, and eyes.
[b]Central nervous system.
[c]Includes sacrum and coccyx.

Please note NCCI data previously published in Injury Facts used data from the Detailed Claim Information file.
The current year's data is from the workers' compensation statistical plan and is not comparable to previous years.

DISABLING WORKPLACE INJURIES AND ILLNESSES

The most disabling workplace injuries and illnesses in 2007 amounted to more than $52 billion in direct workers' compensation costs, averaging more than 1 billion dollars per week according to the 2009 Liberty Mutual Safety Index (WSI). WSI combines information from Liberty Mutual, the U.S. Bureau of Labor Statistics, and the National Academy of Social Insurance to identify the top causes of serious workplace injuries. Injury events that cause an employee to miss six or more days from work are considered serious.

The top 10 causes of serious workplace injuries produced about 87% of the entire cost burden of disabling workplace injuries in 2007. Overexertion injuries remained the largest contributor to the overall burden, accounting for $12.7 billion, or 24%, of the total cost. The top five causes—"Overexertion," "Fall on same level," "Fall to lower level," "Bodily motion," and "Struck by object"—were consistent with results

from the previous year and together accounted for 69% of the total burden. The cost of the combined fall categories exceeded that for the "Overexertion" category for the first time since the initiation of WSI in 1998.

Following a four-year cost decline, WSI for 2006 to 2007 exhibited an 8.9% increase in the cost of the most disabling workplace injuries—from $48.6 billion in 2006 to $53.0 billion in 2007. Over the 10-year period from 1998 to 2007, these costs grew to $53.0 billionfrom $37.1 billion, an increase of 42.8%. After adjusting for inflation, the one-year increase was 5.4% and the 10-year increase was 5.8%. Based on these real growth figures, the two fall categories increased the most, with "Fall on same level" increasing 37% and "Fall to lower level" rising 34% over the 10-year period.

Source: 2009 Workplace Safety Index, retrieved Sept. 7, 2010, from www.libertymutual.com/researchinstitute.

WORKERS' COMPENSATION COSTS FOR THE TOP TEN CAUSES OF DISABLING WORKPLACE INJURIES, UNITED STATES, 2007

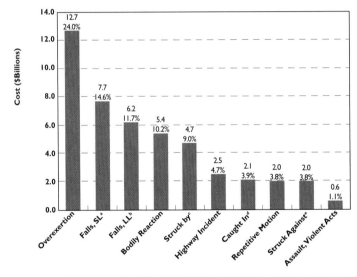

CHANGE IN INFLATION ADJUSTED WORKERS' COMPENSATION COSTS FOR THE TOP TEN CAUSES OF DISABLING WORKPLACE INJURIES, UNITED STATES, 1998-2007

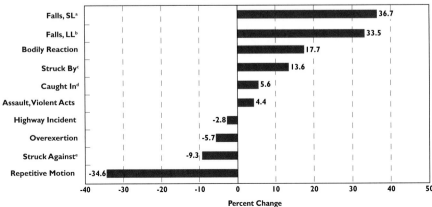

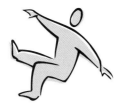

WORKPLACE FALLS

Following highway crashes, falls to a lower level is the second leading fatal workplace event and the fifth leading event resulting in cases with days away from work. In 2008, 593 workers died and another 67,510 were injured. Related to the economic downturn, 2008 fatalities represent more than a 20% decrease from 2007, while nonfatal injuries represent a 13% decrease. Prior to 2008, the number of both fatal and nonfatal falls to a lower level remained relatively stable.

Fatal falls to a lower level typically involve injuries to the head or multiple body parts, while nonfatal injuries most often involve the lower extremities trunk or multiple body parts. The most common nonfatal injuries include sprains and strains, followed by fractures. Falls to a lower level result in dramatically more days away from work than typical injury events. Falls to a lower level cases result in a median of 15 days away from work, compared to eight days across all injury events. In fact, more than 37% of the fall to a lower level cases involving days away from work result in 31 or more lost work days. Falls to a lower level resulting in days away from work most often occur on stairs or steps (27%), followed by ladders (26%). New employees are disproportionably represented, with 31% of nonfatal injuries involving workers with less than one year of service.

By far, construction is the industry most at risk of falls to

a lower level. In 2008, 328 workers in the construction industry died as a result of falls to a lower level, representing 55% of all fall to lower level fatalities. The fall to a lower level fatality rate in this industry is 3.3 per 100,000 workers, more than 6 times the general industry rate of 0.5. Falls to a lower level also represent the single most dangerous injury event within the construction industry, representing 34% of all fatalities. The construction industry also experiences the most nonfatal cases involving days away from work, representing 23% of all nonfatal fall to a lower level cases with 15,560. Thirty-nine percent of these nonfatal cases resulted from falls from ladders (6,140 cases).

Compared with falls to a lower level, falls on the same level tend to result in less severe but more frequent injuries. In 2008, there were 157,680 falls on the same level cases involving days away from work and 92 fatalities. The rate for cases involving days away from work was 16.6 per 10,000 workers, compared to 7.1 for falls to a lower level. Transportation and warehousing has the highest fall on the same level rate with 27.9 per 10,000 workers, followed by retail trade (19.4), and real estate and rental and leasing (19.7).

The following two pages provide injury profiles for both falls to a lower level and falls on the same level.

Source: National Safety Council analysis of Bureau of Labor Statistics data.

FALLS TO A LOWER LEVEL, UNITED STATES, 2003–2008

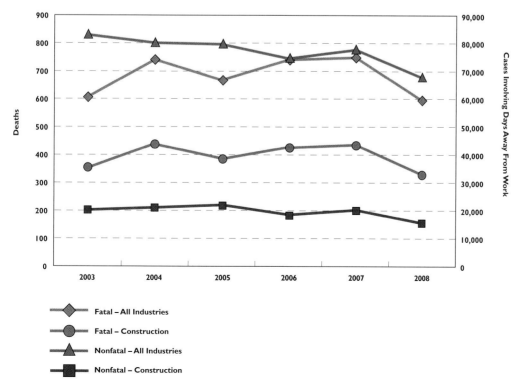

FALL TO LOWER LEVEL

Fall to lower level applies to instances in which the injury was produced by impact between the injured person and the source of injury, the motion producing the contact being that of the person, under the following circumstances:

- The motion of the person and the force of impact were generated by gravity.

- The point of contact with the source of injury was lower than the surface supporting the person at the inception of the fall.

Fall to lower level ranks second behind highway accidents in the number of workplace fatalities, and also is the fifth leading event resulting in cases involving days away from work.

FALL TO LOWER LEVEL NONFATAL OCCUPATIONAL INJURIES AND ILLNESSES INVOLVING DAYS AWAY FROM WORK AND FATAL OCCUPATIONAL INJURIES BY SELECTED WORKERS AND CASE CHARACTERISTICS, UNITED STATES, 2008

Characteristic	Private industry[b,c] nonfatal cases	All industries fatalities
Total	**67,510**	**593**
Sex		
Men	47,840	577
Women	19,080	16
Age		
Under 16	—	—
16 to 19	1,560	5
20 to 24	5,050	36
25 to 34	13,310	77
35 to 44	16,140	111
45 to 54	17,250	167
55 to 64	10,240	115
65 and over	2,280	80
Occupation		
Management, business, and financial	1,960	43
Professional and related	4,170	8
Service	10,600	62
Sales and related	3,920	8
Office and administrative support	4,370	6
Farming, fishing, and forestry	1,290	5
Construction and extractive	14,900	304
Installation, maintenance, and repair	7,350	61
Production	4,900	23
Transportation and material moving	14,000	71
Military occupations	—	—
Race or ethnic origin[d]		
White, non-Hispanic	30,410	399
Black, non-Hispanic	4,810	29
Hispanic	10,870	146
Other, multiple, and not reported	21,420	19
Nature of injury, illness		
Sprains, strains	19,260	—
Fractures	15,320	8
Cuts, lacerations, punctures	1,860	—
Bruises, contusions	8,580	—
Heat burns	—	—
Chemical burns	—	—
Amputations	—	—
Carpal tunnel syndrome	—	—
Tendonitis	40	—
Multiple injuries	7,110	259
Soreness, Pain	5,860	—
Back pain	2,170	—
All other	9,470	321

Characteristic	Private industry[b,c] nonfatal cases	All industries fatalities
Part of body affected		
Head	3,440	249
Eye	20	—
Neck	360	18
Trunk	18,080	51
Back	9,870	11
Shoulder	3,270	—
Upper extremities	8,680	—
Finger	410	—
Hand, except finger	490	—
Wrist	4,190	—
Lower extremities	20,800	11
Knee	6,310	—
Foot, toe	2,910	—
Body systems	80	—
Multiple	15,730	261
All other	330	—
Industry		
Agriculture, forestry, fishing, hunting	1,660	22
Mining	610	11
Construction	15,560	328
Manufacturing	6,860	46
Wholesale trade	3,810	12
Retail trade	7,120	18
Transportation and warehousing	7,490	31
Utilities	450	—
Information	1,760	—
Financial activities	2,310	15
Professional and business services	7,070	56
Education and health services	7,640	—
Leisure and hospitality	3,950	10
Other services	1,220	15
Government	N/A	20

Source: National Safety Council tabulations of Bureau of Labor Statistics data.
Note: Because of rounding and data exclusion of nonclassifiable responses, data may not sum to the totals. Dashes (—) indicate data that do not meet publication guidelines. "N/A" means not applicable.
[a]Days away from work include those that result in days away from work with or without restricted work activity or job transfer.
[b]Excludes farms with less than 11 employees.
[c]Data for mining operators in coal, metal and nonmetal mining and for employees in railroad transportation are provided by BLS by the Mine Safety and Health Administration, U.S. Department of Labor; and the Federal Railroad Administration, U.S. Department of Transportation. Independent mining contractors are excluded from the coal, metal and nonmetal mining industries. MSHA and FRA data do not reflect the changes in OSHA recordkeeping requirements in 2002.
[d]In the fatalities column, non-Hispanic categories include cases with Hispanic origin not reported.

Fall on same level applies to instances in which the injury was produced between the injured person and the source of injury, the motion producing the contact being that of the person, under the following circumstances:

- The motion of the person was generated by gravity following the employee's loss of equilibrium (the person was unable to maintain an upright position).

FALL ON SAME LEVEL

- The point of contact with the source of injury was at the same level or above the surface supporting the person at the inception of the fall.

Fall on same level ranks second behind overexertion in the number of nonfatal injuries involving days away from work but generally is not one of the top 10 events resulting in fatalities.

FALLS ON SAME LEVEL NONFATAL OCCUPATIONAL INJURIES AND ILLNESS INVOLVING DAYS AWAY FROM WORK AND FATAL OCCUPATIONAL INJURIES BY SELECTED WORKER AND CASE CHARACTERISTICS, UNITED STATES, 2008

Characteristic	Private industry [b,c] nonfatal cases	All industries fatalities
Total	157,680	92
Sex		
Men	67,920	70
Women	89,600	22
Age		
Under 16	30	—
16 to 19	3,830	—
20 to 24	10,080	—
25 to 34	25,190	—
35 to 44	31,900	12
45 to 54	42,120	17
55 to 64	33,470	21
65 and over	9,360	37
Occupation		
Management, business, and financial	6,860	17
Professional and related	16,920	—
Service	44,630	31
Sales and related	15,000	6
Office and administrative support	18,130	5
Farming, fishing, and forestry	1,180	—
Construction and extractive	9,540	8
Installation, maintenance, and repair	7,600	8
Production	14,150	5
Transportation and material moving	23,540	9
Military occupations	—	—
Race or ethnic origin [d]		
White, non-Hispanic	72,100	67
Black, non-Hispanic	12,490	9
Hispanic	16,450	11
Other, multiple, and not reported	56,640	5
Nature of injury, illness		
Sprains, strains	46,050	—
Fractures	28,620	18
Cuts, lacerations, punctures	4,350	—
Bruises, contusions	25,080	4
Heat burns	—	—
Chemical burns	—	—
Amputations	20	—
Carpal tunnel syndrome	—	—
Tendonitis	40	—
Multiple injuries	14,290	9
Soreness, Pain	19,350	3
Back pain	3,750	—
All other	19,890	54

Characteristic	Private industry [b,c] nonfatal cases	All industries fatalities
Part of body affected		
Head	8,180	46
Eye	130	—
Neck	1,320	—
Trunk	41,380	13
Back	19,950	5
Shoulder	11,010	—
Upper extremities	23,450	—
Finger	1,420	—
Hand, except finger	2,380	—
Wrist	8,470	—
Lower extremities	46,440	12
Knee	23,760	5
Foot, toe	3,420	—
Body systems	230	—
Multiple	35,800	14
All other	890	—
Industry		
Agriculture, forestry, fishing, hunting	1,490	8
Mining	900	—
Construction	9,160	6
Manufacturing	17,400	12
Wholesale trade	6,980	—
Retail trade	23,620	10
Transportation and warehousing	11,820	5
Utilities	730	—
Information	3,200	—
Financial activities	7,640	—
Professional and business services	14,740	5
Education and health services	37,140	6
Leisure and hospitality	19,040	8
Other services	3,820	6
Government	N/A	20

Source: National Safety Council tabulations of Bureau of Labor Statistics data.
Note: Because of rounding and data exclusion of nonclassifiable responses, data may not sum to the totals. Dashes (—) indicate data that do not meet publication guidelines. "N/A" means not applicable.
[a]Days away from work include those that result in days away from work with or without restricted work activity or job transfer.
[b]Excludes farms with less than 11 employees.
[c]Data for mining operators in coal, metal and nonmetal mining and for employees in railroad transportation are provided by BLS by the Mine Safety and Health Administration, U.S. Department of Labor; and the Federal Railroad Administration, U.S. Department of Transportation. Independent mining contractors are excluded from the coal, metal and nonmetal mining industries. MSHA and FRA data do not reflect the changes in OSHA recordkeeping requirements in 2002.
[d]In the fatalities column, non-Hispanic categories include cases with Hispanic origin not reported.

CAUSES OF WORK-RELATED DEATHS AND INJURIES

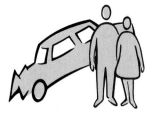

Incidents involving motor vehicles are the leading cause of work-related deaths, followed by contacts with objects or equipment and falls. For nonfatal cases with days away from work, contacts with objects or equipment are the leading causes, followed by overexertion and falls.

WORK-RELATED DEATHS AND INJURIES BY EVENT OR EXPOSURE, UNITED STATES, 2008

Event or exposure	Deaths[a]
Total (all events or exposures)	**5,214**
Contact with object or equipment	937
Struck against object	*12*
Struck by object	*520*
Caught in object or equipment	*302*
Caught in collapsing materials	*100*
Fall	700
Fall to lower level	*593*
Fall on same level	*92*
Bodily reaction and exertion	12
Exposure to harmful substance	439
Contact with electric current	*192*
Contact with temperature extremes	*37*
Exposure to caustic or noxious substances	*130*
Oxygen deficiency	*79*
Drowning	60
Choking on object or substance	9
Transportation accidents	2,130
Motor vehicle accidents	*1,828*
Highway accident	1,215
Nonhighway accident except rail, air, water	284
Pedestrian struck by vehicle, mobile equipment	329
Railway accident	*34*
Water vehicle accident	*76*
Aircraft accident	*191*
Fires, explosions	174
Fires	*94*
Explosions	*80*
Assaults and violent acts	816
By person	*526*
Self-inflicted	*263*
By animal	*25*
Other and nonclassifiable	6

Event or exposure	Cases with days away from work[b]
Total (all events or exposures)	**1,078,140**
Contact with object or equipment	291,880
Struck against object	*70,300*
Struck by object	*152,770*
Caught in object or equipment	*48,610*
Caught in collapsing materials	*620*
Fall	234,840
Fall to lower level	*67,510*
Fall on same level	*157,680*
Bodily reaction and exertion	415,690
Bodily reaction	*119,940*
Bending, climbing, crawling, reaching, twisting	51,310
Slips, trips, loss of balance—without fall	35,420
Overexertion	*250,960*
Overexertion in lifting	129,990
Repetitive motion	*30,920*
Exposure to harmful substance	45,480
Contact with electric current	*2,490*
Contact with temperature extremes	*15,660*
Exposure to caustic or noxious substances	*23,370*
Transportation accidents	48,610
Highway accident	*29,550*
Nonhighway accident except rail, air, water	*8,240*
Pedestrian struck by vehicle, mobile equipment	*8,460*
Railway accident	*190*
Water vehicle accident	*110*
Aircraft accident	*210*
Fires, explosions	2,320
Fires	*930*
Explosions	*1,370*
Assaults and violent acts	22,690
By person	*16,330*
By animal	*6,120*
Other and nonclassifiable	16,640

Source: U.S. Bureau of Labor Statistics.
[a]Includes deaths among all workers.
[b]Includes cases with days away from work among private sector wage and salary workers. Excludes government employees, the self-employed, and unpaid family workers.

DEATHS[a] BY EVENT OR EXPOSURE, UNITED STATES, 2008

0.2% 8.4%
13.4%
18.0%
0.1%
15.7%
3.3%
40.9%

CASES WITH DAYS AWAY FROM WORK[b] BY EVENT OR EXPOSURE, UNITED STATES, 2008

0.2% 2.1% 1.5%
4.5%
4.2%
38.6%
27.1%
21.8%

■ BODILY REACTION AND EXERTION
■ FALL
■ CONTACT WITH OBJECT OR EQUIPMENT
■ OTHER AND NONCLASSIFIABLE

■ ASSAULTS AND VIOLENT ACTS
□ FIRES, EXPLOSIONS
■ TRANSPORTATION ACCIDENTS
■ EXPOSURE TO HARMFUL SUBSTANCE

[a]Includes deaths among all workers.
[b]Includes cases with days away from work among private sector wage and salary workers. Excludes government employees, the self employed, and unpaid family workers.

According to the U.S. Bureau of Labor Statistics, sprains and strains were the most common type of injury involving days away from work in 2008, accounting for 39% of the total 1,078,140 injuries in private industry. Soreness and pain was the second most common type of injury, followed by cuts, lacerations, and punctures. Overall, the education and health services, manufacturing, and retail trade industry sectors had the highest number of injuries, combining to make up 46% of the total.

NUMBER OF NONFATAL OCCUPATIONAL INJURIES AND ILLNESSES INVOLVING DAYS AWAY FROM WORK[a] BY BY NATURE OF INJURY AND INDUSTRY SECTOR, PRIVATE INDUSTRY, UNITED STATES, 2008

| Nature of injury | Private sector[b-d] | Industry sector | | | | | | | | |
		Education & health services	Manufact-uring	Retail trade	Construc-tion	Trans. & ware-housing[d]	Leisure & hospitality	Prof. & business services	Wholesale trade	All other sectors[b,d,e]
Total[c]	1,078,140	182,750	164,940	146,320	120,240	104,120	86,190	85,540	71,880	116,150
Sprains, strains	416,620	89,010	55,470	58,140	39,920	47,590	28,230	30,120	27,060	41,080
Fractures	89,650	10,780	14,610	11,150	13,470	7,880	6,240	7,910	6,000	11,610
Cuts, lacerations, punctures	99,830	5,790	20,500	15,800	17,170	5,140	11,770	7,200	7,190	9,280
Bruises, contusions	93,650	17,040	13,470	14,280	7,870	10,830	7,380	6,700	6,460	9,610
Heat burns	15,630	1,440	2,920	1,370	1,070	960	4,720	400	1,310	1,440
Chemical burns	5,620	480	1,480	590	690	200	650	620	250	650
Amputations	6,230	110	2,720	670	570	250	360	360	390	800
Carpal tunnel syndrome	10,080	870	3,740	740	410	340	680	700	360	2,250
Tendonitis	4,100	790	1,120	520	220	200	400	310	240	310
Multiple injuries	43,960	7,340	6,220	4,460	4,770	4,370	3,550	4,390	3,500	5,380
With fractures	8,840	1,020	1,990	530	1,380	1,120	230	660	950	970
With sprains	16,780	4,100	1,590	2,120	1,110	1,750	1,960	1,600	950	1,580
Soreness, pain	114,030	22,920	12,030	15,970	11,810	12,630	9,640	9,000	8,400	11,640
Back pain	37,140	8,230	3,610	4,800	4,250	4,240	2,380	2,720	3,320	3,600
All other natures	178,740	26,180	30,670	22,620	22,280	13,740	12,560	17,830	10,710	22,130

Source: Bureau of Labor Statistics Occupational Injuries and Illnesses Profile Data, accessed Aug. 23, 2010, from http://data.bls.gov:8080/GQT/servlet/InitialPage.
[a]Days away from work cases include those that result in days away from work with or without job transfer or restriction.
[b]Excludes farms with less than 11 employees.
[c]Data may not sum to row and column totals because of rounding and exclusion of nonclassifiable responses.
[d]Data for transportation and mining do not reflect the changes OSHA made to its recordkeeping requirements that went info effect Jan. 1, 2002; therefore, estimates for these industries are not comparable with estimates for other industries.
[e]Includes Agriculture, Forestry, Fishing, and Hunting; Financial Activities; Information; Mining (including oil and gas extraction); Other Services; and Utilities.

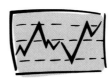

Safety professionals in business and industry often want to compare, or benchmark, the occupational injury and illness incidence rates of their establishments with the national average rates compiled by the U.S. Bureau of Labor Statistics through its annual Survey of Occupational Injuries and Illnesses.[a] The incidence rates published on the following pages are for 2009 and were compiled under the revised OSHA recordkeeping requirements that went into effect in 2002.

Step 1.
The first step in benchmarking is to calculate incidence rates for the establishment. The basic formula for computing incidence rates is (N x $200,000$)/EH, or the number of cases (N) multiplied by $200,000$ then divided by the number of hours worked (EH) by all employees during the time period, where $200,000$ is the base for 100 full-time workers (working 40 hours per week, 50 weeks per year). Because BLS rates are based on reports from entire establishments, both the OSHA 300 Log and the number of hours worked should cover the whole establishment being benchmarked. The hours worked and the log also should cover the same time period (e.g., a month, quarter or full year). The following rates may be calculated:

Total cases—the incidence rate of total OSHA-recordable cases per 200,000 hours worked. For this rate, N is the total number of cases on the OSHA 300 Log.

Cases with days away from work or job transfer or restriction—the incidence rate of cases with days away from work, or job transfer, or restriction. N is the number of cases with a check in column H or column I of the OSHA 300 Log.

Cases with days away from work—the incidence rate of cases with days away from work. N is the number of cases with a check in column H of the OSHA 300 Log.

Cases with job transfer or restriction—the incidence rate of cases with job transfer or restriction, but no days away from work. N is the number of cases with a check in column I of the OSHA 300 Log.

Other recordable cases—the incidence rate of recordable cases without days away from work or job transfer or restriction. N is the number of cases with a check in column J of the OSHA 300 Log.

In the flow chart on the opposite page, post the number of cases to each box in the top row and the number of

employee hours worked in its box. Then use the formula to calculate the rates and write them in the last row of boxes in Step 1.

An alternative approach is to use the Incidence Rate Calculator and Comparison Tool available on the BLS website: *http://data.bls.gov/IIRC/*. This tool will calculate your rate and provide a report comparing your rate to your industry.

Step 2.
After computing one or more of the rates, the next step is to determine the North American Industry Classification System (NAICS) code for the establishment.[b] (NAICS replaced the Standard Industrial Classification code beginning in 2003.) This code is used to find the appropriate BLS rate for comparison. NAICS codes can be found at *www.census.gov/naics*. The website also contains a crosswalk between NAICS and SIC codes. Otherwise, contact a regional BLS office for assistance.

Write the establishment's NAICS code in the box in Step 2 of the flow chart.

Step 3.
Once the NAICS code is known, the national average incidence rates may be found by (a) consulting the table of rates on pages 70-72 (b) visiting the BLS website (*www.bls.gov/iif*) or (c) by calling a regional BLS office. Note that some tables on the website provide incidence rates by size of establishment and rate quartiles within each NAICS code. These rates may be useful for a more precise comparison. Note that the incidence rates for 2001 and earlier years were compiled under the old OSHA recordkeeping requirements in effect at that time. Caution must be used in comparing rates computed for 2002 and later years with earlier years—keeping in mind the differences in recordkeeping requirements.

In the flow chart on the opposite page, post the rates from the BLS survey to the boxes in Step 3. Now compare these with the rates calculated in Step 1.

An alternative way of benchmarking is to compare the current incidence rates for an establishment with its own historical rates to determine if the rates are improving and if progress is satisfactory (using criteria set by the organization).

[a]Bureau of Labor Statistics. (1997). BLS Handbook of Methods. *Washington, DC: U.S. Government Printing Office. (Or on the Internet at www.bls.gov/opub/hom/home.htm)*
[b]Executive Office of the President, Office of Management and Budget. (2002). North American Industry Classification System, United States, 2002. *Springfield, VA: National Technical Information Service.*

BENCHMARKING FLOW CHART

67

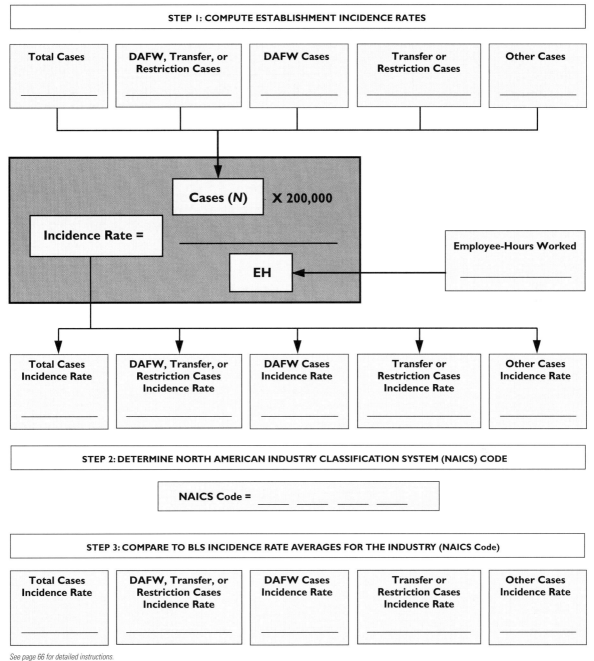

STEP 1: COMPUTE ESTABLISHMENT INCIDENCE RATES

Total Cases · DAFW, Transfer, or Restriction Cases · DAFW Cases · Transfer or Restriction Cases · Other Cases

$$\text{Incidence Rate} = \frac{\text{Cases } (N) \times 200{,}000}{EH}$$

Employee-Hours Worked

Total Cases Incidence Rate · DAFW, Transfer, or Restriction Cases Incidence Rate · DAFW Cases Incidence Rate · Transfer or Restriction Cases Incidence Rate · Other Cases Incidence Rate

STEP 2: DETERMINE NORTH AMERICAN INDUSTRY CLASSIFICATION SYSTEM (NAICS) CODE

NAICS Code = ____ ____ ____ ____

STEP 3: COMPARE TO BLS INCIDENCE RATE AVERAGES FOR THE INDUSTRY (NAICS Code)

Total Cases Incidence Rate · DAFW, Transfer, or Restriction Cases Incidence Rate · DAFW Cases Incidence Rate · Transfer or Restriction Cases Incidence Rate · Other Cases Incidence Rate

See page 66 for detailed instructions.
DAFW = Days away from work

OCCUPATIONAL

NATIONAL SAFETY COUNCIL® INJURY FACTS® 2011 EDITION

TRENDS IN OCCUPATIONAL INCIDENCE RATES

Incidence rates continue recent downward trend

Four of the five private sector occupational injury and illness incidence rates published by the Bureau of Labor Statistics for 2009 decreased from 2008. The incidence rate for total recordable cases was 3.6 per 100 full-time workers in 2009, down nearly 8% from the 2008 rate of 3.9. The incidence rate for total cases with days away from work, job transfer, or restriction was 1.8, a decrease of 10%. The incidence rate for cases with days away from work was 1.1 in 2009, stable from 2008. The incidence rate for cases with job transfer or restriction was 0.8 in 2009, down 11% from 2008. The incidence rate for other recordable cases was 1.8 in 2009, down 5% from 2008.

There have been several changes that affect comparability of incidence rates from year to year. The North American Industry Classification System replaced the Standard Industrial Classification system beginning with the 2003 survey of occupational injuries and illnesses. Revisions to the Occupational Safety and Health Administration's occupational injury and illness recordkeeping requirements that went into effect in 2002. Beginning with 1992, BLS revised its annual survey to include only nonfatal cases and stopped publishing the incidence rate of lost workdays.

OCCUPATIONAL INJURY AND ILLNESS INCIDENCE RATES, PRIVATE INDUSTRY, UNITED STATES, 1988–2009

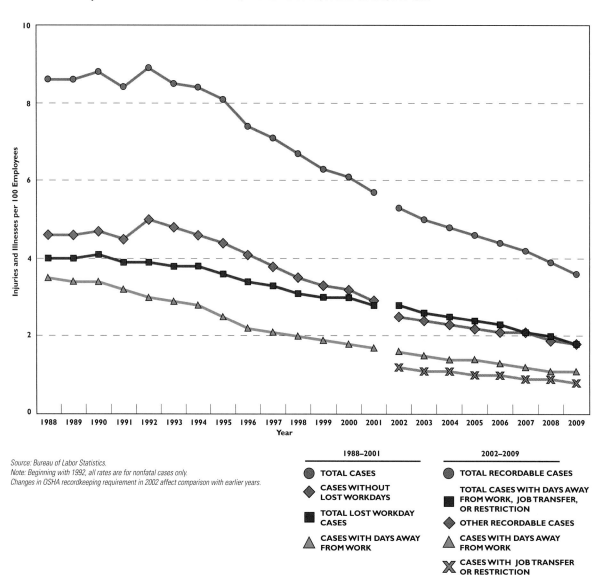

Source: Bureau of Labor Statistics.
Note: Beginning with 1992, all rates are for nonfatal cases only.
Changes in OSHA recordkeeping requirement in 2002 affect comparison with earlier years.

1988–2001	2002–2009
● TOTAL CASES	● TOTAL RECORDABLE CASES
◆ CASES WITHOUT LOST WORKDAYS	■ TOTAL CASES WITH DAYS AWAY FROM WORK, JOB TRANSFER, OR RESTRICTION
■ TOTAL LOST WORKDAY CASES	◆ OTHER RECORDABLE CASES
▲ CASES WITH DAYS AWAY FROM WORK	▲ CASES WITH DAYS AWAY FROM WORK
	✕ CASES WITH JOB TRANSFER OR RESTRICTION

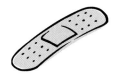

The tables below and on pages 70-72 show results of the 2009 Survey of Occupational Injuries and Illnesses conducted by the Bureau of Labor Statistics, U.S. Department of Labor. The survey collects data on injuries and illnesses (from the OSHA 300 Log) and employee hours worked from a nationwide sample of about 230,000 establishments. The survey excludes private households, the self-employed, and farms with fewer than 11 employees. The incidence rates give the number of cases per 100 full-time workers per year

using 200,000 employee hours as the equivalent. Definitions of the terms are given in the Glossary on page 207.

Beginning with 1992 data, BLS revised its annual survey to include only nonfatal cases and stopped publishing incidence rates of lost workdays. Beginning with 2003 data, BLS adopted the North American Industry Classification System for publication of the incidence rates by industry.

BUREAU OF LABOR STATISTICS ESTIMATES OF NONFATAL OCCUPATIONAL INJURY AND ILLNESS INCIDENCE RATES AND NUMBER OF INJURIES AND ILLNESSES BY INDUSTRY SECTOR, 2009

Industry sector	Total recordable cases	Cases with days away from work, job transfer, or restriction			Other recordable cases
		Total	Cases with days away from work	Cases with job transfer or restriction	
Incidence rate per 100 full-time workers[c]					
All industries (including state and local government)[d]	**3.9**	**1.9**	**1.2**	**0.8**	**2.0**
Private sector[d]	**3.6**	**1.8**	**1.1**	**0.8**	**1.8**
Goods Producing[d]	4.3	2.3	1.2	1.1	2.0
Agriculture, forestry, fishing & hunting[d]	5.3	2.9	1.6	1.2	2.4
Mining	2.4	1.5	1.1	0.4	1.0
Construction	4.3	2.3	1.6	0.7	2.0
Manufacturing	4.3	2.3	1.0	1.3	2.0
Service providing	3.4	1.7	1.0	0.7	1.7
Wholesale trade	3.3	2.0	1.1	0.9	1.3
Retail trade	4.2	2.2	1.2	1.0	2.0
Transportation and warehousing	5.2	3.5	2.3	1.3	1.6
Utilities	3.3	1.8	1.0	0.8	1.5
Information	1.9	1.0	0.7	0.3	0.9
Financial activities	1.5	0.6	0.4	0.2	0.8
Professional and business services	1.8	0.9	0.6	0.3	0.9
Education and health services	5.0	2.2	1.3	1.0	2.7
Leisure and hospitality	3.9	1.6	1.0	0.6	2.3
Other services	2.9	1.4	1.0	0.5	1.5
State and local government[d]	**5.8**	**2.5**	**1.8**	**0.7**	**3.3**
Number of injuries and illnesses (in thousands)					
All industries (including state and local government)[d]	**4,140.7**	**2,041.5**	**1,238.5**	**803.0**	**2,099.2**
Private sector[d]	**3,277.7**	**1,677.4**	**965.0**	**702.4**	**1,610.4**
Goods producing[d]	842.1	457.1	241.3	215.8	385.1
Agriculture, forestry, fishing & hunting[d]	44.9	24.2	13.8	10.4	20.6
Mining	17.7	10.7	7.8	2.9	6.9
Construction	251.0	136.5	92.5	44.0	114.5
Manufacturing	528.6	285.6	127.1	158.5	243.0
Service providing	2,435.6	1,210.3	723.7	486.6	1,225.3
Wholesale trade	185.9	112.2	62.4	49.8	73.7
Retail trade	487.2	254.3	137.0	117.3	233.0
Transportation and warehousing	206.9	141.0	90.7	50.3	65.9
Utilities	18.4	10.0	5.6	4.4	8.4
Information	49.3	25.1	17.0	8.1	24.2
Financial activities	104.6	45.6	30.3	15.4	58.9
Professional and business services	246.9	122.7	80.6	42.0	124.2
Education and health services	708.4	318.5	183.3	135.2	389.9
Leisure and hospitality	340.6	138.0	87.7	50.3	202.6
Other services	87.4	43.0	29.0	13.9	44.5
State and local government[d]	**862.9**	**374.1**	**273.5**	**100.6**	**488.8**

Source: Bureau of Labor Statistics

[a]*Industry Sector and two- and three-digit NAICS code totals on pages 70-72 include data for industries not shown separately.*
[b]*North American Industry Classification System, 2002 Edition, for industries shown on pages 70-72.*
[c]*Incidence Rate =* $\dfrac{Number\ of\ injuries\ \&\ illnesses \times 200{,}000}{Total\ hours\ worked\ by\ all\ employees\ during\ period\ covered}$

where 200,000 is the base for 100 full-time workers (working 40 hours per week, 50 weeks per year). The "Total Recordable Cases" rate is based on the number of cases with checkmarks in columns (G), (H), (I), and (J) of the OSHA 300 Log. The "Cases With Days Away From Work, Job Transfer, or Restriction--Total" rate is based on columns (H) and (I). The "Cases With Days Away From Work" rate is based on column (H). The "Cases With Job Transfer or Restriction" rate is based on column (I). The "Other Recordable Cases" rate is based on column (J).
[d]*Excludes farms with less than 11 employees.*
[e]*Data do not meet publication guidelines.*
[f]*Industry scope changed in 2009.*
[g]*Data too small to be displayed.*

OCCUPATIONAL INJURIES
AND ILLNESSES (CONT.)

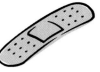

BUREAU OF LABOR STATISTICS ESTIMATES OF NONFATAL OCCUPATIONAL INJURY AND ILLNESS INCIDENCE RATES FOR SELECTED INDUSTRIES, 2009

Industry[a]	NAICS code[b]	Total recordable cases	Incidence rates[c] — Cases with days away from work, job transfer, or restriction — Total	Cases with days away from work	Cases with job transfer or restriction	Other recordable cases
All industries (including state and local gov.)[d]		3.9	1.9	1.2	0.8	2.0
Private sector[e]		3.6	1.8	1.1	0.8	1.8
Goods producing[e]		4.3	2.3	1.2	1.1	2.0
Natural resources and mining[e]		4.0	2.2	1.4	0.8	1.7
Agriculture, forestry, fishing and hunting[e]	11	5.3	2.9	1.6	1.2	2.4
Crop production	111	4.9	2.7	1.5	1.3	2.2
Animal production	112	6.9	3.6	2.0	1.6	3.3
Forestry and logging	113	4.3	1.8	1.6	0.1	2.5
Fishing, hunting, and trapping	114	0.9	0.6	0.4	(e)	0.3
Support activities for agriculture and forestry	115	5.0	2.8	1.6	1.2	2.2
Mining	21	2.4	1.5	1.1	0.4	1.0
Oil and gas extraction	211	1.6	0.9	0.7	0.2	0.7
Mining (except oil and gas)	212	3.2	2.2	1.7	0.5	1.1
Coal mining	2121	4.1	2.8	2.6	0.2	1.3
Metal ore mining	2122	2.6	1.6	1.0	0.7	1.0
Nonmetallic mineral mining and quarrying	2123	2.6	1.7	1.0	0.7	0.9
Support activites for mining	213	2.3	1.3	0.8	0.4	1.0
Construction		4.3	2.3	1.6	0.7	2.0
Construction of buildings	236	3.7	1.9	1.2	0.6	1.8
Residential building construction	2361	3.7	2.1	1.6	(e)	1.6
Nonresidential building construction	2362	3.6	1.7	0.9	0.8	1.9
Heavy and civil engineering construction	237	3.8	2.2	1.4	0.7	1.6
Utility system construction	2371	3.8	2.4	1.7	0.6	1.4
Land subdivision	2372	2.0	0.8	0.5	0.4	1.1
Highway, street and bridge construction	2373	4.6	2.4	1.5	1.0	2.2
Other heavy and civil engineering construction	2379	2.5	1.4	0.9	0.6	1.1
Specialty trade contractors	238	4.6	2.5	1.7	0.8	2.1
Foundation, structure, and building exterior contractors	2381	5.3	3.0	2.0	0.9	2.4
Building equipment contractors	2382	4.6	2.3	1.5	0.8	2.2
Building finishing contractors	2383	4.6	2.7	2.1	0.7	1.8
Other specialty trade contractors	2389	4.0	2.4	1.6	(e)	1.7
Manufacturing		4.3	2.3	1.0	1.3	2.0
Food manufacturing	311	5.7	3.6	1.3	2.3	2.1
Animal food manufacturing	3111	5.0	3.0	1.9	1.1	2.0
Grain and oilseed milling	3112	4.6	2.6	1.3	1.3	2.0
Sugar and confectionery product manufacturing	3113	5.3	3.0	1.2	1.7	2.3
Fruit and vegetable preserving and specialty food manufacturing	3114	5.3	3.0	1.2	1.8	2.3
Dairy product manufacturing	3115	6.6	4.3	2.0	2.3	2.3
Animal slaughtering and processing	3116	6.9	4.6	1.1	3.5	2.3
Seafood product preperation and packaging	3117	6.3	3.5	1.9	1.6	2.8
Bakeries amd tortilla manufacturing	3118	4.3	2.9	1.3	1.6	1.4
Other food manufacturing	3119	4.7	2.8	1.3	1.5	1.9
Beverages and tobacco product manufacturing	312	6.4	4.6	1.7	2.8	1.8
Beverage manufacturing	3121	6.7	4.9	1.8	3.1	1.8
Tobacco manufacturing	3122	3.7	1.9	1.1	0.8	1.8
Textile mills	313	2.9	1.6	0.7	0.9	1.2
Fiber, yarn and thread mills	3131	2.7	1.6	0.5	1.1	1.1
Fabric mills	3132	2.8	1.4	0.7	0.7	1.4
Textile and fabric finishing and fabric coating mills	3133	3.1	2.0	0.9	1.0	1.2
Textile product mills	314	3.7	1.9	0.8	1.1	1.8
Textile furnishings mills	3141	3.3	1.9	0.6	1.3	1.5
Other textile product mills	3149	4.2	1.9	1.0	1.0	2.2
Apparel manufacturing	315	2.6	1.3	0.4	0.9	1.2
Apparel knitting mills	3151	3.3	1.5	0.5	1.1	1.8
Cut and sew apparel manufacturing	3152	2.4	1.3	0.4	0.9	1.1
Apparel accessories and other apparel manufacturing	3159	3.4	1.6	1.1	0.5	1.8
Leather and allied product manufacturing	316	6.2	3.4	0.9	2.5	2.8
Leather and hide tanning and finishing	3161	9.6	7.9	1.7	6.1	1.8
Other leather and allied product manufacturing	3169	4.1	1.7	0.4	1.3	2.4
Wood product manufacturing	321	6.5	3.3	1.8	1.5	3.2
Sawmills and wood preservation	3211	7.0	3.6	2.5	1.1	3.5
Veneer, plywood and engineered wood product manufacturing	3212	4.8	2.4	1.3	1.1	2.4
Other wood product manufacturing	3219	6.9	3.5	1.8	1.8	3.3
Paper manufacturing	322	3.2	1.8	0.9	0.9	1.4
Pulp, paper and paperboard mills	3221	2.7	1.4	0.9	0.6	1.3
Converted paper product manufacturing	3222	3.4	2.0	1.0	1.1	1.4
Printing and related support activities	323	2.7	1.6	0.7	0.9	1.2
Petroleum and coal products manufacturing	324	1.5	0.9	0.5	0.4	0.6
Chemical manufacturing	325	2.3	1.4	0.6	0.7	1.0
Basic chemical manufacturing	3251	1.9	1.1	0.5	0.6	0.8
Resin, synthetic rubber, and artificial and synthetic fibers and filaments manufacturing	3252	2.2	1.4	0.8	0.7	0.8
Pesticide, fertilizer, and other agriculture chemical manufacturing	3253	3.2	1.8	0.9	0.9	1.4
Pharmaceutical and medicine manufacturing	3254	2.0	1.1	0.5	0.6	0.9
Paint, coating, and adhesive manufacturing	3255	2.9	1.9	0.8	1.1	1.0
Soap, cleaning compound, and toilet preparation mfg.	3256	3.2	2.1	0.9	1.1	1.1
Other chemical product and preparation manufacturing	3259	2.6	1.3	0.6	0.7	1.3

See source and footnotes on page 69.

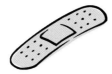

BUREAU OF LABOR STATISTICS ESTIMATES OF NONFATAL OCCUPATIONAL INJURY AND ILLNESS INCIDENCE RATES FOR SELECTED INDUSTRIES, 2009 (Cont.)

Industry[a]	NAICS code[b]	Total recordable cases	Incidence Rates[c]			Other recordable cases
			Cases with days away from work, job transfer, or restriction			
			Total	Cases with days away from work	Cases with job transfer or restriction	
Plastics and rubber products manufacturing	326	4.8	2.7	1.2	1.5	2.1
Plastics product manufacturing	3261	4.6	2.5	1.1	1.4	2.1
Rubber product manufacturing	3262	5.4	3.3	1.5	1.9	2.1
Nonmetallic mineral product manufacturing	327	5.2	3.0	1.6	1.5	2.2
Clay product and refractory manufacturing	3271	5.1	3.1	1.3	1.8	2.0
Glass and glass product manufacturing	3272	5.0	2.8	0.9	2.0	2.2
Cement and concrete product manufacturing	3273	5.4	3.3	1.9	1.4	2.0
Lime and gypsum product manufacturing	3274	2.7	1.6	0.9	0.7	1.2
Other nonmetallic mineral product manufacturing	3279	5.8	2.8	1.7	1.0	3.0
Primary metal manufacturing	331	6.2	3.2	1.5	1.8	2.9
Iron and steel mills and ferroalloy manufacturing	3311	3.4	1.8	0.9	0.9	1.6
Steel product manufacturing from purchased steel	3312	7.6	3.5	1.4	2.1	4.1
Alumina and aluminum production and processing	3313	5.0	2.7	1.2	1.5	2.3
Nonferrous metal (except aluminum) production and processing	3314	5.1	3.0	1.5	1.4	2.1
Foundries	3315	8.7	4.6	2.1	2.5	4.1
Fabricated metal product manufacturing	332	5.5	2.6	1.3	1.3	2.8
Forging and stamping	3321	6.6	3.3	1.7	1.6	3.3
Cutlery and handtool manufacturing	3322	4.7	1.8	1.0	0.8	2.8
Architectural and structural metals manufacturing	3323	6.7	3.3	1.7	1.5	3.4
Boiler, tank, and shipping container manufacturing	3324	5.6	2.8	1.4	1.4	2.8
Hardware manufacturing	3325	4.6	2.5	1.0	1.4	2.1
Spring and wire product manufacturing	3326	4.8	2.3	1.1	1.2	2.5
Machine shops; turned product; and screw, nut, and bolt manufacturing	3327	4.8	2.1	1.0	1.1	2.7
Coating, engraving, heat treating, and allied activities	3328	4.8	2.8	1.3	1.5	2.0
Other fabricated metal product manufacturing	3329	4.7	2.2	1.1	1.1	2.5
Machinery manufacturing	333	4.3	2.0	0.9	1.1	2.3
Agriculture, construction, and mining machinery mfg.	3331	4.9	2.3	1.1	1.2	2.6
Industrial machinery manufacturing	3332	3.8	1.6	0.9	0.7	2.3
Commercial and service machinery manufacturing	3333	3.4	1.9	0.9	1.0	1.5
Ventilation, heating, air-conditioning, and commercial refrigeration equipment manufacturing	3334	5.1	2.5	1.0	1.5	2.6
Metalworking machinery manufacturing	3335	4.4	1.7	0.8	0.9	2.7
Engine, turbine, and power transmission equipment mfg.	3336	3.1	1.5	0.7	0.8	1.5
Other general purpose machinery manufacturing	3339	4.4	2.1	1.0	1.1	2.3
Computer and electronic product manufacturing	334	1.6	0.8	0.4	0.4	0.8
Computer and peripheral equipment manufacturing	3341	0.8	0.4	0.2	0.2	0.5
Communications equipment manufacturing	3342	1.6	0.8	0.4	0.4	0.8
Audio and video equipment manufacturing	3343	1.4	0.6	0.3	0.3	0.8
Semiconductor and other electronic component mfg.	3344	1.8	0.9	0.4	0.5	0.9
Navigational, measuring, electromedical, and control instruments manufacturing	3345	1.8	0.8	0.4	0.4	1.0
Manufacturing and reproducing magnetic and optical media	3346	1.9	1.1	0.5	0.6	0.7
Electrical equipment, appliance, and component mfg.	335	3.5	1.8	0.7	1.1	1.7
Electric lighting equipment manufacturing	3351	4.0	2.0	0.8	1.2	2.0
Household appliance manufacturing	3352	3.3	1.7	0.6	1.1	1.6
Electrical equipment manufacturing	3353	3.6	2.0	0.8	1.2	1.6
Other electrical equipment and component mfg.	3359	3.4	1.6	0.7	0.9	1.7
Transportation equipment manufacturing	336	5.2	2.7	1.1	1.5	2.5
Motor vehicle manufacturing	3361	7.8	3.8	1.3	2.5	4.0
Motor vehicle body and trailer manufacturing	3362	8.2	3.7	1.7	2.1	4.5
Motor vehicle parts manufacturing	3363	5.2	2.6	1.0	1.6	2.6
Aerospace product and parts manufacturing	3364	3.3	1.8	0.7	1.1	1.5
Railroad rolling stock manufacturing	3365	4.1	2.4	1.4	1.0	1.7
Ship and boat building	3366	7.8	4.5	2.5	2.0	3.3
Other transportation equipment manufacturing	3369	4.9	2.4	1.0	1.4	2.4
Furniture and related product manufacturing	337	5.2	2.7	1.3	1.4	2.5
Household and institutional furniture and kitchen cabinet manufacturing	3371	5.3	2.8	1.5	1.4	2.5
Office furniture (including fixtures) manufacturing	3372	5.2	2.4	1.0	1.4	2.8
Other furniture related product manufacturing	3379	4.1	2.5	1.0	1.6	1.5
Miscellaneous manufacturing	339	3.1	1.6	0.7	0.8	1.5
Medical equipment and supplies manufacturing	3391	2.5	1.2	0.5	0.7	1.3
Other miscellaneous manufacturing	3399	3.7	2.0	1.0	1.0	1.7
Service providing		**3.4**	**1.7**	**1.1**	**0.7**	**1.7**
Trade, transportation, and utilities		**4.1**	**2.4**	**1.4**	**1.0**	**1.8**
Wholesale trade	42	3.3	2.0	1.1	0.9	1.3
Merchant wholesalers, durable goods	423	3.1	1.7	1.0	0.7	1.4
Merchant wholesalers, nondurable goods	424	4.3	2.9	1.5	1.4	1.4
Retail trade	44-45	4.2	2.2	1.2	1.0	2.0
Motor vehicle and parts dealers	441	3.8	1.7	1.2	0.5	2.1
Furniture and home furnishings stores	442	4.0	2.3	1.4	0.9	1.7
Electronics and appliance stores	443	1.8	0.8	0.5	0.3	0.9

See source and footnotes on page 69.

OCCUPATIONAL INJURIES
AND ILLNESSES (CONT.)

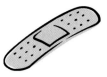

BUREAU OF LABOR STATISTICS ESTIMATES OF NONFATAL OCCUPATIONAL INJURY AND ILLNESS INCIDENCE RATES FOR SELECTED
INDUSTRIES, 2009 (Cont.)

Industry[a]	NAICS code[b]	Incidence rates[c]				
		Total recordable cases	Cases with days away from work, job transfer, or restriction			Other recordable cases
			Total	Cases with days away from work	Cases with job transfer or restriction	
Building material and garden equipment and supplies dealers	444	5.3	3.3	1.5	1.8	2.0
Food and beverage stores	445	5.2	2.8	1.5	1.4	2.3
Health and personal care stores	446	2.3	1.0	0.6	(e)	1.4
Gasoline stations	447	3.4	1.5	1.0	0.4	1.9
Clothing and clothing accessories stores	448	3.0	1.1	0.8	(e)	1.9
Sporting goods, hobby, book, and music stores	451	3.0	1.0	0.6	0.5	2.0
General merchandise stores	452	5.2	3.1	1.4	1.8	2.1
Miscellaneous store retailers	453	4.3	1.6	1.0	0.6	2.7
Nonstore retailers	454	3.6	1.9	1.4	0.6	1.7
Transportation and warehousing	48-49	5.2	3.5	2.3	1.3	1.6
Air transportation	481	8.5	6.5	4.6	1.8	2.1
Rail transportation	482	2.2	1.6	1.4	0.2	0.6
Water transportation	483	2.5	1.7	1.2	0.5	0.8
Truck transportation	484	4.6	3.0	2.3	0.7	1.6
Transit and ground passenger transportation	485	5.0	3.1	2.2	0.9	1.9
Pipeline transportation	486	1.9	0.7	0.5	0.2	1.2
Scenic and sightseeing transportation	487	3.6	2.0	1.8	0.2	1.5
Support activities for transportation	488	4.0	2.7	1.8	0.9	1.3
Couriers and messengers	492	7.2	4.7	2.6	2.0	2.5
Warehousing and storage	493	5.9	4.3	1.7	2.6	1.6
Utilities	22	3.3	1.8	1.0	0.8	1.5
Electric power generation, transmission and distribution	2211	3.0	1.5	0.9	0.6	1.4
Natural gas distribution	2212	4.2	2.5	1.0	1.5	1.7
Water, sewage and other systems	2213	4.1	2.5	1.8	0.7	1.6
Information		**1.9**	**1.0**	**0.7**	**0.3**	**0.9**
Publishing industries (except Internet)	511	1.5	0.7	0.4	(e)	0.7
Motion picture and sound recording industries	512	3.6	0.6	0.4	0.2	3.0
Broadcasting (except Internet)	515	2.0	1.1	0.7	0.4	1.0
Telecommunications	517	2.4	1.5	1.1	0.4	0.9
Data processing, hosting, and related services[f]	518	0.6	0.2	0.1	0.1	0.4
Other information services[f]	519	0.6	0.2	0.2	(g)	0.4
Financial activities		**1.5**	**0.6**	**0.4**	**0.2**	**0.8**
Finance and insurance	52	0.8	0.2	0.2	0.1	0.6
Monetary authorities	521	1.0	0.5	0.3	0.2	0.6
Credit intermediation and related activities	522	1.0	0.2	0.2	0.1	0.8
Securities, commodity contracts, and other financial investments and related activities	523	0.2	0.1	0.1	(g)	0.1
Insurance carriers and related activities	524	0.9	0.3	0.2	0.1	0.6
Funds, trusts, and other financial activities	525	0.7	0.3	0.2	0.1	0.4
Real estate and rental and leasing	53	3.3	1.9	1.2	0.7	1.5
Real estate	531	3.1	1.7	1.2	0.6	1.4
Rental and leasing services	532	3.8	2.3	1.4	0.9	1.5
Lessors of nonfinancial intangible assets (except copyrighted works)	533	0.6	0.2	0.2	(e)	0.4
Professional and business services		**1.8**	**0.9**	**0.6**	**0.3**	**0.9**
Professional, scientific, and technical services	54	1.2	0.5	0.3	0.1	0.7
Management of companies and enterprises	55	1.7	0.8	0.4	0.4	0.9
Administrative and support and waste management and remediation services	56	2.9	1.6	1.1	0.5	1.3
Administrative and support services	561	2.7	1.5	1.0	0.5	1.2
Waste management and remediation services	562	5.2	3.3	1.8	1.4	2.0
Education and health services		**5.0**	**2.2**	**1.3**	**1.0**	**2.7**
Educational services	61	2.4	0.8	0.6	0.2	1.5
Health care and social assistance	62	5.4	2.4	1.4	1.1	2.9
Ambulatory health care services	621	2.7	0.9	0.6	0.3	1.8
Hospitals	622	7.3	2.9	1.6	1.2	4.4
Nursing and residential care facilities	623	8.4	5.0	2.4	2.6	3.4
Social assistance	624	4.0	2.0	1.4	0.6	1.9
Leisure and hospitality		**3.9**	**1.6**	**1.0**	**0.6**	**2.3**
Arts, entertainment, and recreation	71	4.9	2.3	1.3	1.0	2.6
Accommodation and food services	72	3.7	1.5	1.0	0.5	2.3
Accommodation	721	5.0	2.6	1.4	1.1	2.5
Food services and drinking places	722	3.4	1.2	0.9	0.4	2.2
Other services (except public administration)		**2.9**	**1.4**	**1.0**	**0.5**	**1.5**
Repair and maintenance	811	3.8	1.8	1.3	0.5	2.0
Personal and laundry services	812	2.5	1.4	0.8	0.6	1.1
Religious, grantmaking, civic, professional, and similar organizations	813	2.4	1.0	0.7	0.3	1.4
State and local government[d]		**5.8**	**2.5**	**1.8**	**0.7**	**3.3**
State government[d]		**4.6**	**2.3**	**1.8**	**0.5**	**2.3**
Local government[d]		**6.3**	**2.6**	**1.8**	**0.7**	**3.7**

See source and footnotes on page 69.

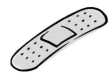

BUREAU OF LABOR STATISTICS ESTIMATES OF NONFATAL OCCUPATIONAL INJURY AND ILLNESS INCIDENCE RATES FOR SELECTED INDUSTRIES, 2009

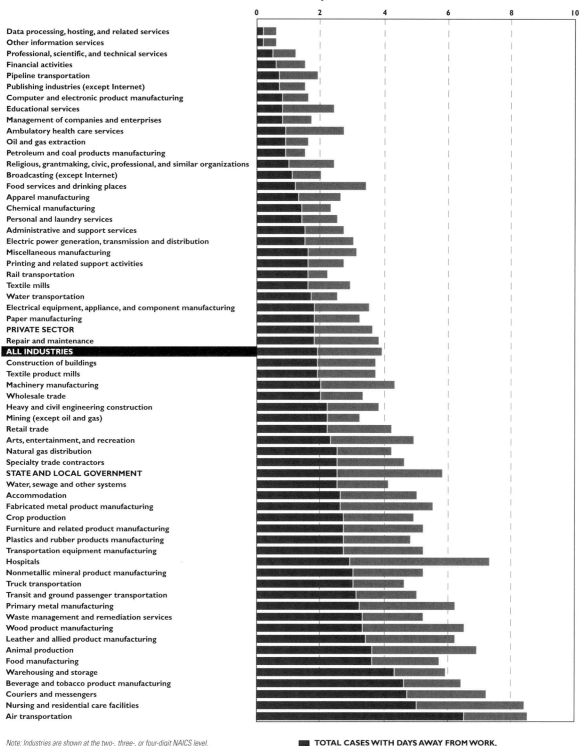

Data processing, hosting, and related services
Other information services
Professional, scientific, and technical services
Financial activities
Pipeline transportation
Publishing industries (except Internet)
Computer and electronic product manufacturing
Educational services
Management of companies and enterprises
Ambulatory health care services
Oil and gas extraction
Petroleum and coal products manufacturing
Religious, grantmaking, civic, professional, and similar organizations
Broadcasting (except Internet)
Food services and drinking places
Apparel manufacturing
Chemical manufacturing
Personal and laundry services
Administrative and support services
Electric power generation, transmission and distribution
Miscellaneous manufacturing
Printing and related support activities
Rail transportation
Textile mills
Water transportation
Electrical equipment, appliance, and component manufacturing
Paper manufacturing
PRIVATE SECTOR
Repair and maintenance
ALL INDUSTRIES
Construction of buildings
Textile product mills
Machinery manufacturing
Wholesale trade
Heavy and civil engineering construction
Mining (except oil and gas)
Retail trade
Arts, entertainment, and recreation
Natural gas distribution
Specialty trade contractors
STATE AND LOCAL GOVERNMENT
Water, sewage and other systems
Accommodation
Fabricated metal product manufacturing
Crop production
Furniture and related product manufacturing
Plastics and rubber products manufacturing
Transportation equipment manufacturing
Hospitals
Nonmetallic mineral product manufacturing
Truck transportation
Transit and ground passenger transportation
Primary metal manufacturing
Waste management and remediation services
Wood product manufacturing
Leather and allied product manufacturing
Animal production
Food manufacturing
Warehousing and storage
Beverage and tobacco product manufacturing
Couriers and messengers
Nursing and residential care facilities
Air transportation

Note: Industries are shown at the two-, three-, or four-digit NAICS level.
Total Cases With Days Away From Work, Job Transfer, or Restriction plus Other Recordable Cases equals Total Recordable Cases.

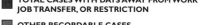 **TOTAL CASES WITH DAYS AWAY FROM WORK, JOB TRANSFER, OR RESTRICTION**

OTHER RECORDABLE CASES

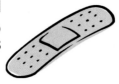
The tables on pages 75-90 present data on the characteristics of injured and ill workers and the injuries and illnesses that affected them. These data indicate how many workers died from on-the-job injuries and how many were affected by nonfatal injuries and illnesses. The data may be used to help set priorities for occupational safety and health programs and for benchmarking.

Fatality information covers only deaths due to injuries and comes from the Bureau of Labor Statistics Census of Fatal Occupational Injuries. The data are for the calendar year 2008 and include wage and salary workers, the self-employed, and unpaid family workers in all types of businesses and industries.

Data on nonfatal cases cover both occupational injuries and illnesses and come from the BLS Survey of Occupational Injuries and Illnesses for 2008. The survey also is used to produce the incidence rates shown on the preceding pages. The estimates on the following pages are the number of cases involving days away from work (with or without days of restricted work activity). The nonfatal cases presented on pages 75-89 do not cover the self-employed or unpaid family workers or federal, state, or local government employees. Nonfatal cases involving state and local government employess are presented on page 90.

Data are presented for the sex, age, occupation, and race or ethnic origin of the worker, and for the nature of injury or illness, the part of body affected, the source of injury or illness, and the event or exposure that produced the injury or illness.

The text at the top of each page describes the kind of establishments that are included in the industry sector and gives the total number of workers in the industry in 2008 and the number working in the private sector.

How to benchmark

Incidence rates, percent distributions, or ranks may be used for benchmarking purposes. The results of the calculations described here may be compared to similar rates, percent distributions, and rankings based on data for a company.

For nonfatal cases incidence rates, multiply the number of cases by 1,000 and then divide by the private sector employment given in the text at the top of the page. This will give the number of cases with days away from work per 1,000 employees per year. For fatality rates, multiply the number of fatalities by 100,000, then divide by the total employment given at the top of the page. This will give the number of deaths per 100,000 employees per year.

To compute percent distributions, divide number of cases for each characteristic by the total number of cases found on the first line of the table. Multiply the quotient by 100 and round to one decimal place. Percent distributions may not add to 100.0% because of unclassifiable cases not shown.

Ranks are determined by arranging the characteristics from largest to smallest within each group, and then numbering consecutively starting with 1 for the largest.

Industry sectors

Page 75 shows nonfatal injury and illness data for the private sector of the economy (excluding government entities) and fatal injury data for all industries (including government). Pages 76-89 present the data for industry sectors based on the North American Industry Classification System. Page 90 presents fatal injury data for all government (employees and nonfatal cases involving state and local government employees).

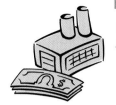

PRIVATE SECTOR / ALL INDUSTRIES

The nonfatal occupational injury and illness data cover only private sector employees and exclude employees in federal, state and local government entities and the self-employed. The fatal injury data cover all workers in both the private sector and government.

There were 146,534,000 people employed in 2008, of which 124,037,000 worked in the private sector.

NUMBER OF NONFATAL OCCUPATIONAL INJURIES AND ILLNESSES INVOLVING DAYS AWAY FROM WORK[a] AND FATAL OCCUPATIONAL INJURIES BY SELECTED WORKER AND CASE CHARACTERISTICS, UNITED STATES, 2008

Characteristic	Private industry [b,c] nonfatal cases	All industries fatalities
Total	**1,078,140**	**5,214**
Sex		
Men	688,790	4,827
Women	384,930	387
Age		
Under 16	130	11
16 to 19	31,010	89
20 to 24	107,880	353
25 to 34	239,580	850
35 to 44	251,490	1,113
45 to 54	261,030	1,292
55 to 64	142,840	920
65 and over	28,420	580
Occupation		
Management, business, and financial	26,310	577
Professional and related	80,790	72
Service	235,340	876
Sales and related	69,410	275
Office and administrative support	80,410	89
Farming, fishing, and forestry	13,510	286
Construction and extractive	120,890	977
Installation, maintenance, and repair	93,880	354
Production	138,890	267
Transportation and material moving	217,070	1,376
Military occupations	—	57
Race or ethnic origin[d]		
White, non-Hispanic	464,500	3,658
Black, non-Hispanic	83,970	532
Hispanic	145,870	804
Other, multiple, and not reported	383,800	220
Nature of injury, illness		
Sprains, strains	416,620	13
Fractures	89,650	38
Cuts, lacerations, punctures	99,830	632
Bruises, contusions	93,650	5
Heat burns	15,630	115
Chemical burns	5,620	—
Amputations	6,230	15
Carpal tunnel syndrome	10,080	
Tendonitis	4,100	—
Multiple injuries	43,960	1,965
Soreness, Pain	114,030	5
Back pain	37,140	—
All other	178,740	2,425

Characteristic	Private industry [b,c] nonfatal cases	All industries fatalities
Part of body affected		
Head	73,270	1,098
Eye	27,450	—
Neck	15,890	138
Trunk	366,710	866
Back	222,290	60
Shoulder	74,100	—
Upper extremities	244,150	18
Finger	95,080	—
Hand, except finger	41,940	—
Wrist	46,660	—
Lower extremities	240,760	57
Knee	91,830	10
Foot, toe	49,390	—
Body systems	15,860	813
Multiple	112,200	2,222
All other	9,290	—
Source of injury, illness		
Chemicals, chemical products	15,220	143
Containers	130,010	75
Furniture, fixtures	42,280	24
Machinery	64,170	381
Parts and materials	106,920	338
Worker motion or position	149,490	6
Floor, ground surfaces	217,420	677
Handtools	50,530	76
Vehicles	91,320	2,253
Health care patient	49,180	—
All other	142,220	1,240
Event or exposure		
Contact with object, equipment	291,880	937
Struck by object	152,770	520
Struck against object	70,300	12
Caught in object, equipment, material	49,240	402
Fall to lower level	67,510	593
Fall on same level	157,680	92
Slips, trips	35,420	—
Overexertion	250,960	5
Overexertion in lifting	129,990	—
Repetitive motion	30,920	—
Exposed to harmful substance	45,480	439
Transportation accidents	48,610	2,130
Highway accident	29,550	1,215
Nonhighway accident, except air, rail, water	8,240	284
Pedestrian, nonpassenger struck by vehicle, mobile equipment	8,460	329
Fires, explosions	2,320	174
Assault, violent act	22,690	816
By person	16,330	526
By other	6,360	290
All other	124,670	27

Source: National Safety Council tabulations of U.S. Bureau of Labor Statistics data.
Note: Because of rounding and data exclusion of nonclassifiable responses, data may not sum to the totals. Dashes (—) indicate data that do not meet publication guidelines.
[a]Days away from work include those that result in days away from work with or without restricted work activity or job transfer.
[b]Excludes farms with fewer than 11 employees.

[c]Data for mining operators in coal, metal, and nonmetal mining and for employees in railroad transportation are provided to BLS by the Mine Safety and Health Administration, U.S. Department of Labor; and the Federal Railroad Administration, U.S. Department of Transportation. Independent mining contractors are excluded from the coal, metal, and nonmetal mining industries. MSHA and FRA data do not reflect the changes in OSHA recordkeeping requirements in 2002.
[d]In fatalities column, non-Hispanic categories include cases with Hispanic origin not reported.

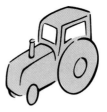

AGRICULTURE, FORESTRY, FISHING, HUNTING

76

The Agriculture, Forestry, Fishing, and Hunting industry sector includes growing crops, raising animals, harvesting timber, and harvesting fish and other animals from a farm, ranch, or their natural habitats, and agricultural support services.

Employment in Agriculture, Forestry, Fishing and Hunting totaled 2,168,000 in 2008, of which 2,102,000 were private sector employees.

NUMBER OF NONFATAL OCCUPATIONAL INJURIES AND ILLNESSES INVOLVING DAYS AWAY FROM WORK[a] AND FATAL OCCUPATIONAL INJURIES BY SELECTED WORKER AND CASE CHARACTERISTICS, UNITED STATES, AGRICULTURE, FORESTRY, FISHING, AND HUNTING, 2008

Characteristic	Nonfatal cases[b]	Fatalities
Total	**16,080**	**672**
Sex		
Men	13,370	648
Women	2,580	24
Age		
Under 16	—	8
16 to 19	610	14
20 to 24	2,110	32
25 to 34	3,910	68
35 to 44	3,680	93
45 to 54	3,200	117
55 to 64	1,800	137
65 and over	370	201
Occupation		
Management, business, and financial	450	327
Professional and related	170	—
Service	420	15
Sales and related	30	—
Office and administrative support	150	—
Farming, fishing, and forestry	11,000	269
Construction and extractive	110	—
Installation, maintenance, and repair	650	8
Production	910	5
Transportation and material moving	2,160	45
Military occupations	—	—
Race or ethnic origin[c]		
White, non-Hispanic	4,290	528
Black, non-Hispanic	340	30
Hispanic	8,340	92
Other, multiple, and not reported	3,110	22
Nature of injury, illness		
Sprains, strains	4,910	—
Fractures	1,770	5
Cuts, lacerations, punctures	1,960	31
Bruises, contusions	1,950	—
Heat burns	110	11
Chemical burns	140	—
Amputations	310	—
Carpal tunnel syndrome	60	—
Tendonitis	50	—
Multiple injuries	610	186
Soreness, Pain	1,440	—
Back pain	*410*	*—*
All other	2,780	435

Characteristic	Nonfatal cases[b]	Fatalities
Part of body affected		
Head	1,420	127
Eye	*620*	*—*
Neck	230	20
Trunk	4,670	166
Back	*2,550*	*10*
Shoulder	*890*	*—*
Upper extremities	3,710	5
Finger	*1,660*	*—*
Hand, except finger	*790*	*—*
Wrist	*390*	*—*
Lower extremities	4,130	8
Knee	*1,290*	*—*
Foot, toe	*930*	*—*
Body systems	240	143
Multiple	1,540	203
All other	140	—
Source of injury, illness		
Chemicals, chemical products	300	—
Containers	1,330	12
Furniture, fixtures	130	—
Machinery	1,090	89
Parts and materials	1,500	20
Worker motion or position	1,780	—
Floor, ground surfaces	2,970	30
Handtools	960	—
Vehicles	1,550	323
Health care patient	—	—
All other	4,330	193
Event or exposure		
Contact with object, equipment	5,520	248
Struck by object	*2,910*	*148*
Struck against object	*1,110*	*—*
Caught in object, equipment, material	*1,080*	*97*
Fall to lower level	1,660	22
Fall on same level	1,490	8
Slips, trips	340	—
Overexertion	1,930	—
Overexertion in lifting	*950*	*—*
Repetitive motion	270	—
Exposed to harmful substance	800	42
Transportation accidents	920	287
Highway accident	*310*	*69*
Nonhighway accident, except air, rail, water	*310*	*144*
Pedestrian, nonpassenger struck by vehicle, mobile equipment	*230*	*24*
Fires, explosions	30	20
Assault, violent act	990	44
By person	*60*	*18*
By other	*930*	*26*
All other	2,120	—

Source: National Safety Council tabulations of U.S. Bureau of Labor Statistics data.
Note: Because of rounding and data exclusion of nonclassifiable responses, data may not sum to the totals. Dashes (—) indicate data that do not meet publication guidelines.
[a] *Days away from work include those that result in days away from work with or without restricted work activity or job transfer.*

[b] *Excludes farms with fewer than 11 employees.*
[c] *In the fatalities column, non-Hispanic categories include cases with Hispanic origin not reported.*

The Mining industry sector includes extraction of naturally occurring mineral solids, such as coal and ores; liquid minerals, such as crude petroleum; and gases, such as natural gas. It also includes quarrying, well operations, beneficiating, other preparation customarily performed at the site, and mining support activities.

Mining employment in 2008 amounted to 819,000 workers, of which 817,000 were private sector employees.

NUMBER OF NONFATAL OCCUPATIONAL INJURIES AND ILLNESSES INVOLVING DAYS AWAY FROM WORK[a] AND FATAL OCCUPATIONAL INJURIES BY SELECTED WORKER AND CASE CHARACTERISTICS, UNITED STATES, MINING, 2008

Characteristic	Nonfatal cases[b]	Fatalities
Total	10,630	176
Sex		
Men	10,390	175
Women	240	—
Age		
Under 16	—	—
16 to 19	230	—
20 to 24	1,670	12
25 to 34	3,780	54
35 to 44	1,850	37
45 to 54	2,150	41
55 to 64	830	23
65 and over	50	8
Occupation		
Management, business, and financial	40	5
Professional and related	120	6
Service	—	—
Sales and related	—	—
Office and administrative support	50	—
Farming, fishing, and forestry	—	—
Construction and extractive	6,380	103
Installation, maintenance, and repair	980	10
Production	930	9
Transportation and material moving	2,110	43
Military occupations	—	—
Race or ethnic origin[c]		
White, non-Hispanic	4,310	141
Black, non-Hispanic	80	7
Hispanic	760	24
Other, multiple, and not reported	5,480	—
Nature of injury, illness		
Sprains, strains	3,560	—
Fractures	1,700	—
Cuts, lacerations, punctures	790	—
Bruises, contusions	810	—
Heat burns	120	8
Chemical burns	50	—
Amputations	190	—
Carpal tunnel syndrome	20	—
Tendonitis	—	—
Multiple injuries	480	79
Soreness, Pain	640	—
Back pain	110	—
All other	2,280	85

Characteristic	Nonfatal cases[b]	Fatalities
Part of body affected		
Head	840	25
Eye	390	—
Neck	170	—
Trunk	2,710	23
Back	1,450	—
Shoulder	570	—
Upper extremities	3,000	—
Finger	1,660	—
Hand, except finger	230	—
Wrist	210	—
Lower extremities	2,850	—
Knee	1,130	—
Foot, toe	380	—
Body systems	90	36
Multiple	930	89
All other	30	—
Source of injury, illness		
Chemicals, chemical products	550	11
Containers	510	6
Furniture, fixtures	20	—
Machinery	1,160	20
Parts and materials	2,380	25
Worker motion or position	390	—
Floor, ground surfaces	2,040	12
Handtools	620	—
Vehicles	1,090	66
Health care patient	—	—
All other	1,860	31
Event or exposure		
Contact with object, equipment	5,250	51
Struck by object	2,960	32
Struck against object	930	—
Caught in object, equipment, material	1,280	18
Fall to lower level	610	11
Fall on same level	900	—
Slips, trips	140	—
Overexertion	2,130	—
Overexertion in lifting	840	—
Repetitive motion	50	—
Exposed to harmful substance	330	21
Transportation accidents	280	71
Highway accident	170	42
Nonhighway accident, except air, rail, water	40	8
Pedestrian, nonpassenger struck by vehicle, mobile equipment	50	11
Fires, explosions	50	18
Assault, violent act	60	—
By person	—	—
By other	50	—
All other	830	—

Source: National Safety Council tabulations of U.S. Bureau of Labor Statistics data.
Note: Because of rounding and data exclusion of nonclassifiable responses, data may not sum to the totals. Dashes (—) indicate data that do not meet publication guidelines.
[a]Days away from work include those that result in days away from work with or without restricted work activity or job transfer.

[b]Data for mining operators in coal, metal, and nonmetal mining are provided to BLS by the Mine Safety and Health Administration, U.S. Department of Labor. Independent mining contractors are excluded from the coal, metal, and nonmetal mining industries. MSHA data do not reflect the changes in OSHA recordkeeping requirements in 2002.
[c]In the fatalities column, non-Hispanic categories include cases with Hispanic origin not reported.

CONSTRUCTION

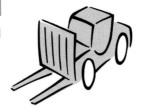

The Construction industry sector includes establishments engaged in construction of buildings, heavy construction other than buildings, and specialty trade contractors such as plumbing, electrical, carpentry, etc.

In 2008, employment in the Construction industry totaled 10,974,000 workers, of which 10,531,000 were private sector employees.

NUMBER OF NONFATAL OCCUPATIONAL INJURIES AND ILLNESSES INVOLVING DAYS AWAY FROM WORK[a] AND FATAL OCCUPATIONAL INJURIES BY SELECTED WORKER AND CASE CHARACTERISTICS, UNITED STATES, CONSTRUCTION, 2008

Characteristic	Nonfatal cases	Fatalities
Total	**120,240**	**975**
Sex		
Men	117,240	963
Women	2,980	12
Age		
Under 16	—	—
16 to 19	2,410	19
20 to 24	13,540	78
25 to 34	35,940	198
35 to 44	31,260	227
45 to 54	25,090	261
55 to 64	9,710	141
65 and over	1,010	50
Occupation		
Management, business, and financial	1,910	62
Professional and related	660	—
Service	1,250	6
Sales and related	750	—
Office and administrative support	630	—
Farming, fishing, and forestry	—	—
Construction and extractive	94,660	749
Installation, maintenance, and repair	10,820	66
Production	4,370	27
Transportation and material moving	5,050	60
Military occupations	—	—
Race or ethnic origin[b]		
White, non-Hispanic	66,810	645
Black, non-Hispanic	4,850	54
Hispanic	25,360	252
Other, multiple, and not reported	23,220	24
Nature of injury, illness		
Sprains, strains	39,920	—
Fractures	13,470	—
Cuts, lacerations, punctures	17,170	27
Bruises, contusions	7,870	—
Heat burns	1,070	12
Chemical burns	690	—
Amputations	570	—
Carpal tunnel syndrome	410	—
Tendonitis	220	—
Multiple injuries	4,770	391
Soreness, Pain	11,810	—
Back pain	*4,250*	—
All other	22,280	538

Characteristic	Nonfatal cases	Fatalities
Part of body affected		
Head	9,980	236
Eye	*5,510*	—
Neck	1,510	21
Trunk	38,210	121
Back	*23,640*	*6*
Shoulder	*5,950*	—
Upper extremities	27,430	—
Finger	*11,910*	—
Hand, except finger	*5,670*	—
Wrist	*3,980*	—
Lower extremities	30,580	8
Knee	*11,360*	—
Foot, toe	*6,680*	—
Body systems	1,590	173
Multiple	10,380	416
All other	560	—
Source of injury, illness		
Chemicals, chemical products	1,630	22
Containers	5,580	16
Furniture, fixtures	2,340	7
Machinery	7,420	118
Parts and materials	27,930	105
Worker motion or position	15,890	—
Floor, ground surfaces	22,920	324
Handtools	10,500	11
Vehicles	6,600	218
Health care patient	—	—
All other	18,500	154
Event or exposure		
Contact with object, equipment	42,970	201
Struck by object	*25,250*	*108*
Struck against object	*9,250*	—
Caught in object, equipment, material	*4,520*	*92*
Fall to lower level	15,560	328
Fall on same level	9,160	6
Slips, trips	3,810	—
Overexertion	21,310	—
Overexertion in lifting	*11,040*	—
Repetitive motion	1,500	—
Exposed to harmful substance	4,850	132
Transportation accidents	4,320	241
Highway accident	*2,650*	*113*
Nonhighway accident, except air, rail, water	*690*	*39*
Pedestrian, nonpassenger struck by vehicle, mobile equipment	*880*	*73*
Fires, explosions	450	26
Assault, violent act	310	38
By person	*140*	*16*
By other	*160*	*22*
All other	15,990	—

Source: National Safety Council tabulations of U.S. Bureau of Labor Statistics data.
Note: Because of rounding and data exclusion of nonclassifiable responses, data may not sum to the totals. Dashes (—) indicate data that do not meet publication guidelines.

[a]Days away from work include those that result in days away from work with or without restricted work activity or job transfer.
[b]In the fatalities column, non-Hispanic categories include cases with Hispanic origin not reported.

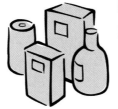

MANUFACTURING

The Manufacturing industry sector includes establishments engaged in the mechanical or chemical transformation of materials, substances, or components into new products. It includes durable and nondurable goods such as food, textiles, apparel, lumber, wood products, paper and paper products, printing, chemicals and pharmaceuticals, petroleum and coal products, rubber and plastics products, metals and metal products, machinery, electrical equipment, and transportation equipment.

Manufacturing employment in 2008 consisted of 15,903,000 workers, of which 15,789,000 were private sector employees.

NUMBER OF NONFATAL OCCUPATIONAL INJURIES AND ILLNESSES INVOLVING DAYS AWAY FROM WORK[a] AND FATAL OCCUPATIONAL INJURIES BY SELECTED WORKER AND CASE CHARACTERISTICS, MANUFACTURING, UNITED STATES, 2008

Characteristic	Nonfatal cases	Fatalities
Total	**164,940**	**411**
Sex		
Men	128,780	381
Women	36,020	30
Age		
Under 16	—	—
16 to 19	3,110	8
20 to 24	14,210	28
25 to 34	33,800	59
35 to 44	40,560	78
45 to 54	44,190	122
55 to 64	23,200	89
65 and over	3,800	27
Occupation		
Management, business, and financial	1,640	18
Professional and related	2,300	15
Service	2,870	5
Sales and related	990	12
Office and administrative support	5,930	—
Farming, fishing, and forestry	500	6
Construction and extractive	7,070	20
Installation, maintenance, and repair	11,970	48
Production	102,210	168
Transportation and material moving	29,280	114
Military occupations	—	—
Race or ethnic origin[b]		
White, non-Hispanic	84,550	270
Black, non-Hispanic	12,770	59
Hispanic	25,090	66
Other, multiple, and not reported	42,530	16
Nature of injury, illness		
Sprains, strains	55,470	—
Fractures	14,610	—
Cuts, lacerations, punctures	20,500	33
Bruises, contusions	13,470	—
Heat burns	2,920	24
Chemical burns	1,480	—
Amputations	2,720	—
Carpal tunnel syndrome	3,740	—
Tendonitis	1,120	—
Multiple injuries	6,220	128
Soreness, Pain	12,030	—
Back pain	3,610	—
All other	30,670	221

Characteristic	Nonfatal cases	Fatalities
Part of body affected		
Head	12,520	98
Eye	6,930	—
Neck	1,670	7
Trunk	51,250	58
Back	26,700	—
Shoulder	12,430	—
Upper extremities	54,050	—
Finger	25,170	—
Hand, except finger	8,270	—
Wrist	9,500	—
Lower extremities	31,010	—
Knee	11,220	—
Foot, toe	7,740	—
Body systems	1,660	81
Multiple	11,760	163
All other	1,030	—
Source of injury, illness		
Chemicals, chemical products	3,610	22
Containers	19,640	15
Furniture, fixtures	4,280	—
Machinery	20,540	61
Parts and materials	29,150	47
Worker motion or position	26,710	—
Floor, ground surfaces	22,480	54
Handtools	10,500	8
Vehicles	8,900	116
Health care patient	—	—
All other	18,250	86
Event or exposure		
Contact with object, equipment	60,430	116
Struck by object	27,330	45
Struck against object	11,680	—
Caught in object, equipment, material	17,320	71
Fall to lower level	6,860	46
Fall on same level	17,400	12
Slips, trips	4,170	—
Overexertion	36,220	—
Overexertion in lifting	18,280	—
Repetitive motion	10,970	—
Exposed to harmful substance	8,640	43
Transportation accidents	3,610	104
Highway accident	1,470	58
Nonhighway accident, except air, rail, water	870	12
Pedestrian, nonpassenger struck by vehicle, mobile equipment	1,180	18
Fires, explosions	390	43
Assault, violent act	390	47
By person	190	20
By other	200	27
All other	15,860	—

Source: National Safety Council tabulations of U.S. Bureau of Labor Statistics data.
Note: Because of rounding and data exclusion of nonclassifiable responses, data may not sum to the totals. Dashes (—) indicate data that do not meet publication guidelines.

[a]Days away from work include those that result in days away from work with or without restricted work activity or job transfer.
[b]In the fatalities column, non-Hispanic categories include cases with Hispanic origin not reported.

WHOLESALE TRADE

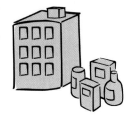

Establishments in Wholesale Trade generally sell merchandise to other businesses. The merchandise includes the outputs of agriculture, mining, manufacturing, and certain information industries such as publishing.

Wholesale Trade employed 4,052,000 people in 2008, of which 4,042,000 were private sector employees.

NUMBER OF NONFATAL OCCUPATIONAL INJURIES AND ILLNESSES INVOLVING DAYS AWAY FROM WORK[a] AND FATAL OCCUPATIONAL INJURIES BY SELECTED WORKER AND CASE CHARACTERISTICS, UNITED STATES, WHOLESALE TRADE, 2008

Characteristic	Nonfatal cases	Fatalities
Total	**71,880**	**180**
Sex		
Men	62,460	172
Women	9,390	8
Age		
Under 16	—	—
16 to 19	1,670	—
20 to 24	7,990	7
25 to 34	16,670	26
35 to 44	16,500	40
45 to 54	17,040	50
55 to 64	9,370	32
65 and over	1,800	23
Occupation		
Management, business, and financial	1,880	10
Professional and related	730	—
Service	850	—
Sales and related	5,670	31
Office and administrative support	4,480	5
Farming, fishing, and forestry	830	—
Construction and extractive	690	—
Installation, maintenance, and repair	9,930	17
Production	6,670	10
Transportation and material moving	40,140	95
Military occupations	—	—
Race or ethnic origin[b]		
White, non-Hispanic	35,210	134
Black, non-Hispanic	5,640	12
Hispanic	11,990	28
Other, multiple, and not reported	19,040	6
Nature of injury, illness		
Sprains, strains	27,060	—
Fractures	6,000	—
Cuts, lacerations, punctures	7,190	16
Bruises, contusions	6,460	—
Heat burns	1,310	—
Chemical burns	250	—
Amputations	390	—
Carpal tunnel syndrome	360	—
Tendonitis	240	—
Multiple injuries	3,500	81
Soreness, Pain	8,400	—
Back pain	3,320	—
All other	10,710	75

Characteristic	Nonfatal cases	Fatalities
Part of body affected		
Head	5,260	40
Eye	1,440	—
Neck	1,090	—
Trunk	26,040	33
Back	16,050	—
Shoulder	5,080	—
Upper extremities	15,170	—
Finger	5,980	—
Hand, except finger	2,530	—
Wrist	2,440	—
Lower extremities	17,090	—
Knee	5,780	—
Foot, toe	4,000	—
Body systems	660	13
Multiple	6,100	88
All other	470	—
Source of injury, illness		
Chemicals, chemical products	670	5
Containers	14,740	—
Furniture, fixtures	1,870	—
Machinery	4,660	12
Parts and materials	8,240	11
Worker motion or position	8,940	—
Floor, ground surfaces	10,530	15
Handtools	2,270	—
Vehicles	11,370	102
Health care patient	—	—
All other	8,200	28
Event or exposure		
Contact with object, equipment	22,360	34
Struck by object	11,040	18
Struck against object	5,830	—
Caught in object, equipment, material	4,490	16
Fall to lower level	3,810	12
Fall on same level	6,980	—
Slips, trips	1,860	—
Overexertion	19,010	—
Overexertion in lifting	10,580	—
Repetitive motion	1,500	—
Exposed to harmful substance	1,990	—
Transportation accidents	5,730	94
Highway accident	2,990	69
Nonhighway accident, except air, rail, water	1,060	9
Pedestrian, nonpassenger struck by vehicle, mobile equipment	1,220	11
Fires, explosions	640	6
Assault, violent act	260	24
By person	140	14
By other	130	10
All other	7,740	—

Source: National Safety Council tabulations of U.S. Bureau of Labor Statistics data.
Note: Because of rounding and data exclusion of nonclassifiable responses, data may not sum to the totals. Dashes (—) indicate data that do not meet publication guidelines.

[a]Days away from work include those that result in days away from work with or without restricted work activity or job transfer.
[b]In the fatalities column, non-Hispanic categories include cases with Hispanic origin not reported.

RETAIL TRADE

Establishments in Retail Trade generally sell merchandise in small quantities for personal or household consumption. This sector includes both store and nonstore retailers.

Retail Trade employed 16,533,000 people in 2008, of which 16,418,000 were private sector employees.

NUMBER OF NONFATAL OCCUPATIONAL INJURIES AND ILLNESSES INVOLVING DAYS AWAY FROM WORK[a] AND FATAL OCCUPATIONAL INJURIES BY SELECTED WORKER AND CASE CHARACTERISTICS, UNITED STATES, RETAIL TRADE, 2008

Characteristic	Nonfatal cases	Fatalities
Total	**146,320**	**301**
Sex		
Men	82,640	260
Women	63,630	41
Age		
Under 16	20	—
16 to 19	7,450	6
20 to 24	18,940	21
25 to 34	30,480	38
35 to 44	29,200	56
45 to 54	31,810	80
55 to 64	19,740	63
65 and over	5,950	36
Occupation		
Management, business, and financial	2,110	8
Professional and related	1,850	—
Service	14,400	17
Sales and related	52,520	184
Office and administrative support	18,390	8
Farming, fishing, and forestry	250	—
Construction and extractive	2,460	5
Installation, maintenance, and repair	15,760	20
Production	6,730	—
Transportation and material moving	31,770	57
Military occupations	—	—
Race or ethnic origin[b]		
White, non-Hispanic	61,090	196
Black, non-Hispanic	7,520	39
Hispanic	12,210	28
Other, multiple, and not reported	65,500	38
Nature of injury, illness		
Sprains, strains	58,140	—
Fractures	11,150	—
Cuts, lacerations, punctures	15,800	125
Bruises, contusions	14,280	—
Heat burns	1,370	—
Chemical burns	590	—
Amputations	670	—
Carpal tunnel syndrome	740	—
Tendonitis	520	—
Multiple injuries	4,460	78
Soreness, Pain	15,970	—
Back pain	4,800	—
All other	22,620	89

Characteristic	Nonfatal cases	Fatalities
Part of body affected		
Head	10,210	88
Eye	3,230	—
Neck	1,930	11
Trunk	50,380	71
Back	31,520	—
Shoulder	10,090	—
Upper extremities	33,410	—
Finger	13,470	—
Hand, except finger	5,350	—
Wrist	6,300	—
Lower extremities	32,380	—
Knee	11,990	—
Foot, toe	8,260	—
Body systems	1,790	22
Multiple	14,560	103
All other	1,650	—
Source of injury, illness		
Chemicals, chemical products	1,520	8
Containers	27,990	5
Furniture, fixtures	8,820	—
Machinery	9,370	—
Parts and materials	11,150	17
Worker motion or position	19,180	—
Floor, ground surfaces	29,100	27
Handtools	7,100	11
Vehicles	12,540	95
Health care patient	—	—
All other	17,100	133
Event or exposure		
Contact with object, equipment	43,000	30
Struck by object	24,320	22
Struck against object	10,250	—
Caught in object, equipment, material	5,590	5
Fall to lower level	7,120	18
Fall on same level	23,620	10
Slips, trips	4,350	—
Overexertion	38,000	—
Overexertion in lifting	23,140	—
Repetitive motion	3,460	—
Exposed to harmful substance	3,650	9
Transportation accidents	4,250	83
Highway accident	2,120	62
Nonhighway accident, except air, rail, water	690	—
Pedestrian, nonpassenger struck by vehicle, mobile equipment	1,260	14
Fires, explosions	250	7
Assault, violent act	1,510	143
By person	980	117
By other	530	26
All other	17,110	—

Source: National Safety Council tabulations of U.S. Bureau of Labor Statistics data.
Note: Because of rounding and data exclusion of nonclassifiable responses, data may not sum to the totals. Dashes (—) indicate data that do not meet publication guidelines.

[a]Days away from work include those that result in days away from work with or without restricted work activity or job transfer.
[b]In the fatalities column, non-Hispanic categories include cases with Hispanic origin not reported.

TRANSPORTATION AND WAREHOUSING

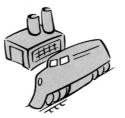

This industry sector includes transportation of cargo and passengers, warehousing and storage of goods, scenic and sightseeing transportation, and support activities related to transportation by rail, highway, air, water, or pipeline.

Employment in the Transportation and Warehousing industry sector totaled 6,501,000 in 2008, of which 5,298,000 were private sector employees.

NUMBER OF NONFATAL OCCUPATIONAL INJURIES AND ILLNESSES INVOLVING DAYS AWAY FROM WORK[a] AND FATAL OCCUPATIONAL INJURIES BY SELECTED WORKER AND CASE CHARACTERISTICS, UNITED STATES, TRANSPORTATION AND WAREHOUSING,[b] 2008

Characteristic	Nonfatal cases	Fatalities
Total	**104,120**	**796**
Sex		
Men	79,210	771
Women	21,480	25
Age		
Under 16	—	—
16 to 19	1,640	—
20 to 24	7,240	21
25 to 34	18,450	101
35 to 44	27,480	201
45 to 54	29,960	231
55 to 64	15,660	171
65 and over	2,900	65
Occupation		
Management, business, and financial	350	8
Professional and related	190	—
Service	6,330	9
Sales and related	620	—
Office and administrative support	12,110	9
Farming, fishing, and forestry	180	—
Construction and extractive	1,040	—
Installation, maintenance, and repair	7,180	25
Production	1,940	—
Transportation and material moving	74,020	738
Military occupations	—	—
Race or ethnic origin[c]		
White, non-Hispanic	29,170	561
Black, non-Hispanic	5,450	127
Hispanic	7,450	73
Other, multiple, and not reported	62,050	35
Nature of injury, illness		
Sprains, strains	47,590	—
Fractures	7,880	—
Cuts, lacerations, punctures	5,140	63
Bruises, contusions	10,830	—
Heat burns	960	31
Chemical burns	200	—
Amputations	250	—
Carpal tunnel syndrome	340	—
Tendonitis	200	—
Multiple injuries	4,370	409
Soreness, Pain	12,630	—
Back pain	4,240	—
All other	13,740	284

Characteristic	Nonfatal cases	Fatalities
Part of body affected		
Head	5,470	115
Eye	1,470	—
Neck	2,200	17
Trunk	40,610	119
Back	22,330	6
Shoulder	10,200	—
Upper extremities	16,960	—
Finger	4,350	—
Hand, except finger	3,310	—
Wrist	3,290	—
Lower extremities	26,420	6
Knee	9,460	—
Foot, toe	5,160	—
Body systems	740	82
Multiple	10,950	454
All other	770	—
Source of injury, illness		
Chemicals, chemical products	730	25
Containers	22,210	6
Furniture, fixtures	2,100	—
Machinery	2,460	8
Parts and materials	9,420	22
Worker motion or position	14,080	—
Floor, ground surfaces	18,800	34
Handtools	1,540	6
Vehicles	20,930	615
Health care patient	160	—
All other	9,980	78
Event or exposure		
Contact with object, equipment	22,930	72
Struck by object	11,450	38
Struck against object	6,360	—
Caught in object, equipment, material	3,400	33
Fall to lower level	7,490	31
Fall on same level	11,820	5
Slips, trips	3,640	—
Overexertion	28,320	—
Overexertion in lifting	13,330	—
Repetitive motion	1,610	—
Exposed to harmful substance	2,150	31
Transportation accidents	11,590	578
Highway accident	7,670	423
Nonhighway accident, except air, rail, water	1,730	13
Pedestrian, nonpassenger struck by vehicle, mobile equipment	1,510	66
Fires, explosions	60	—
Assault, violent act	810	72
By person	470	55
By other	340	17
All other	13,710	—

Source: National Safety Council tabulations of U.S. Bureau of Labor Statistics data.
Note: Because of rounding and data exclusion of nonclassifiable responses, data may not sum to the totals. Dashes (—) indicate data that do not meet publication guidelines.
[a]Days away from work include those that result in days away from work with or without restricted work activity or job transfer.

[b]Data for employees in railroad transportation are provided to BLS by the Federal Railroad Administration, U.S. Department of Transportation. FRA data do not reflect the changes in OSHA recordkeeping requirements in 2002.
[c]In the fatalities column, non-Hispanic categories include cases with Hispanic origin not reported.

UTILITIES

The Utilities sector includes establishments that provide electric power generation, transmission, and distribution; natural gas distribution; steam supply; water treatment and distribution; and sewage collection, treatment, and disposal.

The Utilities sector employed 1,225,000 people in 2008, of which all 890,000 were private sector employees.

NUMBER OF NONFATAL OCCUPATIONAL INJURIES AND ILLNESSES INVOLVING DAYS AWAY FROM WORK[a] AND FATAL OCCUPATIONAL INJURIES BY SELECTED WORKER AND CASE CHARACTERISTICS, UNITED STATES, UTILITIES, 2008

Characteristic	Nonfatal cases	Fatalities
Total	5,890	37
Sex		
Men	5,310	37
Women	580	—
Age		
Under 16	—	—
16 to 19	20	—
20 to 24	340	—
25 to 34	1,200	6
35 to 44	1,420	15
45 to 54	1,890	11
55 to 64	890	—
65 and over	60	—
Occupation		
Management, business, and financial	60	—
Professional and related	260	—
Service	120	—
Sales and related	60	—
Office and administrative support	900	—
Farming, fishing, and forestry	—	—
Construction and extractive	950	6
Installation, maintenance, and repair	2,390	21
Production	860	—
Transportation and material moving	260	—
Military occupations	—	—
Race or ethnic origin[b]		
White, non-Hispanic	2,360	27
Black, non-Hispanic	190	—
Hispanic	160	5
Other, multiple, and not reported	3,180	—
Nature of injury, illness		
Sprains, strains	2,930	—
Fractures	440	—
Cuts, lacerations, punctures	230	—
Bruises, contusions	280	—
Heat burns	110	—
Chemical burns	30	—
Amputations	20	—
Carpal tunnel syndrome	70	—
Tendonitis	30	—
Multiple injuries	170	10
Soreness, Pain	460	—
Back pain	160	—
All other	1,120	25

Characteristic	Nonfatal cases	Fatalities
Part of body affected		
Head	300	—
Eye	110	—
Neck	60	—
Trunk	2,030	—
Back	1,140	—
Shoulder	580	—
Upper extremities	950	—
Finger	250	—
Hand, except finger	170	—
Wrist	190	—
Lower extremities	1,720	—
Knee	840	—
Foot, toe	230	—
Body systems	170	21
Multiple	620	13
All other	40	—
Source of injury, illness		
Chemicals, chemical products	90	—
Containers	260	—
Furniture, fixtures	50	—
Machinery	270	—
Parts and materials	690	16
Worker motion or position	1,290	—
Floor, ground surfaces	1,170	—
Handtools	390	—
Vehicles	460	7
Health care patient	—	—
All other	1,040	12
Event or exposure		
Contact with object, equipment	1,040	6
Struck by object	510	—
Struck against object	320	—
Caught in object, equipment, material	120	—
Fall to lower level	450	—
Fall on same level	730	—
Slips, trips	390	—
Overexertion	1,080	—
Overexertion in lifting	390	—
Repetitive motion	200	—
Exposed to harmful substance	460	21
Transportation accidents	300	6
Highway accident	190	—
Nonhighway accident, except air, rail, water	40	—
Pedestrian, nonpassenger struck by vehicle, mobile equipment	20	—
Fires, explosions	30	—
Assault, violent act	110	—
By person	30	—
By other	80	—
All other	1,100	—

Source: National Safety Council tabulations of U.S. Bureau of Labor Statistics data.
Note: Because of rounding and data exclusion of nonclassifiable responses, data may not sum to the totals. Dashes (—) indicate data that do not meet publication guidelines.

[a]Days away from work include those that result in days away from work with or without restricted work activity or job transfer.
[b]In the fatalities column, non-Hispanic categories include cases with Hispanic origin not reported.

INFORMATION

The Information sector includes establishments that (a) produce and distribute information and cultural products (b) provide the means to transmit or distribute these products, as well as data or communications and (c) process data. Included are both traditional and Internet publishing and broadcasting, motion pictures and sound recordings, telecommunications, Internet service providers, web search portals, data processing, and information services.

The Information sector employed 3,481,000 people in 2008, of which 3,285,000 were private sector employees.

NUMBER OF NONFATAL OCCUPATIONAL INJURIES AND ILLNESSES INVOLVING DAYS AWAY FROM WORK[a] AND FATAL OCCUPATIONAL INJURIES BY SELECTED WORKER AND CASE CHARACTERISTICS, UNITED STATES, INFORMATION, 2008

Characteristic	Nonfatal cases	Fatalities
Total	**18,070**	**47**
Sex		
Male	12,980	39
Female	5,090	8
Age		
Under 16	—	—
16 to 19	320	—
20 to 24	900	—
25 to 34	3,670	7
35 to 44	5,340	11
45 to 54	4,560	13
55 to 64	2,360	7
65 and over	430	—
Occupation		
Management, business, and financial	670	—
Professional and related	2,800	—
Service	750	10
Sales and related	790	—
Office and administrative support	2,820	—
Farming, fishing, and forestry	—	—
Construction and extractive	220	—
Installation, maintenance, and repair	7,040	10
Production	1,510	—
Transportation and material moving	1,460	14
Military occupations	—	—
Race or ethnic origin[b]		
White, non-Hispanic	5,580	34
Black, non-Hispanic	870	5
Hispanic	810	5
Other, multiple, and not reported	10,810	—
Nature of injury, illness		
Sprains, strains	7,650	—
Fractures	1,370	—
Cuts, lacerations, punctures	930	10
Bruises, contusions	1,260	—
Heat burns	60	—
Chemical burns	20	—
Amputations	80	—
Carpal tunnel syndrome	380	—
Tendonitis	110	—
Multiple injuries	1,100	15
Soreness, Pain	1,930	—
Back pain	520	—
All other	3,190	20

Characteristic	Nonfatal cases	Fatalities
Part of body affected		
Head	850	12
Eye	250	—
Neck	340	—
Trunk	5,690	7
Back	3,480	—
Shoulder	1,410	—
Upper extremities	3,480	—
Finger	990	—
Hand, except finger	570	—
Wrist	920	—
Lower extremities	4,790	—
Knee	2,020	—
Foot, toe	710	—
Body systems	270	8
Multiple	2,490	18
All other	160	—
Source of injury, illness		
Chemicals, chemical products	110	—
Containers	1,460	—
Furniture, fixtures	720	—
Machinery	1,070	—
Parts and materials	1,060	—
Worker motion or position	3,560	—
Floor, ground surfaces	4,820	8
Handtools	380	—
Vehicles	1,760	23
Health care patient	—	—
All other	2,970	12
Event or exposure		
Contact with object, equipment	3,680	—
Struck by object	1,570	—
Struck against object	1,190	—
Caught in object, equipment, material	750	—
Fall to lower level	1,760	—
Fall on same level	3,200	—
Slips, trips	680	—
Overexertion	3,140	—
Overexertion in lifting	1,420	—
Repetitive motion	950	—
Exposed to harmful substance	550	—
Transportation accidents	1,250	22
Highway accident	950	17
Nonhighway accident, except air, rail, water	120	—
Pedestrian, nonpassenger struck by vehicle, mobile equipment	130	—
Fires, explosions	—	—
Assault, violent act	200	12
By person	90	6
By other	110	6
All other	2,670	—

Source: National Safety Council tabulations of U.S. Bureau of Labor Statistics data.
Note: Because of rounding and data exclusion of nonclassifiable responses, data may not sum to the totals. Dashes (—) indicate data that do not meet publication guidelines.

[a]Days away from work include those that result in days away from work with or without restricted work activity or job transfer.
[b]In the fatalities column, non-Hispanic categories include cases with Hispanic origin not reported.

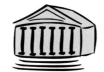

Financial Activities includes the Finance and Insurance sector and the Real Estate and Rental and Leasing sector. Included are banks and other savings institutions; securities and commodities brokers, dealers, exchanges, and services; insurance carriers, brokers, and agents; real estate operators, developers, agents, and brokers; and establishments that rent and lease goods such as automobiles, computers, and household and industrial machinery and equipment.

Financial Activities had 10,227,000 workers in 2008, of which 10,003,000 were private sector employees.

NUMBER OF NONFATAL OCCUPATIONAL INJURIES AND ILLNESSES INVOLVING DAYS AWAY FROM WORKª AND FATAL OCCUPATIONAL INJURIES BY SELECTED WORKER AND CASE CHARACTERISTICS, UNITED STATES, FINANCIAL ACTIVITIES, 2008

Characteristic	Nonfatal cases	Fatalities
Total	**35,010**	**106**
Sex		
Mem	19,480	82
Women	15,530	24
Age		
Under 16	—	—
16 to 19	490	—
20 to 24	2,820	8
25 to 34	7,050	13
35 to 44	7,730	21
45 to 54	10,080	24
55 to 64	4,990	20
65 and over	1,670	19
Occupation		
Management, business, and financial	3,720	30
Professional and related	1,180	—
Service	6,800	8
Sales and related	2,270	24
Office and administrative support	9,120	6
Farming, fishing, and forestry	—	—
Construction and extractive	1,450	—
Installation, maintenance, and repair	5,400	9
Production	410	—
Transportation and material moving	4,390	24
Military occupations	—	—
Race or ethnic origin[b]		
White, non-Hispanic	14,580	80
Black, non-Hispanic	2,810	14
Hispanic	5,310	9
Other, multiple, and not reported	12,310	—
Nature of injury, illness		
Sprains, strains	12,400	—
Fractures	4,090	—
Cuts, lacerations, punctures	1,960	28
Bruises, contusions	3,040	—
Heat burns	210	—
Chemical burns	80	—
Amputations	170	—
Carpal tunnel syndrome	1,150	—
Tendonitis	80	—
Multiple injuries	1,610	38
Soreness, Pain	3,850	—
Back pain	880	—
All other	6,360	35

Characteristic	Nonfatal cases	Fatalities
Part of body affected		
Head	2,300	21
Eye	800	—
Neck	610	—
Trunk	12,490	19
Back	7,330	—
Shoulder	2,160	—
Upper extremities	6,410	—
Finger	2,160	—
Hand, except finger	560	—
Wrist	2,020	—
Lower extremities	6,940	—
Knee	2,530	—
Foot, toe	2,210	—
Body systems	1,180	13
Multiple	4,470	48
All other	620	—
Source of injury, illness		
Chemicals, chemical products	370	—
Containers	2,880	—
Furniture, fixtures	2,450	—
Machinery	2,220	5
Parts and materials	2,650	—
Worker motion or position	5,660	—
Floor, ground surfaces	9,310	14
Handtools	1,450	—
Vehicles	2,990	36
Health care patient	100	—
All other	3,950	43
Event or exposure		
Contact with object, equipment	6,970	7
Struck by object	4,050	—
Struck against object	1,160	—
Caught in object, equipment, material	1,150	—
Fall to lower level	2,310	15
Fall on same level	7,640	—
Slips, trips	930	—
Overexertion	6,520	—
Overexertion in lifting	3,760	—
Repetitive motion	2,550	—
Exposed to harmful substance	1,590	5
Transportation accidents	1,870	35
Highway accident	1,000	27
Nonhighway accident, except air, rail, water	150	—
Pedestrian, nonpassenger struck by vehicle, mobile equipment	570	—
Fires, explosions	20	—
Assault, violent act	860	41
By person	740	34
By other	120	7
All other	3,750	—

Source: National Safety Council tabulations of U.S. Bureau of Labor Statistics data.
Note: Because of rounding and data exclusion of nonclassifiable responses, data may not sum to the totals. Dashes (—) indicate data that do not meet publication guidelines.

ªDays away from work include those that result in days away from work with or without restricted work activity or job transfer.
[b]In the fatalities column, non-Hispanic categories include cases with Hispanic origin not reported.

PROFESSIONAL AND BUSINESS SERVICES

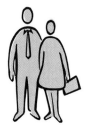

The Professional and Business Services sector includes legal, accounting, architectural, engineering, computer, consulting, research, advertising, photographic, translation and interpretation, veterinary, and other professional scientific and technical services. Also included are business management and administrative and support activities, and waste management and remediation services.

Professional and Business Services employed 15,541,000 people in 2008, of which 15,149,000 were private sector employees.

NUMBER OF NONFATAL OCCUPATIONAL INJURIES AND ILLNESSES INVOLVING DAYS AWAY FROM WORK[a] AND FATAL OCCUPATIONAL INJURIES BY SELECTED WORKER AND CASE CHARACTERISTICS, UNITED STATES, PROFESSIONAL AND BUSINESS SERVICES, 2008

Characteristic	Nonfatal cases	Fatalities
Total	**85,540**	**403**
Sex		
Mem	56,080	377
Women	29,040	26
Age		
Under 16	—	—
16 to 19	1,660	—
20 to 24	8,910	49
25 to 34	19,920	73
35 to 44	20,800	87
45 to 54	18,580	91
55 to 64	11,090	70
65 and over	1,890	30
Occupation		
Management, business, and financial	4,070	16
Professional and related	6,680	18
Service	32,820	220
Sales and related	1,720	8
Office and administrative support	11,350	9
Farming, fishing, and forestry	400	—
Construction and extractive	3,110	31
Installation, maintenance, and repair	6,100	14
Production	5,320	11
Transportation and material moving	13,420	73
Military occupations	—	—
Race or ethnic origin[b]		
White, non-Hispanic	32,360	239
Black, non-Hispanic	7,830	40
Hispanic	16,860	111
Other, multiple, and not reported	28,490	13
Nature of injury, illness		
Sprains, strains	30,120	—
Fractures	7,910	—
Cuts, lacerations, punctures	7,200	42
Bruises, contusions	6,700	—
Heat burns	400	—
Chemical burns	620	—
Amputations	360	—
Carpal tunnel syndrome	700	—
Tendonitis	310	—
Multiple injuries	4,390	150
Soreness, Pain	9,000	—
Back pain	2,720	—
All other	17,830	201

Characteristic	Nonfatal cases	Fatalities
Part of body affected		
Head	6,060	85
Eye	1,540	—
Neck	1,380	10
Trunk	25,140	64
Back	15,340	5
Shoulder	4,490	—
Upper extremities	17,970	—
Finger	6,710	—
Hand, except finger	3,060	—
Wrist	3,580	—
Lower extremities	20,610	6
Knee	7,910	—
Foot, toe	3,450	—
Body systems	2,270	76
Multiple	10,890	159
All other	1,220	—
Source of injury, illness		
Chemicals, chemical products	1,180	9
Containers	9,360	7
Furniture, fixtures	2,690	—
Machinery	3,780	30
Parts and materials	5,230	17
Worker motion or position	11,060	—
Floor, ground surfaces	21,300	66
Handtools	3,800	13
Vehicles	8,550	146
Health care patient	630	—
All other	15,600	111
Event or exposure		
Contact with object, equipment	20,120	77
Struck by object	9,840	45
Struck against object	5,600	—
Caught in object, equipment, material	3,430	29
Fall to lower level	7,070	56
Fall on same level	14,740	5
Slips, trips	2,860	—
Overexertion	14,670	—
Overexertion in lifting	8,160	—
Repetitive motion	2,340	—
Exposed to harmful substance	3,680	52
Transportation accidents	6,420	146
Highway accident	4,260	90
Nonhighway accident, except air, rail, water	1,450	14
Pedestrian, nonpassenger struck by vehicle, mobile equipment	600	31
Fires, explosions	160	6
Assault, violent act	3,090	55
By person	1,330	28
By other	1,760	27
All other	10,390	6

Source: National Safety Council tabulations of U.S. Bureau of Labor Statistics data.
Note: Because of rounding and data exclusion of nonclassifiable responses, data may not sum to the totals. Dashes (—) indicate data that do not meet publication guidelines.

[a]Days away from work include those that result in days away from work with or without restricted work activity or job transfer.
[b]In the fatalities column, non-Hispanic categories include cases with Hispanic origin not reported.

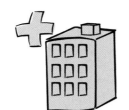

EDUCATIONAL AND HEALTH SERVICES

Educational services includes instruction and training through schools, colleges, universities, and training centers. Health services includes ambulatory health care facilities; hospitals; nursing and residential care facilities; and social assistance for individuals, families and communities.

Educational and Health Services employed 31,402,000 people in 2008, of which 20,401,000 were private sector employees.

NUMBER OF NONFATAL OCCUPATIONAL INJURIES AND ILLNESSES INVOLVING DAYS AWAY FROM WORK[a] AND FATAL OCCUPATIONAL INJURIES BY SELECTED WORKER AND CASE CHARACTERISTICS, UNITED STATES, EDUCATIONAL AND HEALTH SERVICES, 2008

Characteristic	Nonfatal cases	Fatalities
Total	**182,750**	**141**
Sex		
Men	36,650	93
Women	145,980	48
Age		
Under 16	—	—
16 to 19	2,770	—
20 to 24	15,670	10
25 to 34	36,710	25
35 to 44	40,830	36
45 to 54	48,450	25
55 to 64	30,230	27
65 and over	5,800	17
Occupation		
Management, business, and financial	6,690	—
Professional and related	59,040	—
Service	96,030	92
Sales and related	400	—
Office and administrative support	10,250	—
Farming, fishing, and forestry	40	—
Construction and extractive	930	—
Installation, maintenance, and repair	3,170	—
Production	1,910	5
Transportation and material moving	3,960	31
Military occupations	—	—
Race or ethnic origin[b]		
White, non-Hispanic	76,690	117
Black, non-Hispanic	26,560	11
Hispanic	14,730	9
Other, multiple, and not reported	64,770	—
Nature of injury, illness		
Sprains, strains	89,010	—
Fractures	10,780	—
Cuts, lacerations, punctures	5,790	20
Bruises, contusions	17,040	—
Heat burns	1,440	—
Chemical burns	480	—
Amputations	110	—
Carpal tunnel syndrome	870	—
Tendonitis	790	—
Multiple injuries	7,340	75
Soreness, Pain	22,920	—
Back pain	8,230	—
All other	26,180	43

Characteristic	Nonfatal cases	Fatalities
Part of body affected		
Head	9,170	15
Eye	2,640	—
Neck	3,750	—
Trunk	72,440	14
Back	49,610	—
Shoulder	12,670	—
Upper extremities	28,860	—
Finger	7,560	—
Hand, except finger	4,090	—
Wrist	7,630	—
Lower extremities	36,950	—
Knee	16,480	—
Foot, toe	5,290	—
Body systems	3,280	25
Multiple	26,610	81
All other	1,700	—
Source of injury, illness		
Chemicals, chemical products	2,650	10
Containers	10,030	—
Furniture, fixtures	9,840	—
Machinery	3,580	—
Parts and materials	2,290	—
Worker motion or position	24,470	—
Floor, ground surfaces	44,430	9
Handtools	2,470	—
Vehicles	8,470	82
Health care patient	48,150	—
All other	19,890	30
Event or exposure		
Contact with object, equipment	24,450	—
Struck by object	12,730	—
Struck against object	7,620	—
Caught in object, equipment, material	2,800	—
Fall to lower level	7,640	—
Fall on same level	37,140	6
Slips, trips	7,250	—
Overexertion	58,920	—
Overexertion in lifting	26,110	—
Repetitive motion	3,010	—
Exposed to harmful substance	7,750	17
Transportation accidents	5,240	80
Highway accident	4,270	19
Nonhighway accident, except air, rail, water	360	—
Pedestrian, nonpassenger struck by vehicle, mobile equipment	310	7
Fires, explosions	80	—
Assault, violent act	11,290	31
By person	10,680	17
By other	610	14
All other	19,980	—

Source: National Safety Council tabulations of U.S. Bureau of Labor Statistics data.
Note: Because of rounding and data exclusion of nonclassifiable responses, data may not sum to the totals. Dashes (—) indicate data that do not meet publication guidelines.

[a]Days away from work include those that result in days away from work with or without restricted work activity or job transfer.
[b]In the fatalities column, non-Hispanic categories include cases with Hispanic origin not reported.

LEISURE AND HOSPITALITY

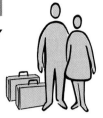

The Leisure sector includes establishments that provide arts, entertainment, and recreation experiences such as theatre, dance, music, and spectator sports, museums, zoos, amusement and theme parks, casinos, golf courses, ski areas, marinas, and fitness and sports centers. The

Hospitality sector includes hotels and other traveler accommodations, food services, and drinking places.

The Leisure and Hospitality sector employed 12,767,000 people in 2008, of which 12,350,000 were private sector employees.

NUMBER OF NONFATAL OCCUPATIONAL INJURIES AND ILLNESSES INVOLVING DAYS AWAY FROM WORK[a] AND FATAL OCCUPATIONAL INJURIES BY SELECTED WORKER AND CASE CHARACTERISTICS, UNITED STATES, LEISURE AND HOSPITALITY, 2008

Characteristic	Nonfatal cases	Fatalities
Total	**86,190**	**238**
Sex		
Mem	42,040	204
Women	44,110	34
Age		
Under 16	50	—
16 to 19	7,800	13
20 to 24	10,500	27
25 to 34	19,840	43
35 to 44	17,930	49
45 to 54	16,870	45
55 to 64	9,410	34
65 and over	2,160	26
Occupation		
Management, business, and financial	1,900	41
Professional and related	3,330	—
Service	66,410	152
Sales and related	3,010	6
Office and administrative support	2,110	6
Farming, fishing, and forestry	70	—
Construction and extractive	680	5
Installation, maintenance, and repair	2,430	10
Production	2,050	—
Transportation and material moving	4,150	17
Military occupations	—	—
Race or ethnic origin[b]		
White, non-Hispanic	30,830	156
Black, non-Hispanic	7,270	32
Hispanic	12,850	38
Other, multiple, and not reported	35,240	12
Nature of injury, illness		
Sprains, strains	28,230	—
Fractures	6,240	—
Cuts, lacerations, punctures	11,770	99
Bruises, contusions	7,380	—
Heat burns	4,720	—
Chemical burns	650	—
Amputations	360	—
Carpal tunnel syndrome	680	—
Tendonitis	400	—
Multiple injuries	3,550	41
Soreness, Pain	9,640	—
Back pain	2,380	—
All other	12,560	93

Characteristic	Nonfatal cases	Fatalities
Part of body affected		
Head	5,430	59
Eye	1,460	—
Neck	590	15
Trunk	25,150	65
Back	15,710	9
Shoulder	5,630	—
Upper extremities	25,500	—
Finger	10,520	—
Hand, except finger	5,170	—
Wrist	4,780	—
Lower extremities	19,040	—
Knee	7,280	—
Foot, toe	2,980	—
Body systems	1,660	32
Multiple	8,100	66
All other	720	—
Source of injury, illness		
Chemicals, chemical products	1,290	8
Containers	12,110	—
Furniture, fixtures	5,840	—
Machinery	4,440	9
Parts and materials	1,670	12
Worker motion or position	11,500	—
Floor, ground surfaces	22,370	19
Handtools	6,660	15
Vehicles	3,430	56
Health care patient	100	—
All other	14,610	118
Event or exposure		
Contact with object, equipment	24,340	17
Struck by object	14,120	9
Struck against object	6,570	—
Caught in object, equipment, material	2,410	6
Fall to lower level	3,950	10
Fall on same level	19,040	8
Slips, trips	4,030	—
Overexertion	13,550	—
Overexertion in lifting	8,070	—
Repetitive motion	1,530	—
Exposed to harmful substance	7,370	17
Transportation accidents	1,660	54
Highway accident	680	16
Nonhighway accident, except air, rail, water	610	23
Pedestrian, nonpassenger struck by vehicle, mobile equipment	280	7
Fires, explosions	120	—
Assault, violent act	1,730	127
By person	1,430	94
By other	300	33
All other	8,860	

Source: National Safety Council tabulations of U.S. Bureau of Labor Statistics data.
Note: Because of rounding and data exclusion of nonclassifiable responses, data may not sum to the totals. Dashes (—) indicate data that do not meet publication guidelines.

[a]Days away from work include those that result in days away from work with or without restricted work activity or job transfer.
[b]In the fatalities column, non-Hispanic categories include cases with Hispanic origin not reported.

The Other Services sector includes repair and maintenance of equipment and machinery and personal and household goods, personal care and laundry services, and religious, grant making, civic, professional and similar organizations.

The Other Services sector employed 7,005,000 people in 2008, of which 6,962,000 were private sector employees.

NUMBER OF NONFATAL OCCUPATIONAL INJURIES AND ILLNESSES INVOLVING DAYS AWAY FROM WORK[a] AND FATAL OCCUPATIONAL INJURIES BY SELECTED WORKER AND CASE CHARACTERISTICS, UNITED STATES, OTHER SERVICES (EXCEPT PUBLIC ADMINISTRATION), 2008

Characteristic	Nonfatal cases	Fatalities
Total	30,470	178
Sex		
Men	22,160	158
Women	8,280	20
Age		
Under 16	—	—
16 to 19	820	—
20 to 24	3,050	8
25 to 34	8,160	32
35 to 44	6,920	36
45 to 54	7,160	50
55 to 64	3,570	25
65 and over	510	24
Occupation		
Management, business, and financial	810	18
Professional and related	1,470	—
Service	6,270	50
Sales and related	590	—
Office and administrative support	2,100	—
Farming, fishing, and forestry	30	—
Construction and extractive	1,120	—
Installation, maintenance, and repair	10,060	73
Production	3,090	12
Transportation and material moving	4,900	16
Military occupations	—	—
Race or ethnic origin[b]		
White, non-Hispanic	16,680	118
Black, non-Hispanic	1,790	24
Hispanic	3,960	25
Other, multiple, and not reported	8,040	11
Nature of injury, illness		
Sprains, strains	9,630	—
Fractures	2,240	—
Cuts, lacerations, punctures	3,410	37
Bruises, contusions	2,270	—
Heat burns	830	5
Chemical burns	330	—
Amputations	30	—
Carpal tunnel syndrome	570	—
Tendonitis	40	—
Multiple injuries	1,410	50
Soreness, Pain	3,320	—
Back pain	*1,520*	—
All other	6,400	83

Characteristic	Nonfatal cases	Fatalities
Part of body affected		
Head	3,450	49
Eye	*1,060*	—
Neck	360	9
Trunk	9,910	33
Back	*5,460*	—
Shoulder	*1,950*	—
Upper extremities	7,250	—
Finger	*2,690*	—
Hand, except finger	*2,180*	—
Wrist	*1,420*	—
Lower extremities	6,230	—
Knee	*2,540*	—
Foot, toe	*1,390*	—
Body systems	260	24
Multiple	2,810	60
All other	190	—
Source of injury, illness		
Chemicals, chemical products	510	—
Containers	1,910	—
Furniture, fixtures	1,120	—
Machinery	2,120	7
Parts and materials	3,570	15
Worker motion or position	4,990	—
Floor, ground surfaces	5,180	20
Handtools	1,910	—
Vehicles	2,680	75
Health care patient	30	—
All other	5,970	54
Event or exposure		
Contact with object, equipment	8,820	32
Struck by object	*4,690*	*23*
Struck against object	*2,430*	—
Caught in object, equipment, material	*900*	*9*
Fall to lower level	1,220	15
Fall on same level	3,820	6
Slips, trips	980	—
Overexertion	6,170	—
Overexertion in lifting	*3,910*	—
Repetitive motion	960	—
Exposed to harmful substance	1,660	11
Transportation accidents	1,170	48
Highway accident	*810*	*32*
Nonhighway accident, except air, rail, water	*120*	—
Pedestrian, nonpassenger struck by vehicle, mobile equipment	*210*	*12*
Fires, explosions	40	18
Assault, violent act	1,090	48
By person	*60*	*34*
By other	*1,030*	*14*
All other	4,550	—

Source: National Safety Council tabulations of U.S. Bureau of Labor Statistics data.
Note: Because of rounding and data exclusion of nonclassifiable responses, data may not sum to the totals. Dashes (—) indicate data that do not meet publication guidelines.

[a]Days away from work include those that result in days away from work with or without restricted work activity or job transfer.
[b]In the fatalities column, non-Hispanic categories include cases with Hispanic origin not reported.

GOVERNMENT

Government includes public employees at all levels from federal (civilian and military) to state, county and municipal.

Total government employment was 22,497,000 in 2008, of which 18,682,000 were state and local government employees.

NUMBER OF NONFATAL OCCUPATIONAL INJURIES AND ILLNESSES INVOLVING DAYS AWAY FROM WORK[a] AND FATAL OCCUPATIONAL INJURIES BY SELECTED WORKER AND CASE CHARACTERISTICS, UNITED STATES, GOVERNMENT, 2008

Characteristic	State and local government nonfatal cases[b]	All government fatalities
Total	**277,680**	**544**
Sex		
Men	159,340	459
Women	117,920	85
Age		
Under 16	40	—
16 to 19	1,710	10
20 to 24	11,730	47
25 to 34	50,940	106
35 to 44	72,650	126
45 to 54	80,410	127
55 to 64	46,740	76
65 and over	7,770	52
Occupation		
Management, business, and financial	6,630	24
Professional and related	56,120	20
Service	138,960	289
Sales and related	1,040	—
Office and administrative support	15,440	28
Farming, fishing, and forestry	620	—
Construction and extractive	14,770	46
Installation, maintenance, and repair	13,000	20
Production	4,840	6
Transportation and material moving	25,630	47
Military occupations	—	57
Race or ethnic origin[c]		
White, non-Hispanic	105,090	407
Black, non-Hispanic	22,750	74
Hispanic	14,290	38
Other, multiple, and not reported	135,550	25
Nature of injury, illness		
Sprains, strains	115,970	6
Fractures	17,450	7
Cuts, lacerations, punctures	11,730	99
Bruises, contusions	26,990	—
Heat burns	2,410	5
Chemical burns	600	—
Amputations	640	—
Carpal tunnel syndrome	1,860	—
Tendonitis	630	—
Multiple injuries	15,340	229
Soreness, Pain	33,160	—
Back pain	8,760	—
All other	50,900	195

Characteristic	State and local government nonfatal cases[b]	All government fatalities
Part of body affected		
Head	18,680	126
Eye	5,530	—
Neck	4,110	12
Trunk	83,210	72
Back	47,160	11
Shoulder	19,300	—
Upper extremities	45,600	—
Finger	12,960	—
Hand, except finger	8,340	—
Wrist	9,370	—
Lower extremities	70,190	12
Knee	31,180	—
Foot, toe	9,630	—
Body systems	7,420	63
Multiple	46,070	256
All other	2,400	—
Source of injury, illness		
Chemicals, chemical products	3,250	11
Containers	16,070	—
Furniture, fixtures	10,250	—
Machinery	6,320	18
Parts and materials	10,540	21
Worker motion or position	44,600	—
Floor, ground surfaces	66,950	43
Handtools	6,290	—
Vehicles	27,890	288
Health care patient	17,440	—
All other	42,430	155
Event or exposure		
Contact with object, equipment	47,990	39
Struck by object	23,790	25
Struck against object	14,910	—
Caught in object, equipment, material	4,540	13
Fall to lower level	15,810	20
Fall on same level	49,580	20
Slips, trips	10,430	—
Overexertion	50,230	—
Overexertion in lifting	24,510	—
Repetitive motion	5,610	—
Exposed to harmful substance	12,210	30
Transportation accidents	18,550	276
Highway accident	14,490	171
Nonhighway accident, except air, rail, water	—	8
Pedestrian, nonpassenger struck by vehicle, mobile equipment	—	50
Fires, explosions	740	19
Assault, violent act	25,380	131
By person	22,970	73
By other	2,410	58
All other	41,140	7

Source: National Safety Council tabulations of U.S. Bureau of Labor Statistics data.
Note: Because of rounding and data exclusion of nonclassifiable responses, data may not sum to the totals. Dashes (—) indicate data that do not meet publication guidelines.
[a]Days away from work include those that result in days away from work with or without restricted work activity or job transfer.

[b]Data for government entities is limited to state and local governments in the national BLS Survey of Occupational Injuries and Illnesses.
[c]In the fatalities column, non-Hispanic categories include cases with Hispanic origin not reported.

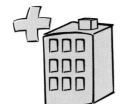

OCCUPATIONAL HEALTH

More than 35,000 new skin diseases or disorders cases were diagnosed in 2009.

Approximately 224,500 occupational illnesses were recognized or diagnosed by employers in 2009 according to the Bureau of Labor Statistics. The all industry illness data published by BLS now includes data for state and local governments in addition to the private sector. The overall incidence rate of occupational illness for all workers was 21.3 per 10,000 full-time workers. The highest overall incidence rates for all illnesses were for state and local government and manufacturing at 39.1 and 39.0 cases per 10,000 full-time workers, respectively—each more than double the private industry rate of 18.3. Workers in state and local government also had the highest incidence rates for respiratory conditions and "all other occupational illnesses." Workers in agriculture, forestry, fishing, and hunting had the highest rate for skin diseases and disorders, utilities had the highest rate for poisoning, and manufacturing had the highest rate for hearing loss.

State and local government and manufacturing accounted for more than one-quarter of all new illness cases in 2009. Skin diseases or disorders were the most common illness with 35,400 new cases, followed by hearing loss with 21,700, respiratory conditions with 21,500, and poisonings with 3,200.

The table below shows the number of occupational illnesses and the incidence rate per 10,000 full-time workers as measured by the 2009 BLS survey. To convert these to incidence rates per 100 full-time workers, which are comparable to other published BLS rates, divide the rates in the table by 100. The BLS survey records illnesses only for the year in which they are recognized or diagnosed as work-related. Because only recognized cases are included, the figures underestimate the incidence of occupational illness.

NONFATAL OCCUPATIONAL ILLNESS INCIDENCE RATES AND NUMBER OF ILLNESSES BY TYPE OF ILLNESS AND INDUSTRY SECTOR, 2009

Industry sector	All illnesses	Skin diseases, disorders	Respiratory conditions	Poisoning	Hearing loss	All other occupational illnesses
Incidence rate per 10,000 full-time workers						
All industries (including state and local government)[a]	21.3	3.4	2.0	0.3	2.1	13.5
Private sector[a]	18.3	2.9	1.6	0.2	2.2	11.5
Goods producing[a]	29.1	3.8	1.3	0.2	7.9	15.8
Agriculture, forestry, fishing & hunting[a]	24.7	7.1	2.3	0.6	1.1	13.5
Mining[b,c]	7.8	0.8	0.7	([d])	2.0	4.4
Construction	11.6	3.4	1.2	0.3	0.2	6.5
Manufacturing	39.0	4.0	1.4	0.2	12.4	21.1
Service providing	15.3	2.6	1.7	0.2	0.6	10.3
Wholesale trade	7.9	1.8	0.7	0.1	0.6	4.8
Retail trade	10.6	1.8	1.2	0.2	0.2	7.3
Transportation and warehousing	17.4	1.1	1.6	0.3	4.0	10.4
Utilities	32.6	6.7	0.4	1.2	12.0	12.2
Information	12.3	0.9	0.7	0.1	0.7	9.9
Financial activities	9.4	1.0	0.8	([d])	([d])	7.4
Professional and business services	9.2	2.2	0.7	0.3	0.5	5.6
Education and health services	32.0	5.2	3.6	0.2	0.1	22.9
Leisure and hospitality	11.9	3.1	1.1	0.3	0.1	7.3
Other services	([d])	1.9	([d])	0.2	0.2	([d])
State and local government[a]	39.1	([d])	4.6	0.8	1.5	25.9
Number of illnesses (in thousands)						
All industries (including state and local government)[a]	224.5	35.4	21.5	3.2	21.7	142.7
Private sector[a]	166.2	25.9	14.6	2.0	19.5	104.2
Goods producing[a]	57.3	7.5	2.7	0.4	15.5	31.2
Agriculture, forestry, fishing & hunting[a]	2.1	0.6	0.2	([e])	0.1	1.1
Mining[b,c]	0.6	0.1	([e])	([d])	0.1	0.3
Construction	6.8	2.0	0.7	0.2	0.1	3.8
Manufacturing	47.9	4.9	1.7	0.2	15.2	25.9
Service providing	108.9	18.4	11.9	1.6	4.0	73.0
Wholesale trade	4.5	1.0	0.4	0.1	0.3	2.7
Retail trade	12.3	2.0	1.4	0.2	0.2	8.4
Transportation and warehousing	7.0	0.4	0.7	0.1	1.6	4.2
Utilities	1.8	0.4	([e])	0.1	0.7	0.7
Information	3.2	0.2	0.2	([e])	0.2	2.6
Financial activities	6.8	0.7	0.6	([d])	([d])	5.4
Professional and business services	12.5	2.9	0.9	0.4	0.7	7.5
Education and health services	45.4	7.4	5.0	0.3	0.1	32.5
Leisure and hospitality	10.3	2.7	1.0	0.2	0.1	6.4
Other services	([d])	0.6	([d])	0.1	0.1	([d])
State and local government[a]	58.3	([d])	6.9	1.2	2.2	38.5

Source: Bureau of Labor Statistics, U.S. Department of Labor. Components may not add to totals due to rounding.
[a]*Excludes farms with less than 11 employees.*
[b]*Data for mining do not reflect the changes OSHA made to its recordkeeping requirements that went into effect Jan. 1, 2002; therefore, estimates for this industry are not comparable with estimates for other industries.*
[c]*Mining includes quarrying and oil and gas extraction.*
[d]*Data do not meet publication guidelines.*
[e]*Data too small to be displayed.*

OCCUPATIONAL

NATIONAL SAFETY COUNCIL® INJURY FACTS® 2011 EDITION

91

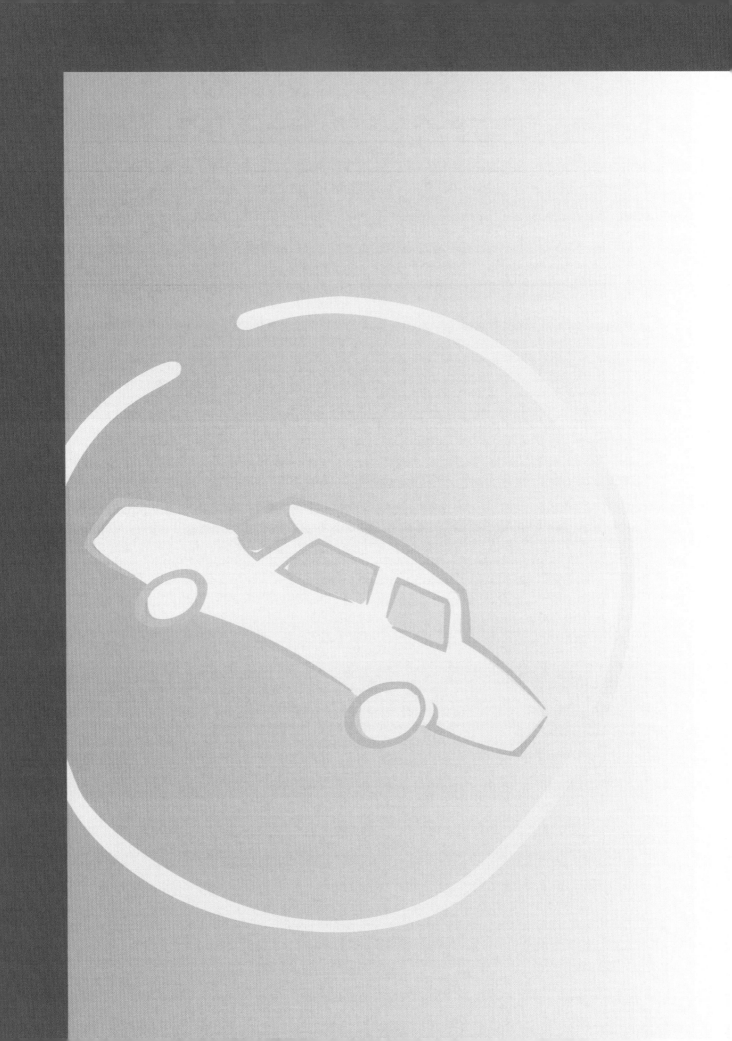

MAJOR CONTRIBUTING FACTORS TO MOTOR VEHICLE DEATHS, UNITED STATES, 2009

33,808
Police-Reported Motor Vehicle Deaths

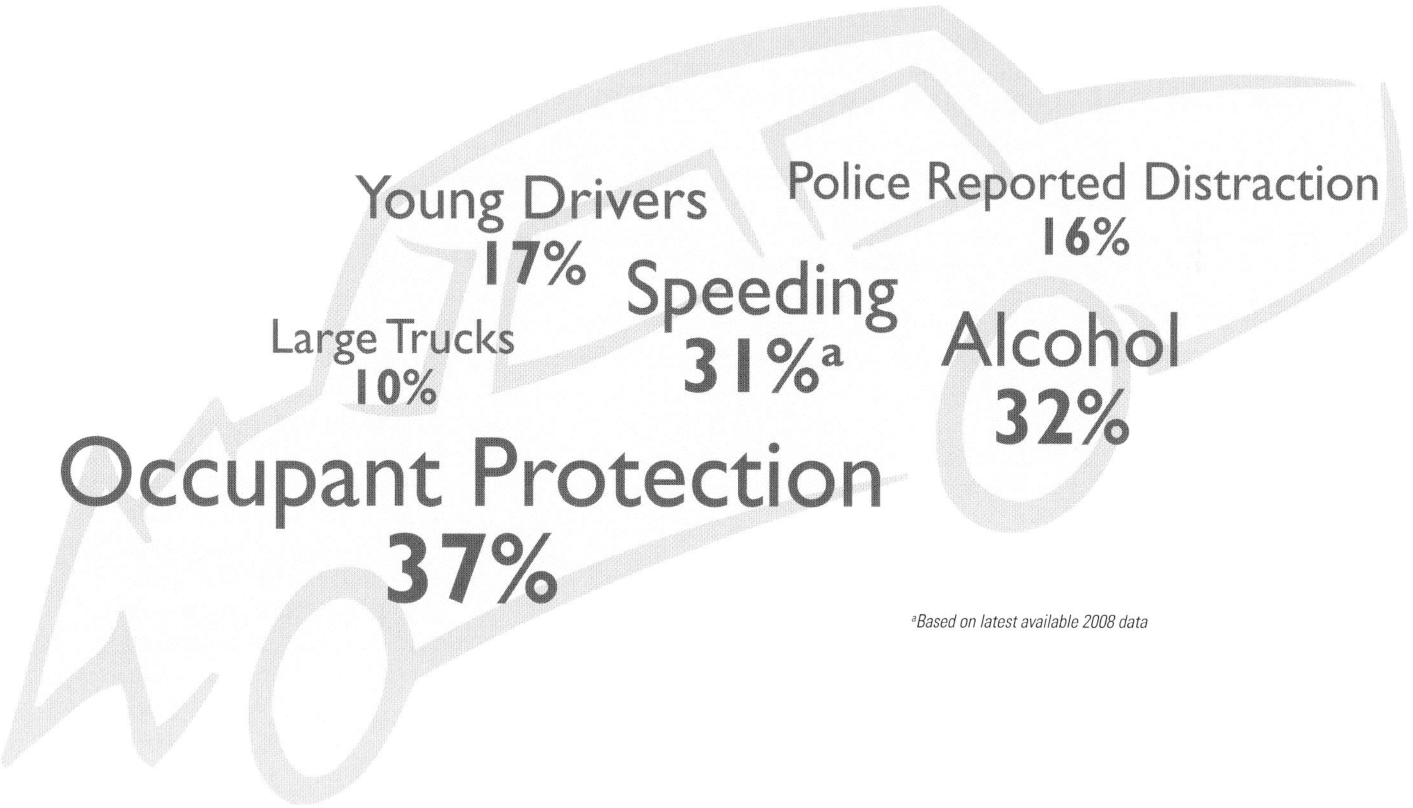

Young Drivers
17%

Police Reported Distraction
16%

Large Trucks
10%

Speeding
31%[a]

Alcohol
32%

Occupant Protection
37%

[a]Based on latest available 2008 data

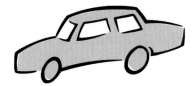

Between 1912 and 2009, motor vehicle deaths per 10,000 registered vehicles were reduced 95%, from 33 to less than 2. In 1912, there were 3,100 fatalities when the number of registered vehicles totaled only 950,000. In 2009, there were 35,900 fatalities, but registrations soared to 259 million. While mileage data were not available in 1912, the 2009 mileage death rate of 1.21 per 100,000,000 vehicle miles was down 10% from the revised 2008 rate of 1.34, and is the lowest on record.

Beginning with this edition of *Injury Facts,* the concept of medically consulted injury has been adopted to replace disabling injury as the measure of nonfatal injuries. A medically consulted injury is an injury serious enough that a medical professional was consulted. Medically consulted injuries reported in this edition are not comparable to previous disabling injury estimates. Please see the Technical Appendix for a detailed description of this change. Medically consulted injuries in motor vehicle accidents totaled 3,500,000 in 2009, and total motor vehicle costs were estimated at $244.7 billion. Costs include wage and productivity losses, medical expenses, administrative expenses, motor vehicle property damage, and employer costs.

Motor vehicle deaths decreased 10% from 2008 to 2009 following a similar 10% decrease from 2007 to 2008. Miles traveled was up less than 0.5%, the number of registered vehicles increased 1%, and the population increased 1%. As a result, the mileage death rate, registration death rate and the population death rate each were down 10% from 2008 to 2009.

Compared with 1999, 2009 motor vehicle deaths decreased by about 15%. However, mileage, registration, and population death rates were all sharply lower in 2009 compared to 1999 (see chart on next page).

The word "accident" may be used in this section as well as the word "crash." When used, "accident" has a specific meaning as defined in the *Manual on Classification of Motor Vehicle Traffic Accidents, ANSI D16.1-2007.* "Crash" is generally used by the National Highway Traffic Safety Administration to mean the same as accident, but it is not formally defined.

Deaths 35,900
Medically consulted injuries 3,500,000
Cost . . . .$244.7 billion
Motor vehicle mileage . . . . .2,979 billion
Registered vehicles in the United States 258,800,000
Licensed drivers in the United States 211,000,000
Death rate per 100,000,000 vehicle miles 1.21
Death rate per 10,000 registered vehicles 1.39
Death rate per 100,000 population 11.70

MOTOR VEHICLE ACCIDENT OUTCOMES, UNITED STATES, 2009

Severity	Deaths or injuries	Accidents or crashes	Drivers (vehicles) involved
Fatal (within 1 year)	35,900	32,700	48,000
Medically consulted injury	3,500,000	2,400,000	4,200,000
Property damage (including unreported) and nondisabling injury		8,400,000	14,200,000
Total		**10,800,000**	**18,400,000**
Fatal (within 30 days)	33,808	30,797	45,218
Injury (disabling and nondisabling)	2,217,000	1,517,000	2,684,000
Police-reported property damage		3,957,000	6,681,000
Total		**5,505,000**	**9,410,000**

Source: National Safety Council estimates (top half) and National Highway Traffic Safety Administration (bottom half, except for "Drivers (vehicles) involved," which are National Safety Council estimates).

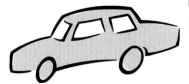

TRAVEL, DEATHS AND DEATH RATES, UNITED STATES, 1925–2009

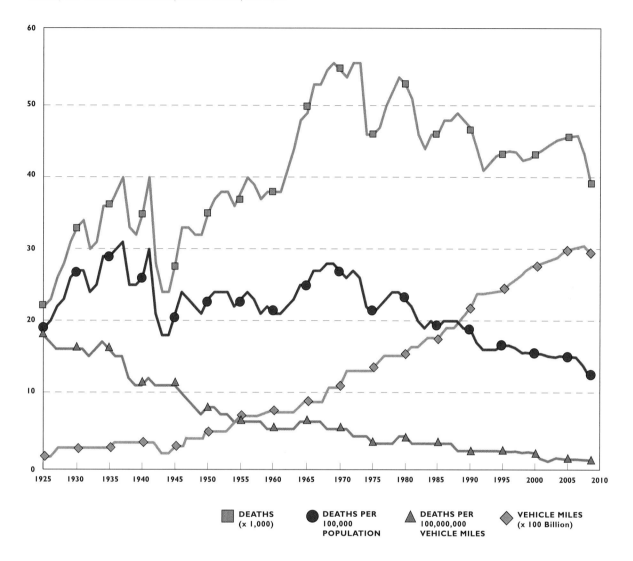

| ■ DEATHS
(x 1,000) | ● DEATHS PER
100,000
POPULATION | ▲ DEATHS PER
100,000,000
VEHICLE MILES | ◆ VEHICLE MILES
(x 100 Billion) |

DEATHS DUE TO MOTOR VEHICLE ACCIDENTS, 2009

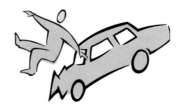

TYPE OF ACCIDENT AND AGE OF VICTIM

All motor vehicle accidents

Includes deaths involving mechanically or electrically powered highway-transport vehicles in motion (except those on rails), both on and off the highway or street.

	Total	Change from 2008	Death rate[a]
Deaths	35,900	−10%	11.7
Nonfatal injuries[b]	3,500,000		

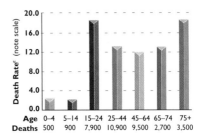

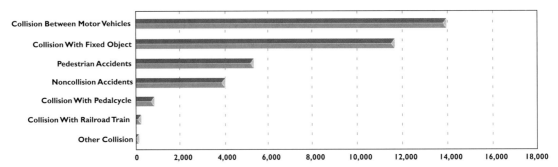

Collision between motor vehicles

Includes deaths from collisions of two or more motor vehicles. Motorized bicycles and scooters, trolley buses, and farm tractors or road machinery traveling on highways are motor vehicles.

	Total	Change from 2008	Death rate[a]
Deaths	13,900	−10%	4.5
Nonfatal injuries[b]	2,610,000		

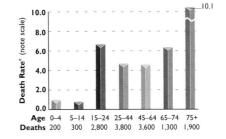

Collision with fixed object

Includes deaths from collisions in which the first harmful event is the striking of a fixed object such as a guardrail, abutment, impact attenuator, etc.

	Total	Change from 2008	Death rate[a]
Deaths	11,600	−10%	3.8
Nonfatal injuries[b]	500,000		

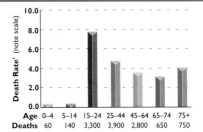

Pedestrian accidents

Includes all deaths of people struck by motor vehicles, either on or off a street or highway, regardless of the circumstances of the accident.

	Total	Change from 2008	Death rate[a]
Deaths	5,300	−7%	1.7
Nonfatal injuries[b]	120,000		

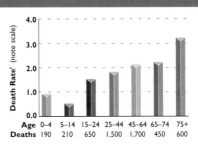

See footnotes on page 97.

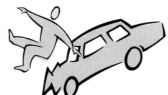

Noncollision accidents

Includes deaths from accidents in which the first injury or damage-producing event was an overturn, jackknife, or other type of noncollision.

	Total	Change from 2008	Death rate^a
Deaths	4,000	−11%	1.3
Nonfatal injuries^b	160,000		

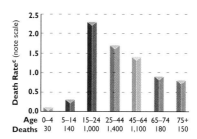

Collision with pedalcycle

Includes deaths of pedalcyclists and motor vehicle occupants from collisions between pedalcycles and motor vehicles on streets, highways, private driveways, parking lots, etc.

	Total	Change from 2008	Death rate^a
Deaths	800	−11%	0.3
Nonfatal injuries^b	100,000		

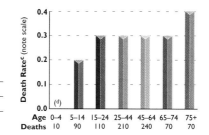

Collision with railroad train

Includes deaths from collisions of motor vehicles (moving or stalled) and railroad vehicles at public or private grade crossings. In other types of accidents, classification requires motor vehicle to be in motion.

	Total	Change from 2008	Death rate^a
Deaths	200	0%	0.1
Nonfatal injuries^b	1,000		

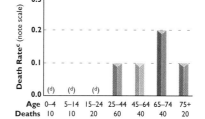

Other collision

Includes deaths from motor vehicle collisions not specified in other categories above. Most of the deaths arose out of accidents involving animals or animal-drawn vehicles.

	Total	Change from 2008	Death rate^a
Deaths	100	0%	(^d)
Nonfatal injuries^b	9,000		

Note: Procedures and benchmarks for estimating deaths by type of accident and age were changed in 1990. Estimates for 1987 and later years are not comparable to earlier years. The noncollision and fixed object categories were most affected by the changes.
^aDeaths per 100,000 population.
^bNonfatal injury is defined as medically consulted injuries and is not comparable to estimates provided in earlier editions that used the definition of disabling injury. Please see the Technical Appendix for more information regarding medically consulted injuries.
^cDeath per 100,000 population in each age group.
^dDeath rate was less than 0.05.

98

Motor vehicle crashes were the leading cause of death for people between the ages of 2 and 35 in 2007. Motor vehicle crashes also were the leading cause of unintentional injury (accidental) death for people for each single year of age from 1 to 33, for age 35, and from ages 56 to 71.

Occupant protection. Safety belt use was 85% overall in 2010, statistically unchanged from the 84% use rate in 2009. Forty-nine states and the District of Columbia have mandatory safety belt use laws in effect, with the laws in 31 states and the District of Columbia allowing standard (primary) enforcement. In 2010, safety belt use was significantly higher in states with standard (primary) enforcement (88%) than in states with secondary enforcement or no safety belt use law (76%). More than half (53%) of the passenger vehicle occupants killed in 2009 were unrestrained, and safety belt use was significantly lower among occupants 16-24 years old than for other age groups. Reported helmet use rates for fatally injured motorcyclists in 2009 were 69% for operators and 55% for passengers, compared with the corresponding rates of 64% and 54%, respectively, in 2008.

Alcohol. From 2008 to 2009, traffic fatalities in alcohol-impaired crashes as a percentage of total traffic fatalities increased by 0.8% to 32.1%. Overall, 10,839 people were killed in alcohol-impaired crashes in 2009, a reduction of more than 7% from 2008. Thirty-three states showed decreases in the number of alcohol-impaired driving fatalities from 2008 to 2009. All states and the District of Columbia have age-21 drinking laws and have created a threshold by law, making it illegal to drive while alcohol impaired.

Speeding. Excessive speed was a factor in 31% of all traffic fatalities in 2008, down from 32% in 2007. The total number of fatal crashes attributed to speeding declined by 10% from 2007 to 2008, but the percentage of speeding-related fatalities among overall fatalities remained essentially unchanged. It has been estimated that speeding-related crashes cost the nation more than $40 billion annually. A recent study using data from states that record "driving too fast for conditions" and "in excess of posted speed limit" separately found that more severe crashes are more often associated with exceeding the posted speed limit, while less severe crashes are associated with driving too fast for conditions.

Distracted driving. Recent epidemiological studies have found cell phone use while driving is associated with a slightly more than fourfold increase in crash risk. The results also showed no significant difference between handheld and hands-free phone use. A review of 33 cell phone driving studies concluded cell phone use while driving increases driver reaction time by about 0.25 second. The National Safety Council estimates 23% of all traffic crashes are associated with drivers using cell phones and texting (21% cell phones and 2% texting). Although the research cited above indicates there is no safety advantage of hands-free over handheld cell phone use, the 14 states that have implemented bans impacting all drivers have focused on handheld bans.

Large trucks. In 2009, 3,380 fatalities resulted from traffic crashes involving a large truck (gross vehicle weight rating greater than 10,000 pounds), a 20% decline from 4,245 in 2008. Although the majority of these deaths (75%) were occupants of vehicles other than the large truck, a decline in the number of fatalities among other vehicle occupants was primarily responsible for the overall decline in deaths from crashes involving a large truck. Large trucks were more likely to be involved in a multiple-vehicle fatal crash than passenger vehicles – 82% versus 58%, respectively, in 2008.

Motorcycles. Fatalities and nonfatal injuries among motorcycle riders and passengers each increased 80% between 1999 and 2009, from 2,483 to 4,462 and from 50,000 to 90,000, respectively. However, the number of motorcycle fatalities in 2009 was 16% less than in 2008 and injuries decreased 6.3%. The latest available mileage data show motorcycle travel was up 28% to 13.6 billion miles in 2007, resulting in a 61% increase in the death rate between 1999 and 2007, from 23.46 to 37.86 deaths per 100 million miles traveled. The mileage death rate for motorcyclists was 37 times greater than for passenger car occupants in 2007.

Young drivers. There were 5,623 fatalities in crashes involving young drivers ages 15-20 in 2009, a 13% decrease from 2008 and the eighth consecutive yearly decline. Motor vehicle crashes, however, remain the No. 1 cause of death for U.S. teens. Fatalities of young drivers account for more than two-fifths of the overall fatalities associated with young driver crashes; the remainder includes the passengers of young drivers, occupants of other vehicles, and nonoccupants. Periods of decreasing young driver-related fatalities between 1988 and 1992 and beginning in 2003 to the present appear to coincide with the implementation of age-21 drinking laws and improvements in Graduated Driver Licensing laws, respectively.

Pedestrians. There were about 5,300 pedestrian deaths and 120,000 medically consulted injuries in motor vehicle accidents in 2009. The majority (about 60%) of pedestrian deaths and injuries occurred when pedestrians improperly crossed roadways or intersections or darted/ran into streets. Pedestrians age 15 and older were more likely to cross improperly, while those in younger age groups were more likely to dart/run into the roadway.

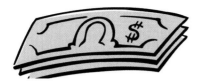

There are two methods commonly used to measure the costs of motor vehicle crashes. One is the *economic cost* framework and the other is the *comprehensive cost* framework.

Economic costs may be used by a community or state to estimate the economic impact of motor vehicle crashes that occurred within its jurisdiction in a given time period. It is a measure of the productivity lost and expenses incurred because of the crashes. Economic costs, however, should not be used for cost-benefit analysis because they do not reflect what society is willing to pay to prevent a statistical fatality or injury.

There are five economic cost components: (a) wage and productivity losses, which include wages, fringe benefits, household production, and travel delay; (b) medical expenses, including emergency service costs; (c) administrative expenses, which include the administrative cost of private and public insurance plus police and legal costs; (d) motor vehicle damage, including the value of damage to property; and (e) uninsured employer costs for crashes involving workers.

The information below shows the average economic costs in 2009 per death (*not* per fatal crash), per injury (*not* per injury crash), and per property damage crash.

ECONOMIC COSTS, 2009

Death **$1,290,000**

Nonfatal disabling injury **$68,100**

    Incapacitating injury[a] $67,800

    Non-incapacitating evident injury[a] $21,900

    Possible injury[a] $12,400

Property damage crash (including minor injuries) **$8,200**

Comprehensive costs include not only the economic cost components, but also a measure of the value of lost quality of life associated with the deaths and injuries; that is, what society is willing to pay to prevent them. The values of lost quality of life were obtained through empirical studies of what people actually pay to reduce their safety and health risks, such as through the purchase of airbags or smoke detectors. Comprehensive

costs should be used for cost-benefit analysis, but because the lost quality of life represents only a dollar equivalence of intangible qualities, they do not represent real economic losses and should not be used to determine the economic impact of past crashes.

The information below shows the average comprehensive costs in 2009 on a per person basis.

COMPREHENSIVE COSTS, 2009

Death **$4,300,000**

    Incapacitating injury[a] $216,800

    Non-incapacitating evident injury[a] $55,300

    Possible injury[a] $26,300

No injury **$2,400**

Source: National Safety Council estimates (see the Technical Appendix) and Children's Safety Network Economics and Insurance Resource Center, Pacific Institute for Research and Evaluation.
Note: The National Safety Council's cost-estimating procedures were extensively revised for the 1993 edition and additional revisions were made for the 2005-2006 edition. The costs are not comparable to those of prior years.
[a]Manual on Classification of Motor Vehicle Traffic Accidents, ANSI D16.1-2007 *(7th ed.). (2007). Itasca, IL: National Safety Council.*

STATE LAWS

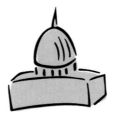

No state has yet passed a total ban on cell phone use while driving, while 14 have bans on handheld devices. Mandatory breath alcohol ignition interlock device laws are in effect in 12 states for first-time driving under the influence convictions. Mandatory safety belt use laws are in effect in 49 states plus the District of Columbia (D.C.), of which 24 states and D.C. have primary enforcement for all seating positions. Graduated Diver Licensing is in effect in some form in nearly all states and D.C., yet relatively few have optimum laws. Please see pages 114-115 for further details regarding young driver issues.

STATE LAWS

State	Distracted driving laws			Alcohol law	Mandatory safety belt use law		Graduated Licensing Laws				
	Total cell phone ban	Total text messaging ban	Additional novice driver restriction[b]	Alcohol ignition interlock device[c]	Enforcement	Seating positions covered by law	Minimum instructional permit period[g]	Minimum hours of supervised driving[h]	No passengers under 20	10 p.m. or earlier night-time driving restrictions	Unrestricted license minimum age[i]
Alabama	no	no	cell phone & texting	no	primary	front	6 mo.	none	no	no	17 yrs.
Alaska	no	yes	no	yes	primary	all	6 mo.	40/10	yes	no	16 yrs, 6 mo.
Arizona	no	no	no	yes	secondary	front[f]	6 mo.	none	no	no	16 yrs, 6 mo.
Arkansas	no	yes	cell phone	yes	primary	front	6 mo.	none	no	no	18 yrs.
California	no[a]	yes	cell phone	no	primary	all	6 mo.	50/10	yes	no	17 yrs.
Colorado	no	yes	cell phone	yes	secondary	front	12 mo.	50/10	yes	no	17 yrs.
Connecticut	no[a]	yes	cell phone	no	primary	front	4 mo.	40/0	yes	no	17 yrs, 4 mo.
Delaware	no[a]	yes	cell phone	yes[d]	primary	all	6 mo.	50/10	no	yes	17 yrs.
Dist. of Columbia	no[a]	yes	cell phone	no	primary	all	6 mo.	40/10	yes	no	18 yrs.
Florida	no	no	no	yes[d]	primary	front[f]	12 mo.	50/10	no	no	18 yrs.
Georgia	no	yes	cell phone	no	primary	front[f]	12 mo.	40/6	yes	no	18 yrs.
Hawaii	no	no	no	yes	primary	front[f]	6 mo.	50/10	no	no	17 yrs.
Idaho	no	no	no	no	secondary	all	6 mo.	50/10	no	yes	16 yrs.
Illinois	no[a]	yes	cell phone	yes	primary	front[f]	9 mo.	50/10	no	no	18 yrs.
Indiana	no	no	cell phone & texting	no	primary	all	6 mo.	50/10	yes	yes	18 yrs.
Iowa	no	yes	cell phone	no	primary	front	6 mo.	20/2	no	no	17 yrs.
Kansas	no	yes	cell phone	yes[d]	primary	all	12 mo.	50/10	no	yes	16 yrs, 6 mo.
Kentucky	no	yes	cell phone	no	primary	all	6 mo.	60/10	no	no	17 yrs.
Louisiana	no	yes	cell phone	yes	primary	all	6 mo.	50/15	no	no	17 yrs.
Maine	no	no	cell phone & texting	no	primary	all	6 mo.	35/5	yes	no	16 yrs, 6 mo.
Maryland	no[a]	yes	cell phone	no	primary	front	9 mo.	60/10	no	no	18 yrs.
Massachusetts	no	yes	cell phone	yes[e]	secondary	all	6 mo.	40/–	no	no	18 yrs.
Michigan	no[a]	yes	no	no	primary	front	6 mo.	50/10	no	no	17 yrs.
Minnesota	no	yes	cell phone	no	primary	all	6 mo.	30/10	no	no	17 yrs.
Mississippi	no	no	texting	no	primary	front	12 mo.	none	no	no	16 yrs, 6 mo.
Missouri	no	no	texting	yes[e]	secondary	front	6 mo.	40/10	no	no	17 yrs, 11 mo.
Montana	no	no	no	yes[e]	secondary	all	6 mo.	50/10	no	no	16 yrs.
Nebraska	no	yes	cell phone	yes	secondary	front	6 mo.	none	no	no	17 yrs.
Nevada	no	no	no	no	secondary	all	6 mo.	50/10	no	yes	18 yrs.
New Hampshire	no	yes	no	yes[e]	no law	no law	none	40/10	no	no	17 yrs, 1 mo.
New Jersey	no[a]	yes	cell phone	yes[d,e]	primary	all	6 mo.	none	no	no	18 yrs.
New Mexico	no	no	no	yes	primary	all	6 mo.	50/10	no	no	16 yrs, 6 mo.
New York	no[a]	yes	no	yes	primary	front	6 mo.	50/15	no	yes	17 yrs.
North Carolina	no	yes	cell phone	yes[d,e]	primary	all	12 mo.	none	no	yes	16 yrs, 6 mo.
North Dakota	no[a]	no	no	no	secondary	front	6 mo.	none	no	no	16 yrs.
Ohio	no	no	no	no	secondary	front[f]	6 mo.	50/10	no	no	18 yrs.
Oklahoma	no	no	handheld & texting	yes[e]	primary	front	6 mo.	50/10	no	yes	16 yrs, 6 mo.
Oregon	no[a]	yes	cell phone	yes[e]	primary	all	6 mo.	50/–	yes	no	17 yrs.
Pennsylvania	no[a]	no	no	no	secondary	front[f]	6 mo.	50/–	no	no	17 yrs.
Rhode Island	no	yes	cell phone	no	secondary	all	6 mo.	50/10	no	no	17 yrs, 6 mo.
South Carolina	no	no	no	yes[e]	primary	all	6 mo.	40/10	no	yes	16 yrs, 6 mo.
South Dakota	no	no	no	no	secondary	front	3 mo.	none	no	yes	16 yrs.
Tennessee	no	yes	cell phone	no	primary	front	6 mo.	50/10	no	no	17 yrs.
Texas	no	no	cell phone & texting	yes[e]	primary	all	6 mo.	20/10	no	no	17 yrs.
Utah	no[a]	yes	no	yes	secondary	all	6 mo.	40/10	yes	no	17 yrs.
Vermont	no	yes	cell phone	no	secondary	all	12 mo.	40/10	yes	no	16 yrs, 6 mo.
Virginia	no	yes	cell phone	yes[d]	secondary	front	9 mo.	45/15	no	no	18 yrs.
Washington	no[a]	yes	cell phone	yes	primary	all	6 mo.	50/10	yes	no	17 yrs.
West Virginia	no	no	cell phone & texting	yes[d]	secondary	front[f]	6 mo.	none	yes	yes	17 yrs.
Wisconsin	no	yes	no	yes[d]	primary	all	6 mo.	30/10	no	no	16 yrs, 9 mo.
Wyoming	no	yes	no	yes[d]	secondary	all	10 days	50/10	no	no	16 yrs, 6 mo.

Source: Governors Highway Safety Association data retrieved from www.ghsa.org/; Insurance Institute for Highway Safety data retrieved from www.iihs.org/; Mothers Against Drunk Driving data retrieved from www.madd.org/. All data retrieved on July 29, 2010.
[a] Statewide handheld ban.
[b] Restrictions specific to novice drivers in addition to any other all-driver ban.
[c] Instuments designed to prevent drivers from starting their cars when breath alcohol content is at or above a set point.
[d] Mandatory with a conviction for a BAC of at least 0.15 versus the lower limit of 0.08 found in other mandatory states.
[e] Mandatory with repeat convictions or upon reinstatement.
[f] Required for certain ages at all seating positions.
[g] Minimum instructional periods often include time spent in driver's education classes.
[h] Figures shown as follows: Total hours/Nighttime hours. For example, 25/5 means 25 hours of supervised driving, 5 of which must be at night. When states (AL, AZ, CT, NE, OR, WV) have lower requirements if drivers education is taken, the lower requirement is reflected in the table.
[i] Minimum age to obtain unrestricted license provided driver is crash and violation free. Alcohol restrictions still apply at least until 21.

Safety belt use was 85% overall in 2010, statistically unchanged from the 84% use rate in 2009 and much higher than the 71% use rate in 2000. These results are from the National Occupant Protection Use Survey, conducted annually by the National Highway Traffic Safety Administration, which includes the observation of drivers and right-front passengers of passenger vehicles with no commercial or governmental markings.

A significant increase in safety belt use for occupants traveling on expressways was observed from 2009 to 2010, with the use rate increasing from 89% to 91%. Other significant increases in safety belt use observed during this period were among occupants traveling in moderately dense traffic (83% to 92%), in rural areas (81% to 83%), during weekdays (83% to 85%), and during weekday rush hours (84% to 86%).

In 2010, safety belt use was significantly higher for drivers (86%) than right-front passengers (83%), for occupants in states with primary enforcement laws (88%) than those with secondary enforcement laws or no safety belt use law (76%), for occupants traveling on expressways (91%) than on surface streets (82%), those traveling in fast traffic (88%) rather than medium (85%) or slow (80%) traffic, and people traveling in moderately dense traffic (92%) rather than heavy (90%) or light (85%) traffic.

Results from the NOPUS Controlled Intersection Study show that in 2009 safety belt use continued to be lower among occupants 16-24 years old than other age groups, while use among occupants age 70 and older was higher than other age groups. Safety belt use also continued to be lower among males (81%) than females (87%). Although black occupants showed a significant increase in safety belt use from 75% to 79% from 2008 to 2009, their use rate continued to be lower than occupants of other race groups. Overall, drivers with no passengers were less likely to use safety belts (83%) in 2009 than those with at least one passenger (87%). Similarly, drivers with no passengers were less likely to use safety belts than drivers with young passengers less than 8 years old (88%), passengers 8 and older (87%), or a mixture of the two age groups (90%). Drivers ages 16-24 were less likely to wear safety belts

(80%) when all passengers were in the same age group than when driving alone or with at least one passenger not in their age group.

Rear-safety belt use was 70% in 2009, statistically unchanged from 74% in 2008. In the 21 states and District of Columbia that required safety belt use in all seating positions, rear-safety belt use was significantly higher at 78% compared to 64% in states that required only front seat use.

Child restraint use. Restraint use by child passengers less than 8 was 88% in 2009, statistically unchanged from 87% in 2008. In 2009, 99% of infants, 99% of children 1-3 years old, and 90% of children ages 4-7 rode in the rear seat. Child passengers in the Midwest showed a significant 5 percentage point increase in safety belt use from 2008 to 2009. Safety belt use by the driver strongly influences the restraint status of child passengers. When the driver was belted, 91% of child passengers younger than 8 were restrained, compared to only 66% of children when the driver was unbelted. By type of vehicle, child restraint use was highest in vans and SUVs (93%), somewhat lower in passenger cars (84%), and lowest in pickup trucks (80%). Child passengers in vans and SUVs showed a significant 3 percentage point increase in safety belt use from 2008 to 2009.

Children 4-7 years old should be restrained in a front-facing safety seat or booster seat, depending on the child's height and weight. The National Survey of the Use of Booster Seats found booster seat use in 2009 for children 4-7 years old was 41%, statistically unchanged from the 2008 rate of 43%. However, the survey also found as many as 45% of children in this age group were not properly restrained (32% in safety belts and 13% unrestrained) in 2009. The 2009 NSUBS also found restraint use among children ages 1-3 increased from 92% to 96% from 2008 to 2009, while restraint use rate for children younger than 13 remained unchanged at 89%.

Source: Pickrell, T. M., and Ye, T. J. (2010). Seat belt use in 2010 – overall results. Traffic Safety Facts Research Note, DOT HS 811 378. Washington, DC: National Highway Traffic Safety Administration.
Pickrell, T. M., and Ye, T. J. (2010). Occupant Restraint Use in 2009 – Results from the National Occupant Protection Use Survey Controlled Intersection Study (DOT HS 811 414). Washington, DC: National Highway Traffic Safety Administration.
Pickrell, T. M., and Ye, T. J. (2010). The 2009 National Survey of the Use of Booster Seats (DOT HS 811 377. Washington, DC: National Highway Traffic Safety Administration.

SEAT BELT USE, UNITED STATES, 2000–2010

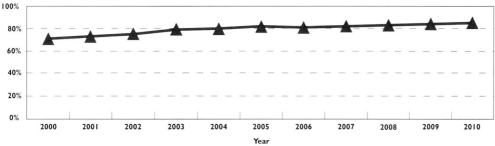

Source: NHTSA, NOPUS.

OCCUPANT PROTECTION

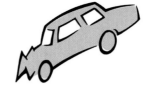

Safety belts

- When used, lap/shoulder safety belts reduce the risk of fatal injury to front seat passenger car occupants by 45% and reduce the risk of moderate-to-critical injury by 50%.

- For light truck occupants, safety belts reduce the risk of fatal injury by 60% and moderate-to-critical injury by 65%.

- Forty-nine states and the District of Columbia have mandatory safety belt use laws in effect, the only exception being New Hampshire. Eighteen of the states with safety belt use laws in effect in 2009 specified secondary enforcement (i.e., police officers are permitted to write a citation only after a vehicle is stopped for some other traffic infraction). Thirty-one states and the District of Columbia had laws that allowed primary enforcement, enabling officers to stop vehicles and write citations whenever they observe violations of the safety belt law. (see page 100 for additional information on state laws.)

- Safety belts saved an estimated 12,713 lives in 2009 among passenger vehicle occupants over 4 years old. An additional 3,688 lives could have been saved in 2009 if all passenger vehicle occupants over age 4 wore safety belts. From 1975 through 2009, an estimated 267,890 lives were saved by safety belts.

- More than half (53%) of the passenger vehicle occupants killed in 2009 were unrestrained (see table below). Nearly two-thirds (62%) of those killed during the night were unrestrained, compared to 44% during the day.

PASSENGER VEHICLE OCCUPANT FATALITIES BY RESTRAINT USE AND TIME OF DAY, UNITED STATES, 2008-2009

Type	2008		2009		Change	Percent change
	Number	Percent	Number	Percent		
Fatalities	25,462	100	23,382	100	-2,080	-8.2
Restraint Used	11,527	45	10,950	47	-577	-5.0
Restraint Not Used	13,935	55	12,432	53	-1,503	-11
Day	12,530	49	11,609	50	-921	-7.4
Restraint Used	6,868	55	6,488	56	-380	-5.5
Restraint Not Used	5,662	45	5,121	44	-541	-9.6
Night	12,733	50	11,593	50	-1,140	-9.0
Restraint Used	4,564	36	4,370	38	-194	-4.3
Restraint Not Used	8,169	64	7,223	62	-946	-12

Source: National Center for Statistics and Analysis. (2010). Traffic Safety Facts Research Note—Highlights of 2009 Motor Vehicle Crashes (DOT HS 811 363) *Washington, DC: National Highway Traffic Safety Administration*

Air bags

- Air bags, combined with lap/shoulder safety belts, offer the best available protection for passenger vehicle occupants. Recent analyses indicate a fatality-reducing effectiveness for air bags of 14% when no safety belt was used and 11% when a safety belt was used in conjunction with air bags.

- Lap/shoulder belts should always be used, even in a vehicle with an air bag. Air bags are a supplemental form of protection and most are designed to deploy only in moderate-to-severe frontal crashes.

- Children in rear-facing child seats should not be placed in the front seat of vehicles equipped with passenger-side air bags. The impact of the deploying air bag could result in injury to the child.

- An estimated 2,381 lives were saved by air bags in 2009 and a total of 29,872 lives were saved from 1987 through 2009.

- Beginning September 1997, all new passenger cars wer required to have driver and passenger side air bags. In 1998, the same requirement went into effect for light trucks.

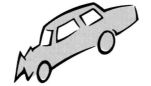

OCCUPANT PROTECTION

Child restraints

- Child restraints saved an estimated 309 lives in 2009 among children under the age of 5. An additional 63 lives of such children could have been saved if all had used child safety seats.

- All states and the District of Columbia have had child restraint use laws in effect since 1985.

- Research has shown that child safety seats reduce fatal injury in passenger cars by 71% for infants (less than 1 year old), and by 54% for toddlers (1-4 years old).

For infants and toddlers in light trucks, the corresponding reductions are 58% and 59%, respectively.

- In 2009, there were 322 occupant fatalities among children age 4 and younger. Of the 298 fatalities among children less than 4 years of age for which restraint use was known, 92 (31%) were totally unrestrained.

- An estimated 9,310 lives have been saved by child restraints from 1975 through 2009.

ESTIMATED NUMBER OF LIVES SAVED BY RESTRAINT SYSTEMS, 1975-2009

Restraint type	1975-2001	2002	2003	2004	2005	2006	2007	2008	2009
Safety belts	150,589	14,264	15,095	15,548	15,688	15,458	15,223	13,312	12,713
Child restraints	6,191	383	447	455	424	427	388	286	309
Air bags	9,415	2,324	2,519	2,660	2,752	2,824	2,800	2,557	2,381

Source: 1975-2003 data: National Center for Statistics and Analysis. (2009). Traffic Safety Facts 2008 Data—Occupant Protection (DOT HS 811 160). Washington, DC: National Highway Traffic Safety Administration; 2004–2007 data: National Center for Statistics and Analysis. (June 2009). Traffic Safety Facts Crash Stats—Lives Saved in 2008 by Restraint Use and Minimum Drinking Age Laws (DOT HS 811 153). Washington, DC: National Highway Traffic Safety Administration; 2008-2009 data: National Center for Statistics and Analysis. (September 2010). Traffic Safety Facts Crash Stats—Lives Saved in 2009 by Restraint Use and Minimum Drinking Age Laws (DOT HS 811 383). Washington, DC: National Highway Safety Traffic Administration

Motorcycle helmets

- Motorcycle helmets are estimated to be 37% effective in preventing fatal injuries to motorcycle riders and 41% effective for motorcylce passengers.

- It is estimated that motorcycle helmets saved the lives of 1,483 motorcyclists in 2009. An additional 732 lives could have been saved in 2009 if all motorcyclists had worn helmets.

- Reported helmet use rates for fatally injured motorcyclists in 2009 were 69% for operators and 55% for passengers, compared with the corresponding rates of 64% and 54%, respectively, in 2008.

- In 2009, 20 states, the District of Columbia, and Puerto Rico required helmet use by all motorcycle

operators and passengers. Helmet use in these states increased significantly, from 78% to 86% in 2009 and remains higher than in states that either required only a subset of motorcyclists to use helmets (such as those under 18), or had no helmet requirement.

- According to the National Occupant Protection Use Survey, use of DOT-compliant helmets was at 67% in 2009, an increase from the 63% use rate observed in 2008.

Source: National Center for Statistics and Analysis. (September 2010). Traffic Safety Facts Crash Stats–Lives Saved in 2009 by Restraint Use and Minimum Drinking Age Laws (DOT HS 811 383). Washington. DC: National Highway Traffic Safety Administration, National Center for Statistics and Analysis. (2008). Traffic Safety Facts 2009 Data–Children (DOT HS 811 387); Traffic Safety Facts Research Note--motorcycle Helmet Use in 2009–Overall Results (DOT HS 811 254). Washington, DC: National Highway Traffic Safety Administration.

ALCOHOL

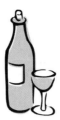

According to studies conducted by the National Highway Traffic Safety Administration, about 10,839 people were killed in alcohol-impaired crashes in 2009, a decline of more than 7% from the 11,711 fatalities in 2008. Alcohol-impaired driving crashes are crashes that involve at least one driver or motorcycle operator with a blood alcohol concentration of 0.08 grams per deciliter or greater. The following data summarizes the extent of alcohol involvement in motor vehicle crashes involving at least one alcohol-impaired driver or MC operator:

- The cost of alcohol-related motor vehicle crashes is estimated by the National Safety Council to be $28.8 billion in 2009.

- Traffic fatalities in alcohol-impaired driving crashes as a percentage of total traffic fatalities increased by 0.8% to 32.1% from 2008 to 2009 and by 2.0% from 1999 to 2009. (See corresponding chart.) In 1999, alcohol-impaired driving fatalities accounted for 30.1% of all traffic deaths.

- The 10,839 fatalities in alcohol-impaired driving crashes in 2009 represent an average of one alcohol-impaired driving fatality every 48 minutes.

- In 2009, about 39% of fatalities associated with alcohol-imparied driving crashes were occupants of passenger cars, 21% were occupants of light trucks/pickups, 15% were occupants of SUVs, 12% were motorcycle operators, 3% were occupants of vans, and fewer than 1% were occupants of large trucks. (See table for further details).

- Since July 1988, all states and the District of Columbia have had a minimum legal drinking age of 21. The impact these laws had on alcohol-related fatalities was dramatic. Among fatally injured drivers ages 16 to 20, the percentage with positive BACs declined from 61% in 1982 to 31% in 1995, a bigger decline than for older age groups. These declines occurred among the ages directly affected by raising the drinking age (ages 18-20) and among young teenagers not directly affected (ages 16-17).

- In 2009, while drivers ages 25-34 constituted 19% of all drivers involved in fatal crashes, they were over-represented among the drivers with BACs of 0.08 g/dL or greater, comprising 27% of such drivers involved in fatal crashes. Drivers ages 21-24 were similarly over-represnted, accounting for 10% of

PERCENT OF ALCOHOL-IMPAIRED DRIVING FATALITIES, UNITED STATES, 1999–2009

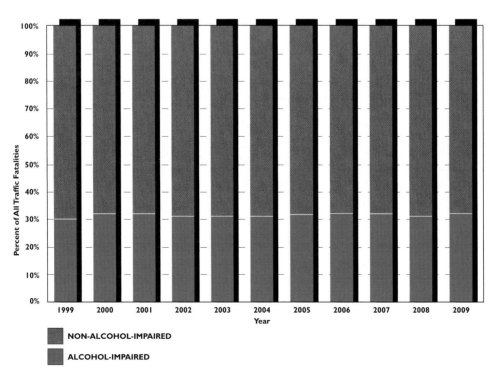

■ NON-ALCOHOL-IMPAIRED

■ ALCOHOL-IMPAIRED

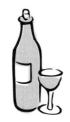

ALCOHOL (CONT.)

ALCOHOL-IMPAIRED DRIVING FATALITIES BY VEHICLE TYPE, UNITED STATES, 2008 AND 2009

	2008	2009	Change	% change
Total	11,711	10,839	-872	-7.4%
Passenger Car	4,679	4,242	-437	-9.3%
Light Truck – Van	337	296	-41	-12%
Light Truck – SUV	1,651	1,576	-75	-4.5%
Light Truck – Pickup	2,316	2,260	-56	-2.4%
Motorcycles	1,561	1,314	-247	-16%
Large Trucks	63	54	-9	-14%

Source:
National Center for Statistics and Analysis (2010). Traffic Safety Facts 2009 Data: Alcohol-Impaired Driving. Washington D.C.: National Highway Traffic Administration.
National Center for Statistics and Analysis. (2010). Research Note: Highlights of 2009 Motor Vehicle Crashes. Washington DC: National Highway Traffic Safety Administration.
McCartt , A.T., Hellinga, L.A., and Kirley, B.B. (2010). The effect of minimum legal drinking age 21 laws on alcohol-related driving in the United States. Journal of Safety Research. (41) 173-181.

drivers in fatal crashes and 16% of those with BACs of 0.08 g/dL or greater. The 35-44 age group also was slightly over-represented, making up 17% of drivers in fatal crashes and 20% of those with BACs of 0.08 g/dL or greater.

- Males continue to comprise the majority (82% in 2009) of all drivers involved in fatal crashes with a BAC of 0.08 g/dL or greater. Both male and female drivers showed a 2% increase in the proportion of drivers involved in fatal crashes who were alcohol-

impaired from 1999 to 2009.

- Thirty-three states showed decreases in the number of alcohol-impaired driving fatalities in 2009, as compared to 2008 (see corresponding chart).

- All states and the District of Columbia now have age-21 drinking laws. In 2009, all states plus the District of Columbia, by law, created a threshold making it illegal to drive with a BAC of 0.08 g/dL or higher.

PERCENT CHANGE IN NUMBER OF ALCOHOL-IMPAIRED DRIVING FATALITIES, BY STATE, 2008–2009

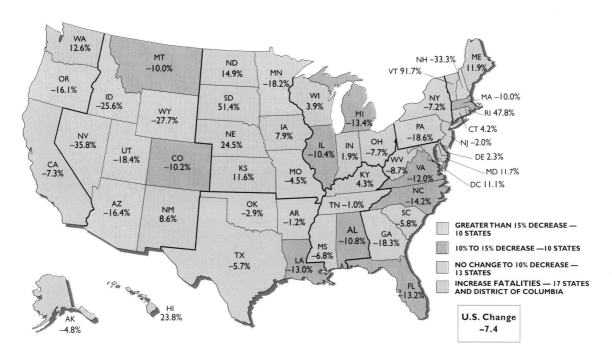

TYPE OF MOTOR VEHICLE ACCIDENT

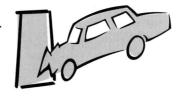

Although motor vehicle deaths occur more often in collisions between motor vehicles than any other type of accident, this type represents only about 39% of the total. Collisions between a motor vehicle and a fixed object were the next most common type, with about 32% of the deaths, followed by pedestrian accidents and noncollisions (rollovers, etc.).

While collisions between motor vehicles accounted for less than half of motor vehicle fatalities, this accident type represented 75% of injuries, 67% of injury accidents, and 70% of all accidents. Single-vehicle accidents involving collisions with fixed objects, pedestrians, and noncollisions, on the other hand,

accounted for a greater proportion of fatalities and fatal accidents compared with less serious accidents. These three accident types made up 58% of both fatalities and fatal accidents, but only 29% or less of injuries, injury accidents, or all accidents.

Of collisions between motor vehicles, angle collisions cause the greatest number of deaths, about 6,700 in 2009 and the greatest number of nonfatal injuries as well as fatal and injury accidents. The table below shows the estimated number of deaths, injuries, fatal accidents, injury accidents, and all accidents for various types of motor vehicle accidents.

MOTOR VEHICLE DEATHS AND INJURIES AND NUMBER OF ACCIDENTS BY TYPE OF ACCIDENT, 2009

Type of accident	Deaths	Nonfatal injuries[a]	Fatal accidents	Injury accidents	All accidents
Total	**35,900**	**3,500,000**	**32,700**	**2,400,000**	**10,800,000**
Collision with—					
Pedestrian	5,300	120,000	3,600	90,000	110,000
Other motor vehicle	13,900	2,610,000	12,700	1,620,000	7,580,000
Angle collision	*6,700*	*1,203,000*	*6,800*	*715,000*	*2,900,000*
Head-on collision	*4,000*	*189,000*	*3,500*	*97,000*	*260,000*
Rear-end collision	*2,100*	*1,078,000*	*1,600*	*716,000*	*3,540,000*
Sideswipe and other two-vehicle collisions	*1,100*	*140,000*	*800*	*92,000*	*880,000*
Railroad train	200	1,000	200	1,000	2,000
Pedalcycle	800	100,000	800	85,000	108,000
Animal, animal-drawn vehicle	100	9,000	100	9,000	550,000
Fixed or other object	11,600	500,000	11,400	465,000	2,150,000
Noncollision	**4,000**	**160,000**	**3,900**	**130,000**	**300,000**

Source: National Safety Council estimates based on data from the National Highway Traffic Safety Administration Fatality Analysis Reporting System and General Estimates System. Procedures for estimating the number of accidents by type were changed for the 1998 edition and are not comparable to estimates in previous editions (see Technical Appendix).
[a] Nonfatal injury is defined as medically consulted injuries and is not comparable to estimates provided in earlier editions that used the definition of disabling injury. Please see the Technical Appendix for more information regarding medically consulted injuries.

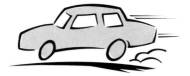

Speeding is one of the major factors contributing to the occurrence of deaths, injuries, and property damage related to motor vehicle crashes. The role of speeding in crash causation can be described in terms of its effect on the driver, vehicle, and road. Excessive-speed driving reduces the amount of time the driver has to react in a dangerous situation to avoid a crash. Speeding increases vehicle stopping distance and reduces the ability of road safety structures such as guardrails, impact attenuators, crash cushions, median dividers, and concrete barriers to protect vehicle occupants in a crash.

The National Highway Traffic Safety Administration estimates that speeding-related crashes[a] cost the nation $40.4 billion in 2000, or 18% of the entire cost of motor vehicle crashes in the United States. This economic loss is equivalent to $110.7 million per day or $4.6 million per hour.

Speeding was a factor in 31% of all traffic fatalities in 2008, killing an average of 32 people per day for a total of 11,674 speeding-related fatalities. The total number of fatal motor vehicle crashes attributable to speeding has not changed appreciably over the last decade, with more than 10,000 occurring every year.

Speeding, as typically reported by NHTSA, combines both "driving too fast for conditions" and "in excess of posted speed limit," as well as other speed-related offenses, including racing. A recent NHTSA study using data from six states whose police accident reports record these components separately found that more severe crashes are more often associated with exceeding

the posted speed limit, while less severe crashes are associated with driving too fast for conditions:

Fatal crashes
- 55% attributed to exceeding posted speed limit
- 45% attributed to driving too fast for conditions

Injury crashes
- 26% attributed to exceeding posted speed limit
- 74% attributed to driving too fast for conditions

Property damage-only
- 18% attributed to exceeding posted speed limit
- 82% attributed to driving too fast for conditions

Alcohol and speeding are a deadly combination, with alcohol involvement highly prevalent among drivers in speeding-related crashes. In 2008, 41% of drivers with a blood alcohol concentration of 0.08 grams per deciliter or higher involved in fatal crashes were speeding, compared with only 15% of drivers with a BAC of 0.00 g/dL involved in fatal crashes. Between midnight and 3 a.m., 72% of speeding drivers involved in fatal crashes were alcohol impaired (see chart). The alcohol/speeding combination was especially prevalent among young drivers between the ages of 21 and 24, where 50% of speeding drivers had a BAC of 0.08 g/dL or higher, compared with only 27% of nonspeeding drivers.

Source: National Center for Statistics and Analysis. (2009). Traffic Safety Facts 2008 Data— Speeding. Washington, DC: National Highway Traffic Safety Administration. DOT HS 811 166. National Center for Statistics and Analysis. (2010). An Analysis of Speeding-Related Crashes: Definitions and the Effects of Road Environments. Washington, DC: National Highway Traffic Safety Administration. DOT HS 811 090.
[a]A crash is considered speeding-related if the driver was charged with a speeding-related offense or if racing, driving too fast for conditions, or exceeding the posted speed limit was indicated as a contributing factor in the crash.

PERCENTAGE OF ALCOHOL-IMPAIRED DRIVERS IN FATAL CRASHES BY SPEEDING STATUS AND TIME OF DAY, UNITED STATES, 2008

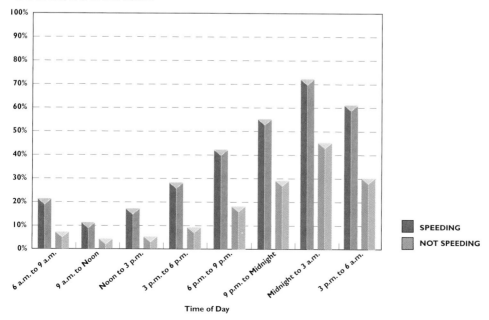

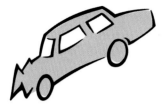

The term distracted driving is not always used consistently. Some reports use the terms inattention and distraction synonymously. While drowsiness and daydreaming can be categorized as inattention, the term distraction as defined by the National Highway Traffic Safety Administration is a specific type of inattention that occurs when drivers divert their attention away from driving to focus on another activity. These distractions can be from electronic sources, such as cell phones or navigation devices, or more conventional distractions, such as interacting with passengers and eating. Distracting tasks can affect drivers in different ways, and can be categorized into the following types:

Visual distraction: Tasks that require the driver to look away from the roadway to visually obtain information.

Manual distraction: Tasks that require the driver to take one hand off the steering wheel and manipulate a device.

Cognitive distraction: The mental workload associated with a task that involves thinking about something other than driving (NHTSA, 2010).

The impact of distraction on driving is determined not only by the type of distraction, but also the frequency and duration of the task. Because of this, even if a task is less distracting, a driver who engages in it frequently or for long durations may increase the crash risk to a level comparable to that of much more difficult tasks performed less often. Text messaging while driving, for example, has been found to pose a greater crash risk than talking on a cell phone. However, because drivers currently talk on cell phones more frequently and for longer durations than they text message, cell phone use accounts for more crashes.

Cell phone driving prevalence
Nationally, about 9% of drivers are using handheld or hands-free cell phones at any given daylight moment. This result from the National Occupant Protection Use

Survey conducted by the NHTSA is the only national estimate of driver cell phone use based on actual driver observations. As shown in the graph below, the percentage of drivers likely to be on either handheld or hands-free cell phones decreased to 9% in 2009 from 11% in 2007 and 2008. The corresponding handheld cell phone use estimate decreased to 5% from 6% of drivers. In addition, the percent of drivers observed manipulating handheld electronic devices decreased to 0.6 percent in 2009 from 1.0 percent in 2008. Among other activities, this observation included text messaging and manipulating devices such as MP3 players.

A national telephone survey conducted by the Insurance Institute for Highway Safety in November and December of 2009 provided detailed driver cell phone usage data. As shown in the graph on the next page, 19% of respondents reported using a cell phone while driving on a daily basis, while an additional 21% reported using a cell phone at least a few times a week. Only 35% of the sample reported never using a cell phone while driving. Males reported greater cell phone use while driving than females. Twenty-four percent of males reported daily cell phone use while driving, compared with 15% of females. In addition, 41% of females reported never using a cell phone while driving, compared with 27% of males. Individuals 25-29 years old reported the highest frequency of cell phone use while driving while respondents age 60 and older reported the least frequent use. Among the 25-29 age group, 39% reported daily cell phone use while driving, but only 20% reported never using a cell phone while driving. The 60 and older age group is the only demographic group with a majority of respondents who reported never using a cell phone while driving.

DRIVER USE OF CELL PHONES, 2002–2009

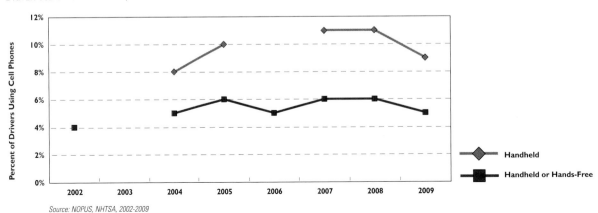

Source: NOPUS, NHTSA, 2002-2009

Cell phone driving risk

Two epidemiological studies have found that cell phone use while driving is associated with approximately a quadrupling of crash risk. Researchers in Western Australia analyzed cell phone records of drivers who went to hospital emergency departments due to injuries sustained in a crash. A second group of researchers in Canada analyzed cell phone records of drivers who reported property damage-only crashes. Both studies compared cell phone use during a 10-minute period prior to the time of the crash and during non-crash periods, and found cell phone use while driving was associated with a slightly more than fourfold increase in crash risk. Results also showed no significant difference between handheld and hands-free phone use.

A review of 33 cell phone driving studies concluded that cell phone conversation while driving increases driver reaction time by about 0.25 second. The use of handheld and hands-free phones results in similar increases in reaction time.

The National Safety Council estimates that 23% of all traffic crashes are associated with drivers using cell phones and text messaging (21% cell phone and 2% text messaging). The percent crash estimates are based on a population attributable risk percent calculation that factors in the relative risk of an activity and the prevalence of the activity. The data inputs for the 21% of crashes associated with cell phones included epidemiological studies that have found cell phone use results in a fourfold increase in the risk of crashes, and NHTSA's NOPUS results show 9% of drivers are talking on cell phones at any given daylight moment. The 2% of crashes associated with text messaging is based on an 8 times relative risk while text messaging estimate and a NOPUS estimate

that about 0.6% of drivers at any given daylight moment are observed manipulating handheld electronic devices. For additional details on the National Safety Council's crash estimates, please visit our website at *www.nsc.org/Pages/NSCestimates16millioncrashescausedby driversusingcellphonesandtexting.aspx.*

State laws

Although research findings indicate there is little to no safety advantage of hands-free over handheld cell phone use, states that have implemented bans impacting all drivers have focused on handheld bans. As of July 2010, 29 states and the District of Columbia have passed total text ban laws. The only state laws banning any use of cell phones while driving are limited to either young drivers or bus drivers. As of July 2010, 28 states and the District of Columbia ban young or novice drivers from using cell phones. See page 100 for additional information regarding state motor vehicle laws.

Braitman, K.A. and McCartt, A.T. (2010). National reported patterns of driver cellphone use. Insurance Institute for Highway Safety. Arlington, VA.

McEvoy, S.P., Stevenson, M.R., McCartt, A.T., Woodward, M., Haworth, C., Palamar, P., and Cercarelli, R. (2005). Role of mobile phones in motor vehicle crashes resulting in hospital attendance: A case-crossover study. British Medical Journal. Online First BMJ, doi:10.1136/bmj.38537.397512.55 (published July 12, 2005).

National Highway Traffic Safety Administration. (2002-2010). Traffic Safety Fact Sheets. Available at www-nrd.nhtsa.dot.gov/cats/index.aspx.

National Highway Traffic Safety Administration (2010). Overview of the national highway traffic safety administration's driver distraction program. DOT HS 811 299.

National Safety Council (2010). Understanding the distracted brain, why driving while using hands-free cellphones is risky behavior. Downloaded on Sept. 1, 2010, from www.nsc.org/safety_road/Distracted_Driving/Pages/distracted_driving.aspx.

Ranney, T.A. (2008, April). Driver distraction: A review of the current state-of-knowledge (Report No. DOT HS 810 787). Washington, DC: National Highway Traffic Safety Administration.

Redelmeier, D.A., and Tibshirani, R.J. (1997). Association between cellular-telephone calls and motor vehicle collisions, New England Journal of Medicine, 336 (7), 453-458.

Young, M.S., Mahfoud, J.M., Walker, G.H., Jenkins, D.P., and Stanton, N.A. (in press). Crash dieting: the effects of eating and drinking on driving performance. Accident Analysis & Prevention.

PERCENT DISTRIBUTION OF FREQUENCY OF CELL PHONE USE WHEN DRIVING BY GENDER AND AGE

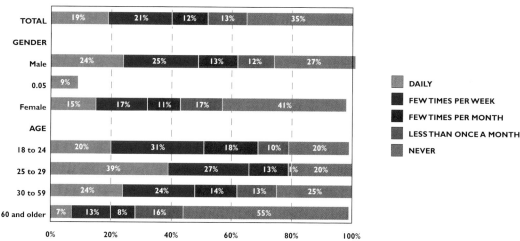

Source: Insurance Institute for Highway Safety (2010). National Reported Patterns of Driver Cellphone Use

IMPROPER DRIVING

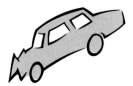

In most motor vehicle accidents, factors are present relating to the driver, vehicle, and road, and it is the interaction of these factors that often sets up a series of events that result in an accident. The table below relates only to the driver, and shows the principal kinds of improper driving in accidents in 2009 as reported by police. The "other improper driving" catergory in the table includes driver inattention—however, see page 108 for a discussion of distracted driving issues.

Exceeding the posted speed limit or driving at an unsafe speed was the most common primary error in fatal accidents. Right-of-way violations predominated in the injury accidents and all accidents catergorics.

While some drivers were under the influence of alcohol or other drugs, this represents the driver's physical condition—not a driving error. See page 104 for a discussion of alcohol involvement in traffic accidents.

Correcting the improper practices listed below could reduce the number of accidents. This does not mean, however, that road and vehicle conditions can be disregarded.

PRIMARY IMPROPER DRIVING REPORTED IN ACCIDENTS, 2009

Kind of improper driving	Fatal accidents	Injury accidents	All accidents
Total	100.0%	100.0%	100.0%
Improper driving	59.5	55.9	54.4
Speed too fast or unsafe	15.7	6.6	5.9
Right of way	10.9	15.1	13.2
Failed to yeild	7.2	10.4	9.6
Disregarded signal	1.5	2.6	1.7
Passed stop sign	2.2	2.1	1.9
Drove left of center	6.9	1.5	1.2
Made improper turn	0.9	2.2	2.0
Improper overtaking	0.9	0.8	1.1
Followed too closely	1.0	6.9	9.3
Other improper driving	23.2	22.8	21.7
No improper driving stated	40.5	44.1	45.6

Source: Based on reports from 18 state traffic authorities. Percents may not add to totals due to rounding.

LARGE TRUCKS

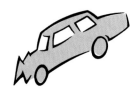

In 2009, 3,380 fatalities resulted from a traffic crash involving a large truck, a 20% decline from 4,245 in 2008. More than 75% of these deaths were occupants of vehicles other than the large truck (see figure below). The overall decrease of 865 fatalities is primarily due to the 600 fewer fatalities of occupants of other vehicles in these crashes. A large truck is one with a gross vehicle weight rating greater than 10,000 pounds.

Large trucks are more likely to be involved in a multiple-vehicle fatal crash than passenger vehicles. In 2008, 82% of large trucks in fatal crashes were in multiple-vehicle crashes, compared with 58% of passenger vehicles.

In 30% of the two-vehicle crashes involving a large truck and another type of vehicle in 2008, both vehicles were impacted in the front. The truck was struck in the rear more than 3 times as often as the other vehicle—19% and 6%, respectively.

FATALITIES IN CRASHES INVOLVING LARGE TRUCKS, UNITED STATES, 2009

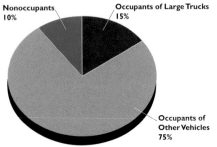

National Center for Statistics and Analysis. (2010). Traffic Safety Facts Research Note: Highlights of 2009 Motor Vehicle Crashes. DOT HS 811 363. Washington, DC: National Highway Traffic Safety Administration. National Center for Statistics and Analysis. (2009). Traffic Safety Facts 2008 Data: Large Trucks. DOT HS 811 158. Washington, DC: National Highway Traffic Safety Administration.

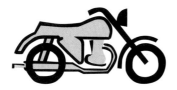

Although motorcycles make up slightly less than 3% of all registered vehicles and only 0.4% of all vehicle miles traveled in the United States, motorcyclists accounted for 13% of total traffic fatalities, 16% of all occupant fatalities, and 4% of all occupant injuries in 2009.

Fatalities among motorcycle riders and passengers increased 80% between 1999 and 2009, from 2,483 to 4,462. Nonfatal injuries increased as well, from 50,000 to 90,000 over the same period. However, the number of motorcycle fatalities in 2009 was 16% less than 2008, and injuries decreased 6.3%.

Exposure also increased. From 1999 to 2008 (the latest year available), the number of registered motorcycles increased more than 90% to 7.8 million from 4.1 million. Miles traveled was up 28%, from 10.6 billion to 13.6 billion in 2007 (latest available data). As a result, the death rate between 1999 to 2007 increased 61%, from 23.46 to 37.86 deaths per 100 million miles traveled.

In 2008, speeding was a factor in 35% of fatal motorcycle crashes, compared with 23% for fatal passenger car crashes.

Twenty-nine percent of motorcycle fatalities involved alcohol-impaired motorcycle operators (BAC >0.08 g/dL), compared to 18% of passenger car fatalities and 11% of large truck fatalities.

Motorcycle helmets were estimated to be 37% effective in preventing fatal injuries to operators and 41% effective for passengers. The National Highway Traffic Safety Administration estimated helmets saved 1,829 motorcyclists' lives in 2008, and an addtional 823 lives could have been saved if all motorcyclists wore helmets.

Although helmet use was down from a high of 71% in 2000, the latest survey showed some improvement, with an increase from 58% in 2007 to 63% in 2008.

In 2010, 20 states and the District of Columbia had laws requiring helmet use by all motorcyclists. Other states either required only a subset of motorcyclists to use helmets (such as those younger than 18), or had no helmet requirement.

A study conducted by the Insurance Institute for Highway Safety found a strong relationship between motorcycle type and driver death rate per 10,000 registered vehicle years. Driver death rates for supersport motorcycles were 4 times as high as those for cruiser/standard motorcycles. Fatally injured supersport drivers were most likely to have been speeding and most likely to have worn helmets, but least likely to have been impaired by alcohol compared with drivers of other motorcycle types. The patterns in driver factors held after accounting for the effects of age and gender. Overall, both supersport and sport/unclad sport drivers have higher-than-average fatality rates, while crusier, touring, and sport touring drivers have average or lower-than-average fatality rates. These trends have been consistent over the six years investigated (see chart).

Source: National Center for Statistics and Analysis (2010). Traffic Safety Facts Research Note: Highlights of 2009 Motor Vehicle Crashes. *DOT HS 811 363. Washington, DC: National Highway Traffic Safety Administration.*

National Center for Statistics and Analysis (2009). Traffic Safety Facts 2008 Data: Motorcycles. *DOT HS 811 159. Washington, DC: National Highway Traffic Safety Administration.*

Insurance Institute for Highway Safety (2010). Helmet use laws. Downloaded on Nov. 30, 2010, from www.iihs.org/laws/HelmetUseOverview.aspx.

Teoh, E.R. and Campbell, M. (2010). Role of motorcycle type in fatal motorcycle crashes. Journal of Safety Research, 41 (6).

MOTORCYCLE DRIVER FATALITY RATE BY MOTORCYCLE TYPE, UNITED STATES, 2003–2008

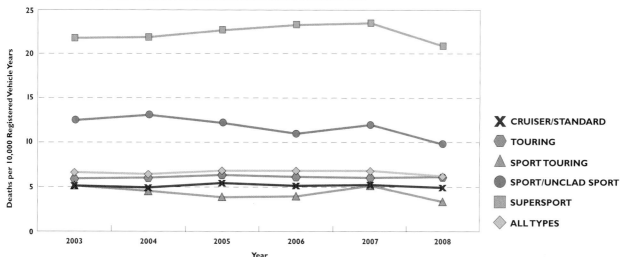

SCHOOL BUS TRANSPORTATION

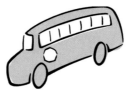

School bus-related crashes killed 118 people nationwide in 2009, according to National Safety Council tabulations of data from the National Highway Traffic Safety Administration.

A school bus-related crash is defined by NHTSA as any crash in which a vehicle, regardless of body design, used as a school bus is directly or indirectly involved, such as a crash involving school children alighting from a vehicle.

From 2004 to 2009, about 73% of the deaths in school bus-related crashes were occupants of vehicles other than the school bus, and 17% were pedestrians. About 4% were school bus passengers, 3% were school bus drivers, and another 3% were pedalcyclists.

Of the 21 pedestrians killed in school bus-related crashes in 2009, 12 were struck by the school bus.

Out of the people injured in school bus-related crashes from 2004 to 2009, about 41% were school bus passengers, 9% were school bus drivers, and another 43% were occupants of other vehicles. The remainder were pedestrians, pedalcyclists, and other or unknown type persons.

Characteristics of school bus transportation

According to School Transportation News, an estimated 444,000-480,000 yellow school buses provide transportation service daily nationwide and travel approximately 4.4 billion miles each school year. Approximately 26 million elementary and secondary school children ride school buses to and from school each day in the United States. That equates to more than 55 million student trips daily—not including student trips for extracurricular activities. This compares to projections from the U.S. Department of Education of enrollments in fall 2009 in grades K-12 of about 49.8 million public school pupils and a projected 5.8 million private school pupils nationwide.

DEATHS AND INJURIES IN SCHOOL BUS-RELATED CRASHES, UNITED STATES, 2004-2009

	2004	2005	2006	2007	2008	2009
Deaths						
Totals	133	134	150	142	153	118
School bus driver	3	5	3	4	4	2
School bus passenger	4	5	5	1	15	1
Pedestrian	30	30	22	19	21	21
Pedalcyclist	3	6	2	6	8	1
Occupant of other vehicle	93	87	118	112	105	93
Other non-occupants	0	1	0	0	0	0
Injuries						
Total	17,000	11,000	13,000	9,000	13,000	13,000
School bus driver	1,000	1,000	2,000	1,000	1,000	1,000
School bus passenger	8,000	4,000	5,000	2,000	6,000	6,000
Pedestrian	1,000	(a)	(a)	(a)	(a)	600
Pedalcyclist	(a)	(a)	(a)	(a)	(a)	(a)
Occupant of other vehicle	7,000	6,000	5,000	5,000	5,000	5,000
Other non-occupants	(a)	(a)	(a)	(a)	(a)	(a)

Source: Deaths for 2004-2008: National Center for Statistics and Analysis (2009). Traffic Safety Facts 2008 Data - School Transportation-Related Crashes. DOT HS 811 165. Washington, DC: National Highway Traffic Safety Administration. Fatality data for 2009 and pedalcyclist deaths are National Safety Council tabulations of Fatality Analysis Reporting System (FARS) data. Injuries: National Center for Statistics and Analysis. (2004-2008). Traffic Safety Facts, 2003-2008 editions. Washington, DC: National Highway Traffic Safety Administration. Injury data for 2009 are National Safety Council tabulations of General Estimates System (GES) data. School bus transportation data accessed Nov. 29, 2010, from School Transportation News at http://stnonline.com/resources/safety/school-bus-safety-data. Student enrollment data from the Digest of Education Statistics: 2009 accessed Nov. 29, 2010, from the National Center for Education Statistics at http://nces.ed.gov/programs/digest/d09/.
[a]Less than 500.

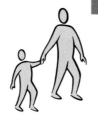

PEDESTRIANS

In 2009, there were an estimated 5,300 pedestrian deaths and 120,000 medically consulted nonfatal injuries[a] to pedestrians in motor vehicle accidents. About 60% of these deaths and injuries occur when pedestrians improperly cross roadways or intersections or dart/run into streets. Playing, working, standing, and so forth, in the roadway accounted for about 12% of pedestrian deaths and injuries, while walking with traffic accounted for over 5%.

The distribution of pedestrian deaths and injuries by action varies for people of different ages.

Darting/running into the road was the leading type of injury or death for the three youngest age groups, varying from 69% for those ages 10-14 years old to more than 80% for those in the 0-4 age group. Improper crossing of the roadway or intersection was the leading type for all age groups from the mid-teens to the oldest adults, ranging from 28% for people ages 20-24 years old to about 54% for those 65 and older.

[a]Nonfatal injury is defined as medically consulted injuries and is not comparable to estimates provided in earlier editions that used the definition of disabling injury. Please see the Technical Appendix for more information regarding medically consulted injuries.

DEATHS AND INJURIES OF PEDESTRIANS BY AGE AND ACTION, 2009

		Age of persons killed or injured							
	Total[a]	0-4	5-9	10-14	15-19	20-24	25-44	45-64	65+
All actions	*100.0%*	*4.2%*	*9.0%*	*13.4%*	*11.4%*	*10.7%*	*20.6%*	*21.1%*	*9.5%*
Totals	**100.0%**	**100.0%**	**100.0%**	**100.0%**	**100.0%**	**100.0%**	**100.0%**	**100.0%**	**100.0%**
Improper crossing of roadway or intersection	30.5%	8.4%	14.5%	19.5%	34.1%	27.6%	28.8%	39.1%	54.1%
Darting or running into roadway	29.5%	80.6%	69.6%	68.6%	22.2%	26.5%	12.8%	12.1%	1.1%
Walking with traffic	5.4%	0.0%	0.5%	0.8%	7.8%	6.9%	8.4%	4.2%	10.6%
Walking against traffic	1.9%	0.0%	0.0%	4.1%	4.4%	1.5%	1.3%	1.1%	2.4%
Playing/working/standing, etc. in roadway	11.7%	5.1%	0.4%	3.7%	4.4%	20.1%	21.0%	16.5%	5.0%
Nonmotorist pushing a vehicle in roadway	0.0%	0.0%	0.0%	0.0%	0.0%	0.0%	0.0%	0.0%	0.0%
Inattentive—talking, eating, etc.	0.9%	0.0%	0.0%	1.0%	0.0%	0.0%	2.8%	0.8%	0.0%
Other action	10.0%	3.7%	14.0%	1.9%	9.6%	4.7%	16.8%	10.7%	10.3%
Unknown action	10.1%	2.2%	1.0%	0.3%	17.6%	12.6%	8.1%	15.5%	16.5%

Source: National Safety Council tabulations of National Highway Traffic Safety Administration General Estimates System (GES) data.
[a]Total includes "Age Unknown."

PEDESTRIAN DEATHS AND DEATH RATES BY SEX AND AGE GROUP, UNITED STATES, 2007

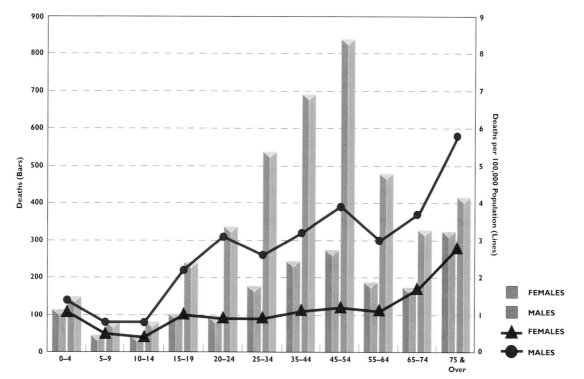

Source: National Safety Council tabulations based on U.S. Census Bureau and National Center for Health Statistics data.

YOUNG DRIVERS

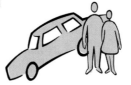

According to the latest data available from the National Highway Traffic Safety Administration, 2009 marked the eighth consecutive year in which the number of teen fatalities in motor vehicle crashes decreased in the United States. However, motor vehicle crashes are still the leading cause of death for U.S. teens. National Center for Health Statistics data indicate more than 1 out of every 3 deaths among 16- to 20-year-olds is caused by a crash. The death toll exceeds 5,500 per year and is equivalent to about 15 deaths a day.

Crashes involving young drivers impact people of all ages. The chart below shows young driver fatalities account for only about half of the overall fatalities associated with young driver crashes. In 2009, there were 2,336 young driver fatalities, 1,447 fatalities of passengers of young drivers, 1,372 fatalities to occupants of all other vehicles, and 468 nonoccupant fatalities. Although the number of deaths has dramatically decreased since 1982, the number of young driver deaths per licensed drivers still is nearly 3 times higher compared to all drivers of passenger vehicles.

HISTORICAL TREND OF YOUNG DRIVER-RELATED FATALITIES, UNITED STATES, 1982–2009

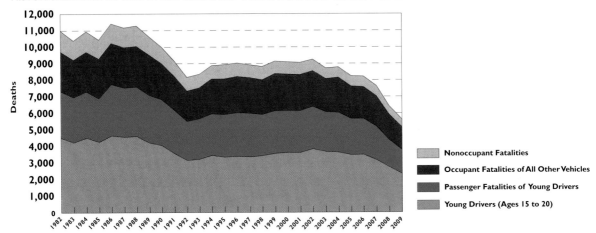

The severity of young driver crashes increases with alcohol involvement. In 2008, two percent of the 15- to 20-year-old drivers involved in property damage-only crashes had been drinking, 4 percent of those involved in crashes resulting in injury had been drinking, and 22 percent of those involved in fatal crashes had been drinking.

Along with alcohol use, other risk factors disproportionately impact young drivers. Safety belt use data for 2008 show young drivers and passengers (ages 16-24) are least likely to use safety belts. Only 79% of young drivers with no passengers use safety belts compared to an 82% average national use rate for all occupants. However, when young drivers are accompanied by at least one passenger not ages 16-24, safety belt usage jumps to 83%.

Young male drivers involved in fatal crashes also are most likely to speed. The proportion of speeding-related fatal crashes decreases with increasing age. In 2008, fully 37% of male drivers ages 15-20 who were involved in fatal crashes were speeding at the time of the crash.

Incidence of crashes related to distractions is 4 times higher among 18-20 year olds, compared to older drivers. The most well-known causes of distraction for drivers include passengers and technology-related factors such as cell phone use and text messaging. Currently, 38 states and the District of Columbia have enacted laws that prohibit young drivers from text messaging while driving, and another 28 states and the District of Columbia restrict the use of cell phones (see page 100 for more information on state motor vehicle laws).

A strategy shown to help prevent young driver crashes is the passage and enforcement of state Graduated Driver Licensing laws. GDL laws allow for a gradual phasing-in of full driving privileges using a three-step process comprised of an initial learner's permit phase; an intermediate, or provisional, license phase; and a full licensure phase.

Not all state GDL laws are equally effective. A recent national study of the impact of state GDL laws found laws rated good were associated with 30 percent lower fatal crash rates among 15-17 year olds, compared with GDL laws rated poor. Laws rated fair yielded fatal crash rates 11% lower.

Although the components of GDL laws vary from state to state, stronger GDL programs consist of five or more of the following components:

1. A minimum age of at least 16 for gaining a learner's permit.
2. A requirement to hold the learner's permit for at least 6 months before gaining a license that allows unsupervised driving.
3. A requirement for certification of at least 30 hours of supervised driving practice during the learner's permit stage.
4. An intermediate stage of licensing with a minimum entry age of at least 16 years and 6 months.
5. A nighttime driving restriction for intermediate license holders, beginning no later than 10 p.m.
6. A passenger restriction for intermediate license holders, allowing no more than one passenger (except family members).
7. A minimum age of 17 for full licensure.

Looking at the adoption of these seven GDL components by states over time shows dramatic advancements in young driver safety. As shown in the chart below, starting in 1991 only 10 states had any laws reflecting GDL components. By 2001, 36 states

and the District of Columbia had laws reflecting one or more GDL components. The latest available data show that by the beginning of 2010 only one state had implemented all seven components and only six states and the District of Columbia had 5-6 GDL components. The majority of states have either three or four components implemented.

In addition to these seven components commonly associated with GDL programs, the National Safety Council recommends additional or more stringent components to be included in comprehensive GDL programs:

- Cell phone use ban
- Text messaging ban
- No passengers younger than 18
- Mandatory safety belt use (primary safety belt laws)

Baker, S.P., Chen, L-H, and Li, G. (2007). National review of graduated driver licensing. Downloaded Aug. 8, 2009, from: www.aaafoundation.org/resources/index.cfm?button=research.
Braitman, K.A., et al. (2008). Crashes of novice teenage drivers: characteristics and contributing factors. Journal of Safety Research, 39, 27–54.
McCartt, A.T., Teoh, E.R., Fields, M., Braitman, K.A., and Hellinga, L.A. (2010). Graduated licensing laws and fatal crashes of teenage drivers: a national study. Traffic Injury Prevention, 11, 240-248.
National Highway Traffic Safety Administration. (2010). Traffic Safety Fact Sheets. Available at www-nrd.nhtsa.dot.gov/cats/index.aspx.
Rice, T.M., et al. (2003). Nighttime driving, passenger transport, and injury crash rates of young drivers. Injury Prevention, 9, 245-250.
Shinar, D., and Compton, R. (2004). Aggressive driving: an observational study of driver, vehicle, and situational variables. Accident Analysis & Prevention, 36 (3), 429-437.

HISTORICAL TREND OF THE NUMBER OF STATES WITH GDL COMPONENTS, 1991–2010

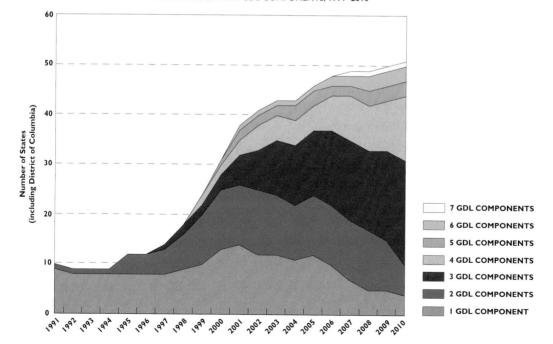

- 7 GDL COMPONENTS
- 6 GDL COMPONENTS
- 5 GDL COMPONENTS
- 4 GDL COMPONENTS
- 3 GDL COMPONENTS
- 2 GDL COMPONENTS
- 1 GDL COMPONENT

Source: National Safety Council analysis of Insurance Institute for Highway Safety data and review of individual state laws.

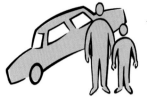

AGE OF DRIVER

The table below shows the total number of licensed drivers and drivers involved in accidents by selected ages and age groups. Also shown is the rate of accident involvement on the basis of the number of drivers in each age group. The fatal accident involvement rates per 100,000 licensed drivers in each age group ranged from a low of 18 for drivers in the 55-64 and 65-74 age groups to a high of 42 for drivers age 18. The all accident involvement rates per 100 drivers in each age group ranged from 4 for drivers ages 65-74 and 75 and older to 23 for drivers age 16.

On the basis of miles driven by each age group, however, involvement rates (not shown in the table) are highest for the youngest and oldest drivers. For drivers age 16 and younger, the fatal involvement rate per 100 million vehicle miles traveled was about 16.3 in 1996, more than 6 times the overall rate of 2.6 for all drivers in passenger vehicles. The rate declines to about 2 for drivers 35-70 years old, and then rises steeply for drivers age 75 and older before reaching a value of 10.2 for drivers in the 85 and older age group. A similar U-shaped curve was found for crash involvement rates.[a]

LICENSED DRIVERS AND NUMBER IN ACCIDENTS BY AGE OF DRIVER, UNITED STATES, 2009

Age group	Licensed drivers		Drivers in...					
			Fatal accidents			All accidents		
	Number	Percent	Number	Percent	Rate[b]	Number	Percent	Rate[c]
Total	211,000,000	100.0%	48,000	100.0%	23	16,500,000	100.0%	8
Younger than 16	658,000	0.3	200	0.4	(d)	250,000	1.5	(d)
16	1,311,000	0.6	500	1.0	38	300,000	1.8	23
17	2,145,000	1.0	700	1.5	33	420,000	2.5	20
18	2,854,000	1.4	1,200	2.5	42	530,000	3.2	19
19	3,358,000	1.6	1,300	2.7	39	520,000	3.1	15
19 and younger	10,326,000	4.9	3,900	8.1	38	2,020,000	12.2	20
20	3,404,000	1.6	1,400	2.9	41	500,000	3.0	15
21	3,447,000	1.6	1,400	2.9	41	490,000	3.0	14
22	3,444,000	1.6	1,200	2.5	35	470,000	2.8	14
23	3,551,000	1.7	1,200	2.5	34	620,000	3.7	17
24	3,619,000	1.7	1,100	2.3	30	400,000	2.4	11
20-24	17,465,000	8.3	6,300	13.1	36	2,480,000	15.0	14
25-34	36,694,000	17.4	8,800	18.3	24	3,270,000	19.8	9
35-44	38,424,000	18.2	7,500	15.6	20	2,910,000	17.6	8
45-54	41,921,000	19.9	8,300	17.3	20	2,750,000	16.7	7
55-64	33,271,000	15.8	5,900	12.3	18	1,710,000	10.4	5
65-74	19,135,000	9.1	3,500	7.3	18	820,000	5.0	4
75 and older	13,764,000	6.5	3,800	7.9	28	540,000	3.3	4

Source: National Safety Council estimates. Drivers in accidents based on data from the National Highway Traffic Safety Administration's Fatality Analysis Reporting System and General Estimates System. Total licensed drivers and age distribution estimated by National Safety Council based on data from the Federal Highway Administration.
Note: Percents may not add to total due to rounding.
[a]Cerrelli, E.C. (1998, January). Crash data and rates for age-sex groups of drivers, 1996. Research Note, Washington, DC: National Center for Statistics & Analysis. Accessed Nov. 5, 2010, at www-nrd.nhtsa.dot.gov/Pubs/98.010.pdf.
[b]Drivers in fatal accidents per 100,000 licensed drivers in each age group.
[c]Drivers in all accidents per 100 licensed drivers in each age group.
[d]Rates for drivers younger than 16 are substantially overstated due to the high proportion of unlicensed drivers involved.

Motor vehicle deaths in 2009 were at their lowest level in February and increased to their highest level in August. In 2009, the highest monthly mileage death rate of 1.28 deaths per 100,000,000 vehicle miles occurred in August. The overall rate for the year was 1.21.

Source: Deaths: National Safety Council estimates. Mileage: Federal Highway Administration, Traffic Volume Trends.

MOTOR VEHICLE DEATHS AND MILEAGE DEATH RATES BY MONTH, 2009

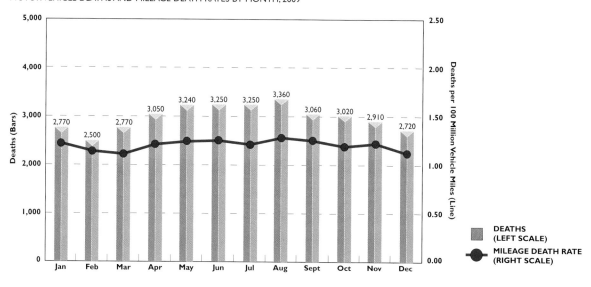

HOLIDAYS

Holidays traditionally are a time of travel for families across the United States. Many choose to travel by automobile, which has the highest fatality rate of any of the major forms of transportation based on fatalities per passenger mile (see page 144). Therefore, their risk of dying in a motor vehicle crash increases. In addition, holidays often are the cause for celebrations that include the drinking of alcohol, which is a major contributing factor in motor vehicle crashes. Nationwide, alcohol-impaired (blood alcohol content of 0.08 g/dL or greater) fatalities in 2009 represented 32% of the total traffic fatalities for the year. The table below shows the number of fatalities for each major holiday period and the percent of those fatalities that were alcohol-impaired.

MOTOR VEHICLE DEATHS AND PERCENT ALCOHOL-IMPAIRED DURING HOLIDAY PERIODS, 2005-2009

| | Holiday period[a] | | | | | | | | | | | |
| | New Year's Day | | Memorial Day | | Independence Day | | Labor Day | | Thanksgiving | | Christmas | |
Year	Deaths[b]	Alcohol-impaired[c] %	Deaths[b]	Alcohol-impaired[c] %	Deaths[b]	Alcohol-impaired[c] %	Deaths[b]	Alcohol-impaired[c] %	Deaths[b]	Alcohol-impaired[c] %	Deaths[b]	Alcohol-impaired[c] %
2005	449 (3)	38	512 (3)	39	565 (3)	44	500 (3)	40	605 (4)	37	383 (3)	40
2006	432 (3)	42	493 (3)	40	629 (4)	37	487 (3)	37	623 (4)	34	379 (3)	42
2007	387 (3)	40	475 (3)	37	184 (1)	45	508 (3)	42	542 (4)	35	454 (3)	38
2008	407 (4)	41	414 (3)	41	472 (3)	43	473 (3)	40	484 (4)	36	409 (4)	34
2009	458 (4)	—	462 (3)	—	398 (3)	—	351 (3)	—	401 (4)	—	248 (3)	—

Source: Deaths: National Safety Council tabulations of National Highway Traffic Safety Administration, Fatality Analysis Reporting System data. Percent alcohol impaired: NHTSA, Traffic Safety Facts, 2008 edition.
Note: Dashes (—) indicate data not available.
[a]The length of the holiday period depends on the day of the week on which the holiday falls. Memorial Day and Labor Day always are 3.25 days; Thanksgiving always is 4.25 days; and New Year's, Independence Day, and Christmas are 3.25 days if the holiday falls Friday through Monday, 4.25 days if on Tuesday or Thursday, and 1.25 days if on Wednesday.
[b]Number in parentheses refers to the number of whole days in the holiday period.
[c]Highest blood alcohol concentration (BAC) among drivers or motorcycle riders involved in the crash was 0.08 grams per deciliter (g/dL) or greater. The holiday periods used to calculate the percentages conform to the NHTSA holiday period definitions that add another quarter day to the periods noted in footnote a.

WORK ZONE DEATHS AND INJURIES

118

In 2009, 667 people were killed and 28,958 were injured in work zone crashes (see table below). Compared to 2008, work zone fatalities and injuries each decreased 7%. Of the 667 people killed in work zones, 510 were in construction zones, 60 were in maintenance zones, 15 were in utility zones, and 82 were in an unknown type of work zone.

From 2000 to 2009, work zone deaths have ranged from 667 to 1,181 and averaged 976 per year.

According to the Governors Highway Safety Association,[a] all states have laws that increase the penalties for speeding or committing other traffic violations while in a construction work zone as of November 2009. The penalties often involve doubled fines, but also can be a fixed dollar amount. In some cases, the penalty is applicable only when workers are present and/or if signs are posted. Currently, 33 states double the fine for speeding or other traffic violations in a work zone. Twenty-three states require workers to be present in the construction zone for the increased penalties to take effect.

[a]Retrieved Nov. 15, 2010, from www.ghsa.org/html/stateinfo/laws/sanctions_laws.html.

PERSONS KILLED AND INJURED IN WORK ZONES, UNITED STATES, 2009

	Total	Vehicle occupants	Pedestrians	Pedalcyclists	Other non-motorists
Killed	667	558	98	8	3
Injured	28,958	27,509	1,301	109	39

Sources: National Safety Council analysis of data from National Highway Traffic Safety Administration Fatality Analysis Reporting System (FARS) and General Estimates Systems (GES).

EMERGENCY VEHICLES

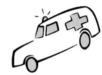

CRASHES INVOLVING EMERGENCY VEHICLES, UNITED STATES, 2009

	Ambulance		Fire truck/car		Police car	
	Total	Emergency use[a]	Total	Emergency use[a]	Total	Emergency use[a]
Emergency vehicles in fatal crashes	29	16	14	9	83	32
Emergency vehicles in injury crashes	959	488	397	182	8,318	4,059
Emergency vehicles in all crashes	3,029	1,404	2,838	1,185	27,524	10,746
Emergency vehicle drivers killed	3	1	1	0	25	12
Emergency vehicle passengers killed	10	5	2	1	3	0
Other vehicle occupants killed	17	9	12	6	43	16
Nonmotorists killed	5	3	3	3	19	5
Total killed in crashes	35	18	18	10	90	33
Total injured in crashes	1,579	918	568	271	14,411	7,628

Sources: National Safety Council analysis of data from National Highway Traffic Safety Administration Fatality Analysis Reporting System (FARS) and General Estimates Systems (GES).
[a]Emergency lights and/or sirens in use.

The National Safety Council and the National Highway Traffic Safety Administration count motor vehicle crash deaths using somewhat different criteria. The Council counts total motor vehicle-related fatalities—both traffic and nontraffic—that occur within one year of the crash. This is consistent with data compiled from death certificates by the National Center for Health Statistics. The Council uses NCHS death certificate data less intentional fatalities as the final count of unintentional deaths from all causes.

NHTSA counts only traffic fatalities that occur within 30 days of the crash in its Fatality Analysis Reporting System. This means the FARS count omits about 800-1,000 motor vehicle-related deaths each year that occur more than 30 days after the crash. Nontraffic fatalities (those that do not occur on public highways; e.g., parking lots, private roads, and driveways), which account for 900-1,900 deaths annually, also are omitted. By using a 30-day cutoff, NHTSA can issue a

"final" count about eight months after the reference year.

Because of the time it takes to process 2.4 million death certificates, NCHS data are not available until about 22 months after the reference year. This means, for example, that this edition of *Injury Facts* includes the 2007 NCHS final counts by cause of death, including motor vehicle crashes, and estimates of the totals for 2008 and 2009. For motor vehicle deaths, these estimates are based on data supplied by traffic authorities in 50 states and the District of Columbia. See the Technical Appendix for more information on estimation procedures.

The graph below shows NCHS death certificate counts of unintentional motor vehicle deaths through 2007 and Council estimates for 2008 and 2009 compared to NHTSA FARS counts of traffic deaths.

MOTOR VEHICLE DEATHS: NSC AND NHTSA, 1992–2009

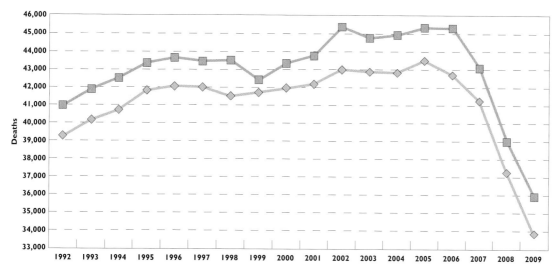

■ NATIONAL SAFETY COUNCIL

◆ NATIONAL HIGHWAY TRAFFIC SAFETY ADMINISTRATION

MOTOR VEHICLE DEATHS AND RATES

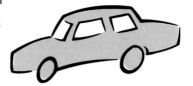

MOTOR VEHICLE DEATHS AND RATES, UNITED STATES, 1913-2009

Year	No. of deaths	Estimated No. of vehicles (millions)	Estimated vehicle miles (billions)	Estimated No. of drivers (millions)	Death rates		
					Per 10,000 motor vehicles	Per 100,000,000 vehicle miles	Per 100,000 population
1913	4,200	1.3	(a)	2.0	33.38	(a)	4.4
1914	4,700	1.8	(a)	3.0	26.65	(a)	4.8
1915	6,600	2.5	(a)	3.0	26.49	(a)	6.6
1916	8,200	3.6	(a)	5.0	22.66	(a)	8.1
1917	10,200	5.1	(a)	7.0	19.93	(a)	10.0
1918	10,700	6.2	(a)	9.0	17.37	(a)	10.3
1919	11,200	7.6	(a)	12.0	14.78	(a)	10.7
1920	12,500	9.2	(a)	14.0	13.53	(a)	11.7
1921	13,900	10.5	(a)	16.0	13.25	(a)	12.9
1922	15,300	12.3	(a)	19.0	12.47	(a)	13.9
1923	18,400	15.1	85	22.0	12.18	21.65	16.5
1924	19,400	17.6	104	26.0	11.02	18.65	17.1
1925	21,900	20.1	122	30.0	10.89	17.95	19.1
1926	23,400	22.2	141	33.0	10.54	16.59	20.1
1927	25,800	23.3	158	34.0	11.07	16.33	21.8
1928	28,000	24.7	173	37.0	11.34	16.18	23.4
1929	31,200	26.7	197	40.0	11.69	15.84	25.7
1930	32,900	26.7	206	40.0	12.32	15.97	26.7
1931	33,700	26.1	216	39.0	12.91	15.60	27.2
1932	29,500	24.4	200	36.0	12.09	14.75	23.6
1933	31,363	24.2	201	35.0	12.96	15.60	25.0
1934	36,101	25.3	216	37.0	14.27	16.71	28.6
1935	36,369	26.5	229	39.0	13.72	15.88	28.6
1936	38,089	28.5	252	42.0	13.36	15.11	29.7
1937	39,643	30.1	270	44.0	13.19	14.68	30.8
1938	32,582	29.8	271	44.0	10.93	12.02	25.1
1939	32,386	31.0	285	46.0	10.44	11.35	24.7
1940	34,501	32.5	302	48.0	10.63	11.42	26.1
1941	39,969	34.9	334	52.0	11.45	11.98	30.0
1942	28,309	33.0	268	49.0	8.58	10.55	21.1
1943	23,823	30.9	208	46.0	7.71	11.44	17.8
1944	24,282	30.5	213	45.0	7.97	11.42	18.3
1945	28,076	31.0	250	46.0	9.05	11.22	21.2
1946	33,411	34.4	341	50.0	9.72	9.80	23.9
1947	32,697	37.8	371	53.0	8.64	8.82	22.8
1948	32,259	41.1	398	55.0	7.85	8.11	22.1
1949	31,701	44.7	424	59.3	7.09	7.47	21.3
1950	34,763	49.2	458	62.2	7.07	7.59	23.0
1951	36,996	51.9	491	64.4	7.13	7.53	24.1
1952	37,794	53.3	514	66.8	7.10	7.36	24.3
1953	37,956	56.3	544	69.9	6.74	6.97	24.0
1954	35,586	58.6	562	72.2	6.07	6.33	22.1
1955	38,426	62.8	606	74.7	6.12	6.34	23.4
1956	39,628	65.2	631	77.9	6.07	6.28	23.7
1957	38,702	67.6	647	79.6	5.73	5.98	22.7
1958	36,981	68.8	665	81.5	5.37	5.56	21.3
1959	37,910	72.1	700	84.5	5.26	5.41	21.5
1960	38,137	74.5	719	87.4	5.12	5.31	21.2
1961	38,091	76.4	738	88.9	4.98	5.16	20.8
1962	40,804	79.7	767	92.0	5.12	5.32	22.0
1963	43,564	83.5	805	93.7	5.22	5.41	23.1
1964	47,700	87.3	847	95.6	5.46	5.63	25.0
1965	49,163	91.8	888	99.0	5.36	5.54	25.4
1966	53,041	95.9	930	101.0	5.53	5.70	27.1
1967	52,924	98.9	962	103.2	5.35	5.50	26.8
1968	54,862	103.1	1,016	105.4	5.32	5.40	27.5
1969	55,791	107.4	1,071	108.3	5.19	5.21	27.7
1970	54,633	111.2	1,120	111.5	4.92	4.88	26.8
1971	54,381	116.3	1,186	114.4	4.68	4.57	26.3
1972	56,278	122.3	1,268	118.4	4.60	4.43	26.9
1973	55,511	129.8	1,309	121.6	4.28	4.24	26.3
1974	46,402	134.9	1,290	125.6	3.44	3.59	21.8
1975	45,853	137.9	1,330	129.8	3.33	3.45	21.3
1976	47,038	143.5	1,412	133.9	3.28	3.33	21.6

See source and footnotes on page 121.

MOTOR VEHICLE DEATHS AND RATES, UNITED STATES, 1913-2009 (Cont.)

Year	No. of deaths	Estimated No. of vehicles (millions)	Estimated vehicle miles (billions)	Estimated No. of drivers (millions)	Death rates		
					Per 10,000 motor vehicles	Per 100,000,000 vehicle miles	Per 100,000 population
1977	49,510	148.8	1,477	138.1	3.33	3.35	22.5
1978	52,411	153.6	1,548	140.8	3.41	3.39	23.6
1979	53,524	159.6	1,529	143.3	3.35	3.50	23.8
1980	53,172	161.6	1,521	145.3	3.29	3.50	23.4
1981	51,385	164.1	1,556	147.1	3.13	3.30	22.4
1982	45,779	165.2	1,592	150.3	2.77	2.88	19.8
1983	44,452	169.4	1,657	154.2	2.62	2.68	19.0
1984	46,263	171.8	1,718	155.4	2.69	2.69	19.6
1985	45,901	177.1	1,774	156.9	2.59	2.59	19.3
1986	47,865	181.4	1,835	159.5	2.63	2.60	19.9
1987	48,290	183.9	1,924	161.8	2.63	2.51	19.9
1988	49,078	189.0	2,026	162.9	2.60	2.42	20.1
1989	47,575	191.7	2,107	165.6	2.48	2.26	19.3
1990	46,814	192.9	2,148	167.0	2.43	2.18	18.8
1991	43,536	192.5	2,172	169.0	2.26	2.00	17.3
1992	40,982	194.4	2,240	173.1	2.11	1.83	16.1
1993	41,893	198.0	2,297	173.1	2.12	1.82	16.3
1994	42,524	201.8	2,360	175.4	2.11	1.80	16.3
1995	43,363	205.3	2,423	176.6	2.11	1.79	16.5
1996	43,649	210.4	2,486	179.5	2.07	1.76	16.5
1997	43,458	211.5	2,562	182.7	2.05	1.70	16.2
1998	43,501	215.0	2,632	185.2	2.02	1.65	16.1
1999	42,401	220.5	2,691	187.2	1.92	1.58	15.5
2000	43,354	225.8	2,747	190.6	1.92	1.58	15.8
2001	43,788	235.3	2,797	191.3	1.86	1.57	15.4
2002	45,380	234.6	2,856	194.3	1.93	1.59	15.8
2003	44,757	236.8	2,890	196.2	1.89	1.55	15.4
2004	44,933	243.0	2,965	199.0	1.85	1.52	15.3
2005	45,343	247.4	2,989	200.5	1.83	1.52	15.3
2006	45,316	250.8	3,014	202.8	1.81	1.50	15.2
2007[b]	43,945	254.4	3,032	205.7	1.73	1.45	14.6
2008[b]	39,700	255.9	2,973	208.3	1.55	1.34	13.1
2009[c]	35,900	258.8	2,979	211.0	1.39	1.21	11.7
Changes							
1999 to 2009	−15%	+17%	+11%	+13%	−28%	−23%	−25%
2008 to 2009	−10%	+1%	+(d)%	+1%	−10%	−10%	−11%

Source: Deaths from National Center for Health Statistics except 1964, 2008, and 2009, which are National Safety Council estimates based on data from the National Highway Traffic Safety Administration's Fatality Analysis Reporting System. See Technical Appendix for comparability. Motor vehicle registrations, mileage, and drivers estimated by Federal Highway Administration except for 2009 registrations and drivers, which are National Safety Council estimates.
[a]*Mileage data inadequate prior to 1923.*
[b]*Revised.*
[c]*Preliminary.*
[d]*Less than 0.5%.*

MOTOR VEHICLE DEATHS BY TYPE OF ACCIDENT

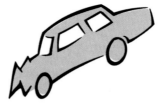

MOTOR VEHICLE DEATHS BY TYPE OF ACCIDENT, UNITED STATES, 1913-2009

| Year | Total deaths | Deaths from collision with... | | | | | | | Deaths from noncollision accidents | Nontraffic deaths[a] |
		Pedestrians	Other motor vehicles	Railroad trains	Streetcars	Pedal-cycles	Animal-drawn vehicle or animal	Fixed objects		
1913	4,200	(b)	(b)	(b)	(b)	(b)	(b)	(b)	(b)	(c)
1914	4,700	(b)	(b)	(b)	(b)	(b)	(b)	(b)	(b)	(c)
1915	6,600	(b)	(b)	(b)	(b)	(b)	(b)	(b)	(b)	(c)
1916	8,200	(b)	(b)	(b)	(b)	(b)	(b)	(b)	(b)	(c)
1917	10,200	(b)	(b)	(b)	(b)	(b)	(b)	(b)	(b)	(c)
1918	10,700	(b)	(b)	(b)	(b)	(b)	(b)	(b)	(b)	(c)
1919	11,200	(b)	(b)	(b)	(b)	(b)	(b)	(b)	(b)	(c)
1920	12,500	(b)	(b)	(b)	(b)	(b)	(b)	(b)	(b)	(c)
1921	13,900	(b)	(b)	(b)	(b)	(b)	(b)	(b)	(b)	(c)
1922	15,300	(b)	(b)	(b)	(b)	(b)	(b)	(b)	(b)	(c)
1923	18,400	(b)	(b)	(b)	(b)	(b)	(b)	(b)	(b)	(c)
1924	19,400	(b)	(b)	1,130	410	(b)	(b)	(b)	(b)	(c)
1925	21,900	(b)	(b)	1,410	560	(b)	(b)	(b)	(b)	(c)
1926	23,400	(b)	(b)	1,730	520	(b)	(b)	(b)	(b)	(c)
1927	25,800	10,820	3,430	1,830	520	(b)	(b)	(b)	(b)	(c)
1928	28,000	11,420	4,310	2,140	570	(b)	(b)	540	8,070	(c)
1929	31,200	12,250	5,400	2,050	530	(b)	(b)	620	9,380	(c)
1930	32,900	12,900	5,880	1,830	480	(b)	(b)	720	9,970	(c)
1931	33,700	13,370	6,820	1,710	440	(b)	(b)	870	9,570	(c)
1932	29,500	11,490	6,070	1,520	320	350	400	800	8,500	(c)
1933	31,363	12,840	6,470	1,437	318	400	310	900	8,680	(c)
1934	36,101	14,480	8,110	1,457	332	500	360	1,040	9,820	(c)
1935	36,369	14,350	8,750	1,587	253	450	250	1,010	9,720	(c)
1936	38,089	15,250	9,500	1,697	269	650	250	1,060	9,410	(c)
1937	39,643	15,500	10,320	1,810	264	700	200	1,160	9,690	(c)
1938	32,582	12,850	8,900	1,490	165	720	170	940	7,350	(c)
1939	32,386	12,400	8,700	1,330	150	710	200	1,000	7,900	(c)
1940	34,501	12,700	10,100	1,707	132	750	210	1,100	7,800	(c)
1941	39,969	13,550	12,500	1,840	118	910	250	1,350	9,450	(c)
1942	28,309	10,650	7,300	1,754	124	650	240	850	6,740	(c)
1943	23,823	9,900	5,300	1,448	171	450	160	700	5,690	(c)
1944	24,282	9,900	5,700	1,663	175	400	140	700	5,600	(c)
1945	28,076	11,000	7,150	1,703	163	500	130	800	6,600	(c)
1946	33,411	11,600	9,400	1,703	174	450	130	950	8,900	(c)
1947	32,697	10,450	9,900	1,736	102	550	150	1,000	8,800	(c)
1948	32,259	9,950	10,200	1,474	83	500	100	1,000	8,950	(c)
1949	31,701	8,800	10,500	1,452	56	550	140	1,100	9,100	838
1950	34,763	9,000	11,650	1,541	89	440	120	1,300	10,600	900
1951	36,996	9,150	13,100	1,573	46	390	100	1,400	11,200	966
1952	37,794	8,900	13,500	1,429	32	430	130	1,450	11,900	970
1953	37,956	8,750	13,400	1,506	26	420	120	1,500	12,200	1,026
1954	35,586	8,000	12,800	1,289	28	380	90	1,500	11,500	1,004
1955	38,426	8,200	14,500	1,490	15	410	90	1,600	12,100	989
1956	39,628	7,900	15,200	1,377	11	440	100	1,600	13,000	888
1957	38,702	7,850	15,400	1,376	13	460	80	1,700	11,800	1,016
1958	36,981	7,650	14,200	1,316	9	450	80	1,650	11,600	929
1959	37,910	7,850	14,900	1,202	6	480	70	1,600	11,800	948
1960	38,137	7,850	14,800	1,368	5	460	80	1,700	11,900	995
1961	38,091	7,650	14,700	1,267	5	490	80	1,700	12,200	1,065
1962	40,804	7,900	16,400	1,245	3	500	90	1,750	12,900	1,029
1963	43,564	8,200	17,600	1,385	10	580	80	1,900	13,800	990
1964	47,700	9,000	19,600	1,580	5	710	100	2,100	14,600	1,123
1965	49,163	8,900	20,800	1,556	5	680	120	2,200	14,900	1,113
1966	53,041	9,400	22,200	1,800	2	740	100	2,500	16,300	1,108
1967	52,924	9,400	22,000	1,620	3	750	100	2,350	16,700	1,165
1968	54,862	9,900	22,400	1,570	4	790	100	2,700	17,400	1,061
1969	55,791	10,100	23,700	1,495	2	800	100	3,900[d]	15,700[d]	1,155
1970	54,633	9,900	23,200	1,459	3	780	100	3,800	15,400	1,140
1971	54,381	9,900	23,100	1,378	2	800	100	3,800	15,300	1,015
1972	56,278	10,300	23,900	1,260	2	1,000	100	3,900	15,800	1,064
1973	55,511	10,200	23,600	1,194	2	1,000	100	3,800	15,600	1,164
1974	46,402	8,500	19,700	1,209	1	1,000	100	3,100	12,800	1,088
1975	45,853	8,400	19,550	979	1	1,000	100	3,130	12,700	1,033
1976	47,038	8,600	20,100	1,033	2	1,000	100	3,200	13,000	1,026

See source and footnotes on page 123.

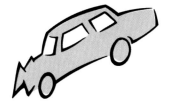

MOTOR VEHICLE DEATHS BY TYPE OF ACCIDENT, UNITED STATES, 1913-2009 (Cont.)

Year	Total deaths	Deaths from collision with...							Deaths from noncollision accidents	Nontraffic deaths[a]
		Pedestrians	Other motor vehicles	Railroad trains	Streetcars	Pedal-cycles	Animal-drawn vehicle or animal	Fixed objects		
1977	49,510	9,100	21,200	902	3	1,100	100	3,400	13,700	1,053
1978	52,411	9,600	22,400	986	1	1,200	100	3,600	14,500	1,074
1979	53,524	9,800	23,100	826	1	1,200	100	3,700	14,800	1,271
1980	53,172	9,700	23,000	739	1	1,200	100	3,700	14,700	1,242
1981	51,385	9,400	22,200	668	1	1,200	100	3,600	14,200	1,189
1982	45,779	8,400	19,800	554	1	1,100	100	3,200	12,600	1,066
1983	44,452	8,200	19,200	520	1	1,100	100	3,100	12,200	1,024
1984	46,263	8,500	20,000	630	0	1,100	100	3,200	12,700	1,055
1985	45,901	8,500	19,900	538	2	1,100	100	3,200	12,600	1,079
1986	47,865	8,900	20,800	574	2	1,100	100	3,300	13,100	998
1987	48,290	7,500[e]	20,700	554	1	1,000[e]	100	13,200[e]	5,200[e]	993
1988	49,078	7,700	20,900	638	2	1,000	100	13,400	5,300	1,054
1989	47,575	7,800	20,300	720	2	900	100	12,900	4,900	989
1990	46,814	7,300	19,900	623	2	900	100	13,100	4,900	987
1991	43,536	6,600	18,200	541	1	800	100	12,600	4,700	915
1992	40,982	6,300	17,600	521	2	700	100	11,700	4,100	997
1993	41,893	6,400	18,300	553	3	800	100	11,500	4,200	994
1994	42,524	6,300	18,900	549	1	800	100	11,500	4,400	1,017
1995	43,363	6,400	19,000	514	(c)	800	100	12,100	4,400	1,032
1996	43,649	6,100	19,600	373	(c)	800	100	12,100	4,600	1,127
1997	43,458	5,900	19,900	371	(c)	800	100	12,000	4,400	1,118
1998	43,501	5,900	19,700	309	(c)	700	100	12,200	4,600	1,310
1999	42,401	6,100	18,600	314	1	800	100	11,800	4,700	1,436
2000	43,354	5,900	19,100	321	(c)	800	100	12,300	4,800	1,360
2001	43,788	6,100	18,800	324	3	800	100	12,800	4,900	1,345
2002	45,380	6,100	19,200	283	(c)	800	100	13,600	5,300	1,315
2003	44,757	6,000	19,300	245	(c)	800	100	13,100	5,200	1,417
2004	44,933	6,000	19,600	253	(c)	900	100	13,000	5,100	1,501
2005	45,343	6,100	19,000	250	(c)	1,000	100	13,600	5,300	1,676
2006	45,316	6,200	18,500	264	(c)	1,000	100	13,900	5,400	1,652
2007[f]	43,945	6,000	17,700	211	(c)	900	100	13,800	5,200	1,914
2008[f]	39,700	5,700	15,400	200	(c)	900	100	12,900	4,500	(c)
2009[g]	35,900	5,300	13,900	200	(c)	800	100	11,600	4,000	(c)
Changes in deaths										
1999 to 2009	−15%	−13%	−25%	−36%	—	0%	0%	−2%	−15%	—
2008 to 2009	−10%	−7%	−10%	0%	—	−11%	0%	−10%	−11%	—

Source: Total deaths from National Center for Health Statistics except 1964, 2008, and 2009, which are National Safety Council estimates based on data from the National Highway Traffic Safety Administration's Fatality Analysis Reporting System. Most totals by type are estimated and may not add to the total deaths. See Technical Appendix for comparability.
[a]See definition, page 207. Nontraffic deaths are included in appropriate accident type totals in table; in 2007, 30% of the nontraffic deaths were pedestrians.
[b]Insufficient data for approximations.
[c]Data not available.
[d]1969-1986 totals are not comparable to previous years.
[e]Procedures and benchmarks for estimating deaths for certain types of accidents were changed for the 1990 edition. Estimates for 1987 and later years are not comparable to earlier years.
[f]Revised.
[g]Preliminary.

MOTOR VEHICLE DEATHS BY AGE

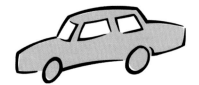

MOTOR VEHICLE DEATHS BY AGE, UNITED STATES, 1913-2009

Year	All ages	Under 5 years	5-14 years	15-24 years	25-44 years	45-64 years	65-74 years	75 & older[a]
1913	4,200	300	1,100	600	1,100	800	300	
1914	4,700	300	1,200	700	1,200	900	400	
1915	6,600	400	1,500	1,000	1,700	1,400	600	
1916	8,200	600	1,800	1,300	2,100	1,700	700	
1917	10,200	700	2,400	1,400	2,700	2,100	900	
1918	10,700	800	2,700	1,400	2,500	2,300	1,000	
1919	11,200	900	3,000	1,400	2,500	2,100	1,300	
1920	12,500	1,000	3,300	1,700	2,800	2,300	1,400	
1921	13,900	1,100	3,400	1,800	3,300	2,700	1,600	
1922	15,300	1,100	3,500	2,100	3,700	3,100	1,800	
1923	18,400	1,200	3,700	2,800	4,600	3,900	2,200	
1924	19,400	1,400	3,800	2,900	4,700	4,100	2,500	
1925	21,900	1,400	3,900	3,600	5,400	4,800	2,800	
1926	23,400	1,400	3,900	3,900	5,900	5,200	3,100	
1927	25,800	1,600	4,000	4,300	6,600	5,800	3,500	
1928	28,000	1,600	3,800	4,900	7,200	6,600	3,900	
1929	31,200	1,600	3,900	5,700	8,000	7,500	4,500	
1930	32,900	1,500	3,600	6,200	8,700	8,000	4,900	
1931	33,700	1,500	3,600	6,300	9,100	8,200	5,000	
1932	29,500	1,200	2,900	5,100	8,100	7,400	4,800	
1933	31,363	1,274	3,121	5,649	8,730	7,947	4,642	
1934	36,101	1,210	3,182	6,561	10,232	9,530	5,386	
1935	36,369	1,253	2,951	6,755	10,474	9,562	5,374	
1936	38,089	1,324	3,026	7,184	10,807	10,089	5,659	
1937	39,643	1,303	2,991	7,800	10,877	10,475	6,197	
1938	32,582	1,122	2,511	6,016	8,772	8,711	5,450	
1939	32,386	1,192	2,339	6,318	8,917	8,292	5,328	
1940	34,501	1,176	2,584	6,846	9,362	8,882	5,651	
1941	39,969	1,378	2,838	8,414	11,069	9,829	6,441	
1942	28,309	1,069	1,991	5,932	7,747	7,254	4,316	
1943	23,823	1,132	1,959	4,522	6,454	5,996	3,760	
1944	24,282	1,203	2,093	4,561	6,514	5,982	3,929	
1945	28,076	1,290	2,386	5,358	7,578	6,794	4,670	
1946	33,411	1,568	2,508	7,445	8,955	7,532	5,403	
1947	32,697	1,502	2,275	7,251	8,775	7,468	5,426	
1948	32,259	1,635	2,337	7,218	8,702	7,190	3,173	2,004
1949	31,701	1,667	2,158	6,772	8,892	7,073	3,116	2,023
1950	34,763	1,767	2,152	7,600	10,214	7,728	3,264	2,038
1951	36,996	1,875	2,300	7,713	11,253	8,276	3,444	2,135
1952	37,794	1,951	2,295	8,115	11,380	8,463	3,472	2,118
1953	37,956	2,019	2,368	8,169	11,302	8,318	3,508	2,271
1954	35,586	1,864	2,332	7,571	10,521	7,848	3,247	2,203
1955	38,426	1,875	2,406	8,656	11,448	8,372	3,455	2,214
1956	39,628	1,770	2,640	9,169	11,551	8,573	3,657	2,268
1957	38,702	1,785	2,604	8,667	11,230	8,545	3,560	2,311
1958	36,981	1,791	2,710	8,388	10,414	7,922	3,535	2,221
1959	37,910	1,842	2,719	8,969	10,358	8,263	3,487	2,272
1960	38,137	1,953	2,814	9,117	10,189	8,294	3,457	2,313
1961	38,091	1,891	2,802	9,088	10,212	8,267	3,467	2,364
1962	40,804	1,903	3,028	10,157	10,701	8,812	3,696	2,507
1963	43,564	1,991	3,063	11,123	11,356	9,506	3,786	2,739
1964	47,700	2,120	3,430	12,400	12,500	10,200	4,150	2,900
1965	49,163	2,059	3,526	13,395	12,595	10,509	4,077	3,002
1966	53,041	2,182	3,869	15,298	13,282	11,051	4,217	3,142
1967	52,924	2,067	3,845	15,646	12,987	10,902	4,285	3,192
1968	54,862	1,987	4,105	16,543	13,602	11,031	4,261	3,333
1969	55,791	2,077	4,045	17,443	13,868	11,012	4,210	3,136
1970	54,633	1,915	4,159	16,720	13,446	11,099	4,084	3,210
1971	54,381	1,885	4,256	17,103	13,307	10,471	4,108	3,251
1972	56,278	1,896	4,258	17,942	13,758	10,836	4,138	3,450
1973	55,511	1,998	4,124	18,032	14,013	10,216	3,892	3,236
1974	46,402	1,546	3,332	15,905	11,834	8,159	3,071	2,555
1975	45,853	1,576	3,286	15,672	11,969	7,663	3,047	2,640
1976	47,038	1,532	3,175	16,650	12,112	7,770	3,082	2,717

See source and footnotes on page 125.

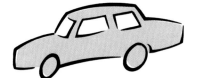

MOTOR VEHICLE DEATHS BY AGE, UNITED STATES, 1913-2009 (Cont.)

Year	All ages	Under 5 years	5-14 years	15-24 years	25-44 years	45-64 years	65-74 years	75 & older[a]
1977	49,510	1,472	3,142	18,092	13,031	8,000	3,060	2,713
1978	52,411	1,551	3,130	19,164	14,574	8,048	3,217	2,727
1979	53,524	1,461	2,952	19,369	15,658	8,162	3,171	2,751
1980	53,172	1,426	2,747	19,040	16,133	8,022	2,991	2,813
1981	51,385	1,256	2,575	17,363	16,447	7,818	3,090	2,836
1982	45,779	1,300	2,301	15,324	14,469	6,879	2,825	2,681
1983	44,452	1,233	2,241	14,289	14,323	6,690	2,827	2,849
1984	46,263	1,138	2,263	14,738	15,036	6,954	3,020	3,114
1985	45,901	1,195	2,319	14,277	15,034	6,885	3,014	3,177
1986	47,865	1,188	2,350	15,227	15,844	6,799	3,096	3,361
1987	48,290	1,190	2,397	14,447	16,405	7,021	3,277	3,553
1988	49,078	1,220	2,423	14,406	16,580	7,245	3,429	3,775
1989	47,575	1,221	2,266	12,941	16,571	7,287	3,465	3,824
1990	46,814	1,123	2,059	12,607	16,488	7,282	3,350	3,905
1991	43,536	1,076	2,011	11,664	15,082	6,616	3,193	3,894
1992	40,982	1,020	1,904	10,305	14,071	6,597	3,247	3,838
1993	41,893	1,081	1,963	10,500	14,283	6,711	3,116	4,239
1994	42,524	1,139	2,026	10,660	13,966	7,097	3,385	4,251
1995	43,363	1,004	2,055	10,600	14,618	7,428	3,300	4,358
1996	43,649	1,035	1,980	10,576	14,482	7,749	3,419	4,408
1997	43,458	933	1,967	10,208	14,167	8,134	3,370	4,679
1998	43,501	921	1,868	10,026	14,095	8,416	3,410	4,765
1999	42,401	834	1,771	10,128	13,516	8,342	3,276	4,534
2000	43,354	819	1,772	10,560	13,811	8,867	3,038	4,487
2001	43,788	770	1,686	10,725	14,020	9,029	2,990	4,568
2002	45,380	733	1,614	11,459	14,169	9,701	3,113	4,591
2003	44,757	766	1,642	10,972	13,794	10,032	2,967	4,584
2004	44,933	778	1,653	10,987	13,699	10,369	2,974	4,473
2005	44,343	763	1,447	10,908	13,987	10,851	3,110	4,277
2006	45,316	728	1,339	11,015	14,025	11,133	2,916	4,160
2007[b]	43,945	675	1,285	10,568	13,457	10,889	2,940	4,131
2008[b]	39,700	500	1,000	9,000	12,300	10,400	2,800	3,700
2009[c]	35,900	500	900	7,900	10,900	9,500	2,700	3,500
Changes in deaths								
1999 to 2009	−15%	−40%	−49%	−22%	−19%	+14%	−18%	−23%
2008 to 2009	−10%	0%	−10%	−12%	−11%	−9%	−4%	−5%

Source: 1913 to 1932 calculated from National Center for Health Statistics data for registration states; 1933 to 1963 and 1965 to 2007 are NCHS totals. All other figures are National Safety Council estimates. See Technical Appendix for comparability.
[a]Includes "age unknown." In 2007, these deaths numbered 9.
[b]Revised.
[c]Preliminary.

MOTOR VEHICLE DEATH RATES BY AGE

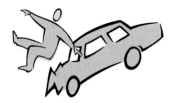

MOTOR VEHICLE DEATH RATES[a] BY AGE, UNITED STATES, 1913-2009

Year	All ages	Under 5 years	5-14 years	15-24 years	25-44 years	45-64 years	65-74 years	75 & older
1913	4.4	2.3	5.5	3.1	3.8	5.3	8.5	
1914	4.8	2.5	5.7	3.5	4.1	6.2	9.3	
1915	6.6	3.5	7.3	5.0	5.6	8.8	13.5	
1916	8.1	4.7	8.6	6.0	7.0	10.7	15.8	
1917	10.0	5.6	10.6	7.4	8.6	12.6	18.6	
1918	10.3	6.9	12.3	7.7	8.3	13.7	21.2	
1919	10.7	7.5	13.9	7.5	8.1	12.4	24.1	
1920	11.7	8.6	14.6	8.7	8.8	13.5	27.0	
1921	12.9	9.0	14.5	9.2	10.2	15.4	31.0	
1922	13.9	9.2	15.0	10.8	11.1	17.2	34.9	
1923	16.5	9.7	15.6	13.4	13.6	21.0	40.5	
1924	17.1	11.1	16.1	14.3	13.7	21.8	43.7	
1925	19.1	11.0	15.6	17.2	15.8	25.0	48.9	
1926	20.1	11.0	15.9	18.6	17.1	26.3	51.4	
1927	21.8	12.8	16.0	20.0	18.8	28.9	56.9	
1928	23.4	12.7	15.5	21.9	20.2	32.4	62.2	
1929	25.7	13.4	15.6	25.6	22.3	35.6	68.6	
1930	26.7	13.0	14.7	27.4	23.9	37.0	72.5	
1931	27.2	13.3	14.5	27.9	24.8	37.4	70.6	
1932	23.6	11.3	12.0	22.6	22.0	32.9	63.6	
1933	25.0	12.0	12.7	24.8	23.4	34.7	63.1	
1934	28.6	11.7	13.0	28.6	27.2	40.7	71.0	
1935	28.6	12.3	12.2	29.2	27.6	39.9	68.9	
1936	29.7	13.2	12.6	30.8	28.2	41.3	70.5	
1937	30.8	13.0	12.7	33.2	28.2	42.0	75.1	
1938	25.1	11.0	10.8	25.4	22.5	34.3	64.1	
1939	24.7	11.2	10.4	26.5	22.6	32.2	60.2	
1940	26.1	11.1	11.5	28.7	23.5	33.9	62.1	
1941	30.0	12.7	12.6	35.7	27.5	37.0	68.6	
1942	21.1	9.5	8.8	25.8	19.2	26.9	44.5	
1943	17.8	9.4	8.6	20.6	16.1	21.9	37.6	
1944	18.3	9.6	9.1	22.5	16.6	21.6	38.2	
1945	21.2	10.0	10.3	27.8	19.7	24.2	44.1	
1946	23.9	11.9	10.8	34.4	21.1	26.4	49.6	
1947	22.8	10.5	9.7	32.8	20.3	25.7	48.2	
1948	22.1	11.0	9.8	32.5	19.8	24.3	39.6	55.4
1949	21.3	10.7	9.0	30.7	19.9	23.4	37.8	53.9
1950	23.0	10.8	8.8	34.5	22.5	25.1	38.8	52.4
1951	24.1	10.9	9.2	36.0	24.7	26.5	39.5	53.0
1952	24.3	11.3	8.7	38.6	24.7	26.7	38.5	50.8
1953	24.0	11.5	8.5	39.1	24.5	25.8	37.7	52.6
1954	22.1	10.4	8.1	36.2	22.6	24.0	33.9	49.0
1955	23.4	10.2	8.0	40.9	24.5	25.2	35.1	47.1
1956	23.7	9.4	8.4	42.9	24.6	25.3	36.2	46.4
1957	22.7	9.2	8.0	39.7	23.9	24.8	34.4	45.5
1958	21.3	9.1	8.1	37.0	22.3	22.6	33.5	42.3
1959	21.5	9.1	7.9	38.2	22.2	23.2	32.3	41.8
1960	21.2	9.6	7.9	37.7	21.7	22.9	31.3	41.1
1961	20.8	9.2	7.6	36.5	21.8	22.5	30.7	40.5
1962	22.0	9.3	8.1	38.4	22.9	23.7	32.2	41.7
1963	23.1	9.8	8.0	40.0	24.3	25.2	32.6	44.3
1964	25.0	10.5	8.8	42.6	26.8	26.6	35.5	45.2
1965	25.4	10.4	8.9	44.2	27.0	27.0	34.6	45.4
1966	27.1	11.4	9.7	48.7	28.5	27.9	35.4	46.2
1967	26.8	11.2	9.5	48.4	27.8	27.1	35.6	45.4
1968	27.5	11.1	10.1	49.8	28.8	27.0	35.1	46.0
1969	27.7	12.0	9.9	50.7	29.1	26.6	34.3	42.0
1970	26.8	11.2	10.2	46.7	27.9	26.4	32.7	42.2
1971	26.3	10.9	10.5	45.7	27.4	24.7	32.4	41.3
1972	26.9	11.1	10.7	47.1	27.4	25.3	32.0	42.6
1973	26.3	11.9	10.5	46.3	27.2	23.6	29.4	39.1
1974	21.8	9.4	8.6	40.0	22.4	18.8	22.6	30.1
1975	21.3	9.8	8.6	38.7	22.1	17.5	21.9	30.1
1976	21.6	9.8	8.4	40.3	21.8	17.6	21.6	30.1

See source and footnotes on page 127.

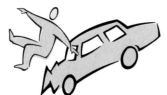

MOTOR VEHICLE DEATH RATES
BY AGE (CONT.)

MOTOR VEHICLE DEATH RATES[a] BY AGE, UNITED STATES, 1913-2009 (Cont.)

Year	All ages	Under 5 years	5-14 years	15-24 years	25-44 years	45-64 years	65-74 years	75 & older
1977	22.5	9.5	8.5	43.3	22.7	18.1	20.9	29.3
1978	23.6	9.9	8.6	45.4	24.6	18.2	21.5	28.7
1979	23.8	9.1	8.3	45.6	25.6	18.4	20.7	28.1
1980	23.4	8.7	7.9	44.8	25.5	18.0	19.1	28.0
1981	22.4	7.4	7.5	41.1	25.2	17.6	19.4	27.5
1982	19.8	7.5	6.7	36.8	21.5	15.5	17.5	25.2
1983	19.0	7.0	6.6	34.8	20.6	15.0	17.2	26.0
1984	19.6	6.4	6.7	36.4	21.0	15.6	18.2	27.7
1985	19.3	6.7	6.9	35.7	20.5	15.4	17.9	27.5
1986	19.9	6.6	7.0	38.5	21.0	15.2	18.1	28.3
1987	19.9	6.6	7.1	37.1	21.3	15.7	18.8	29.1
1988	20.1	6.7	7.1	37.8	21.2	15.9	19.5	30.2
1989	19.3	6.6	6.5	34.6	20.8	15.9	19.4	29.8
1990	18.8	6.0	5.8	34.2	20.4	15.7	18.5	29.7
1991	17.3	5.6	5.6	32.1	18.3	14.2	17.5	28.9
1992	16.1	5.2	5.2	28.5	17.1	13.6	17.6	27.8
1993	16.3	5.5	5.3	29.1	17.3	13.5	16.7	30.0
1994	16.3	5.8	5.4	29.5	16.8	13.9	18.1	29.4
1995	16.5	5.1	5.4	29.3	17.5	14.2	17.6	29.4
1996	16.5	5.4	5.2	29.2	17.3	14.4	18.3	29.0
1997	16.2	4.9	5.1	27.9	17.0	14.7	18.2	29.9
1998	16.1	4.9	4.8	26.9	16.9	14.7	18.5	29.8
1999	15.5	4.4	4.5	26.8	16.3	14.1	18.0	27.8
2000	15.7	4.3	4.5	27.5	16.8	14.5	16.7	27.0
2001	15.4	4.0	4.1	26.8	16.5	14.0	16.3	26.8
2002	15.8	3.7	3.9	28.2	16.8	14.6	17.0	26.5
2003	15.4	3.9	4.0	26.6	16.4	14.6	16.2	26.0
2004	15.3	3.9	4.1	26.4	16.3	14.7	16.1	25.1
2005	15.3	3.8	3.6	25.9	16.6	14.9	16.7	23.6
2006	15.2	3.6	3.3	26.1	16.8	14.9	15.4	22.7
2007[b]	14.6	3.3	3.2	24.9	16.1	14.2	15.2	22.2
2008[b]	13.1	2.4	2.5	21.1	14.7	13.3	14.5	19.7
2009[c]	11.7	2.4	2.2	18.5	13.1	11.9	13.0	18.6
Changes in rates								
1999 to 2009	−24%	−45%	−51%	−31%	−20%	−16%	−28%	−33%
2008 to 2009	−11%	0%	−12%	−12%	−11%	−10%	−10%	−6%

Source: 1913 to 1932 calculated from National Center for Health Statistics data for registration states; 1933 to 1963 and 1965 to 2007 are NCHS totals. All other figures are National Safety Council estimates. See Technical Appendix for comparability.
[a]Death rates are deaths per 100,000 population in each age group that were calculated using population data from the U.S. Census Bureau.
[b]Revised.
[c]Preliminary.

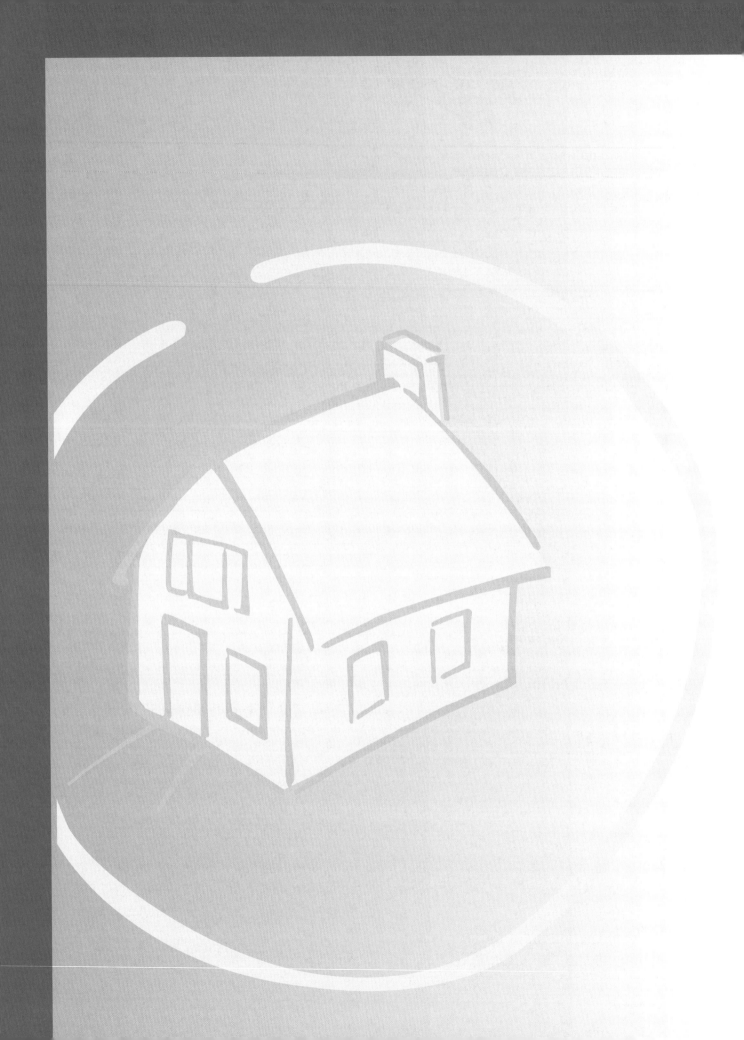

OVERVIEW OF HOME AND COMMUNITY DEATHS, UNITED STATES, 2009

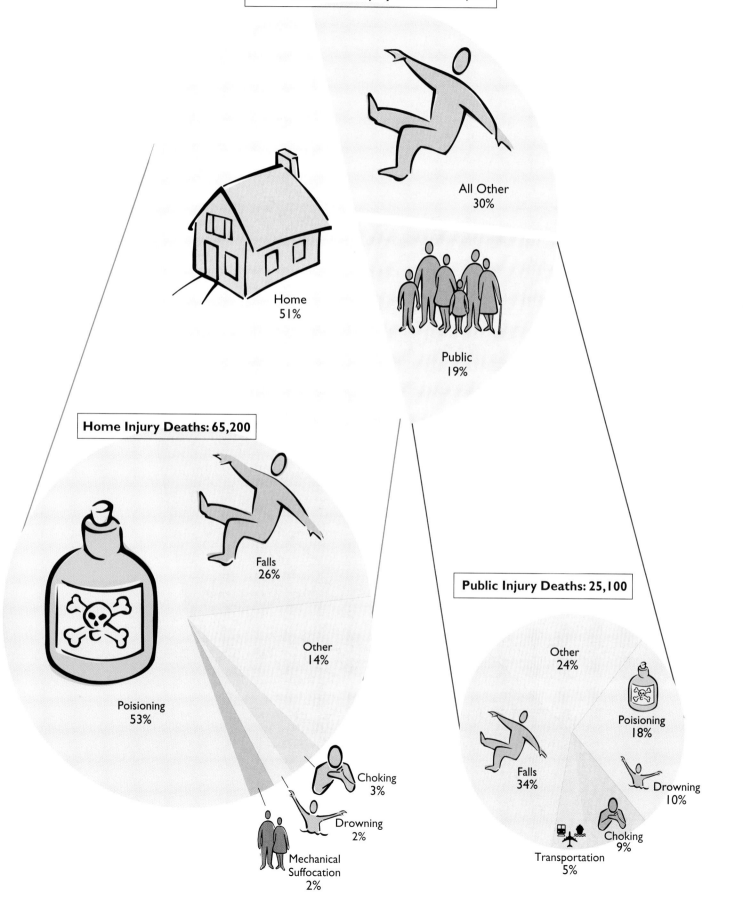

All Unintentional Injury Deaths: 128,200

All Other
30%

Home
51%

Public
19%

Home Injury Deaths: 65,200

Falls
26%

Other
14%

Poisioning
53%

Choking
3%

Drowning
2%

Mechanical
Suffocation
2%

Public Injury Deaths: 25,100

Other
24%

Poisioning
18%

Falls
34%

Drowning
10%

Choking
9%

Transportation
5%

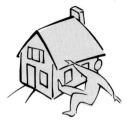

The Home and Community venue is the combination of the Home class and the Public class. Home and Community together with the Occupational and Transportation venues make up the total number of unintentional injuries. Home and Community includes all unintentional injuries that are not work related and do not involve motor vehicles on streets and highways.

In 2009, an estimated 90,300 unintentional injury deaths occurred in the Home and Community venue, or 70% of all unintentional injury deaths that year. The number of deaths was up about 8% from the revised 2008 total of 83,700. An additional 30,500,000 people suffered nonfatal medically consulted injuries. The death rate per 100,000 population was 29.5, 7% higher than the revised 2008 rate.

About 1 out of every 10 people experienced an unintentional injury in the Home and Community venue, and about 1 out of every 3,500 people died from such an injury in 2009. About 42% of the deaths and injuries involved workers while they were off the job.

The graph on the next page shows the five leading causes of unintentional injury deaths in the Home and Community venue and the broad age groups (children, youths and adults, and the elderly) affected by them. This is one way to prioritize issues in this venue. Below is a graph of the trend in deaths and death rates from 1999 to the present. Similar graphs for the Public and Home classes appear on pages 132 and 136.

The National Safety Council adopted the U.S. Bureau of Labor Statistics' Census of Fatal Occupational Injuries count for work-related unintentional injuries beginning with 1992 data. Because of the lower Work class total resulting from this change, adjustments had to be made to the Home and Public classes. Long-term historical comparisons for these three classes should be made with caution. Also, beginning with 1999 data, deaths are classified according to the 10th revision of the International Classification of Diseases. Caution should be used when comparing data classified under the 10th revision with prior revisions. See the Technical Appendix for more information about both changes.

Deaths **90,300**

Medically consulted injuries **30,500,000**

Death rate per 100,000 population **29.5**

Costs . . . . **$300 billion**

HOME AND COMMUNITY DEATHS AND DEATH RATES, UNITED STATES, 1999–2009

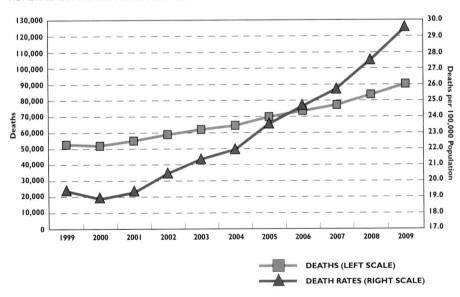

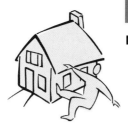

LEADING CAUSES OF UNINTENTIONAL INJURY DEATHS IN HOME AND COMMUNITY, UNITED STATES, 2009

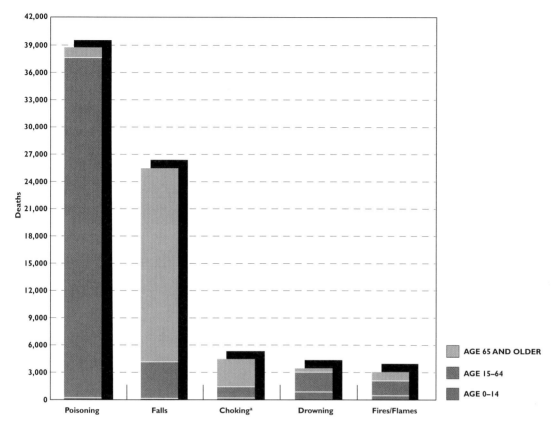

AGE 65 AND OLDER

AGE 15–64

AGE 0–14

ᵃInhalation and ingestion of food or other object that obstructs breathing.

CAUSES OF UNINTENTIONAL INJURY DEATHS IN HOME AND COMMUNITY, UNITED STATES, 2009

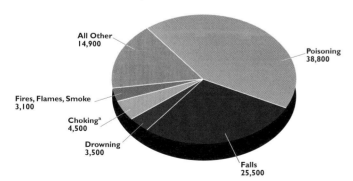

All Other
14,900

Poisoning
38,800

Fires, Flames, Smoke
3,100

Chokingᵃ
4,500

Drowning
3,500

Falls
25,500

ᵃInhalation and ingestion of food or other object that obstructs breathing.

PUBLIC, 2009

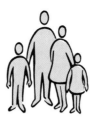

Between 1912 and 2009, public unintentional injury deaths per 100,000 population were reduced 73% to 8.2 (after adjusting for the 1948 change in classification) from 30. In 1912, an estimated 28,000-30,000 people died from public nonmotor vehicle injuries. In 2009, with the population tripled, and travel and recreational activity greatly increased, 25,100 people died of public unintentional injuries and 9,400,000 suffered injuries serious enough to consult a health professional. The public class excludes deaths and injuries involving motor vehicles and people at work or at home.

The number of public unintentional injury deaths was up 2.9% from the revised 2008 figure of 24,400. The death rate per 100,000 population increased from 8.0 to 8.2, or 2%.

With an estimated 9,400,000 medically consulted unintentional injuries occurring in public places and a population of more than 306 million people, about 1 person out of every 32 experienced such an injury, on average.

The Council adopted the Bureau of Labor Statistics' Census of Fatal Occupational Injuries counts for work-related unintentional injuries beginning with 1992 data. This affected long-term historical comparisons for the Work, Home, and Public classes. Beginning with 1999 data, deaths are classified according to the 10th revision of the International Classification of Diseases. Caution should be used when comparing current data with data classified under prior revisions. See the Technical Appendix for more information.

Deaths **25,100**
Medically consulted injuries **9,400,000**
Death rate per 100,000 population **8.2**
Costs . . . . **$108.2 billion**

PUBLIC DEATHS AND DEATH RATES, UNITED STATES, 1999–2009

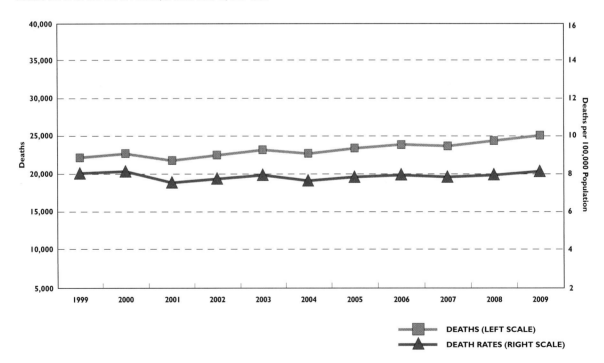

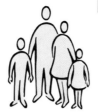

PRINCIPAL TYPES OF PUBLIC UNINTENTIONAL INJURY DEATHS, UNITED STATES, 1987-2009

Year	Total public[a]	Falls	Poisoning	Drowning	Choking[g]	Fires, flames, smoke	Firearms	Air transport	Water transport	Rail transport[b]	Mechanical suffocation
1987	18,400	4,000	800	3,200	1,100	500	600	900	800	400	(c)
1988	18,400	4,100	900	3,100	1,100	500	600	700	800	400	(c)
1989	18,200	4,200	900	3,000	1,000	500	600	800	700	400	(c)
1990	17,400	4,300	900	2,800	1,000	400	500	700	800	400	(c)
1991	17,600	4,500	1,000	2,800	900	400	600	700	700	500	(c)
1992	19,000	4,400	1,700	2,500	1,600	200	400	700	700	600	(c)
1993	19,700	4,600	1,900	2,800	1,500	200	400	600	700	600	(c)
1994	19,600	4,700	2,100	2,400	1,500	200	400	600	600	600	(c)
1995	20,100	5,000	2,000	2,800	1,600	200	300	600	700	500	(c)
1996	21,000	5,300	2,100	2,500	1,700	200	300	700	600	500	(c)
1997	21,700	5,600	2,300	2,600	1,700	200	300	500	600	400	(c)
1998	22,600	6,000	2,300	2,900	1,700	200	300	500	600	500	(c)
1999[d]	22,200	4,800	2,800	2,600	2,000	200	300	500	600	400	500
2000	22,700	5,500	2,900	2,400	2,200	200	200	500	500	400	300
2001	21,800	5,600	2,700	2,400	2,100	200	200	700	500	400	300
2002	22,500	5,900	3,600	2,500	2,200	300	200	500	500	400	300
2003	23,200	6,300	3,400	2,400	2,200	300	200	600	500	400	300
2004	22,700	6,700	3,400	2,400	2,200	200	200	400	500	400	200
2005	23,400	6,800	3,500	2,600	2,100	(c)	(c)	400	500	400	200
2006	23,900	7,200	4,100	2,500	2,100	(c)	(c)	400	400	400	200
2007[e]	23,700	7,600	3,900	2,400	2,200	(c)	(c)	400	400	400	200
2008[e]	24,400	8,100	4,200	2,400	2,200	(c)	(c)	400	400	400	200
2009[f]	25,100	8,600	4,500	2,400	2,200	(c)	(c)	400	400	400	200

Source: National Safety Council estimates based on data from the National Center for Health Statistics and state vital statistics departments. The Council adopted the U.S. Bureau of Labor Statistics' Census of Fatal Occupational Injuries counts for work-related unintentional injuries retroactive to 1992 data. Because of the lower Work class total resulting from this change, several thousand unintentional injury deaths that were classified by the Council as work-related had to be reassigned to the Home and Public classes. For this reason, long-term historical comparisons for these three classes should be made with caution. See the Technical Appendix for an explanation of the methodological changes.
[a]Includes some deaths not shown separately.
[b]Includes subways and elevated trains.
[c]Estimates not available.
[d]In 1999, a revision was made in the International Classification of Diseases. See the Technical Appendix for comparability with earlier years.
[e]Revised.
[f]Preliminary.
[g]Inhalation and ingestion of food or other object that obstructs breathing.

PRINCIPAL TYPES OF PUBLIC UNINTENTIONAL INJURY DEATHS, UNITED STATES, 2009

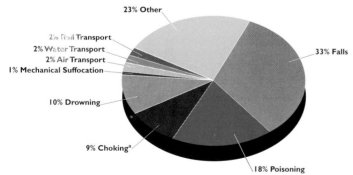

23% Other
2% Rail Transport
2% Water Transport
2% Air Transport
1% Mechanical Suffocation
10% Drowning
9% Choking[a]
18% Poisoning
33% Falls

[a]Inhalation and ingestion of food or other object that obstructs breathing.

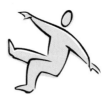

DEATHS DUE TO UNINTENTIONAL PUBLIC INJURIES, 2009

TYPE OF EVENT AND AGE OF VICTIM

All public

Includes deaths in public places and not involving motor vehicles. Most sports, recreation, and transportation deaths are included. Excludes work deaths.

	Total	Change from 2008	Death rate[a]
Deaths	25,100	+3%	8.2

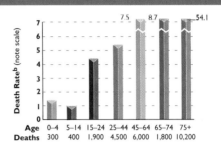

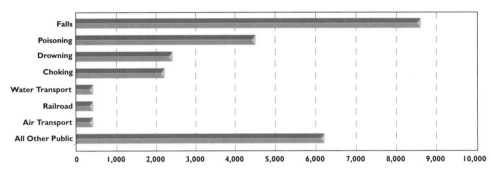

Falls

Includes deaths from falls from one level to another or on the same level in public places. Excludes deaths from falls in moving vehicles.

	Total	Change from 2008	Death rate[a]
Deaths	8,600	+6%	2.8

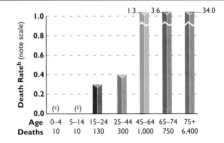

Poisoning

Includes deaths from drugs, medicines, other solid and liquid substances, and gases and vapors. Excludes poisonings from spoiled foods.

	Total	Change from 2008	Death rate[a]
Deaths	4,500	+7%	1.5

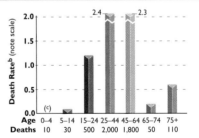

Drowning

Includes drownings of person swimming or playing in water, or falling into water, except on home premises or at work. Excludes drownings involving boats, which are in water transportation.

	Total	Change from 2008	Death rate[a]
Deaths	2,400	0%	0.8

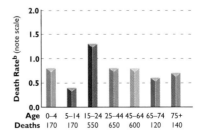

See footnotes on page 135.

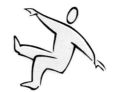

TYPE OF EVENT AND AGE OF VICTIM

Choking

Includes deaths from unintentional ingestion or inhalation of food or other objects resulting in the obstruction of respiratory passages.

	Total	Change from 2008	Death rate[a]
Deaths	2,200	0%	0.7

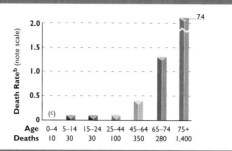

Age	0–4	5–14	15–24	25–44	45–64	65–74	75+
Deaths	10	30	30	100	350	280	1,400

Water transport

Includes deaths in water transport accidents from falls, burns, etc., as well as drownings. Excludes crews and people traveling in the course of employment.

	Total	Change from 2008	Death rate[a]
Deaths	400	0%	0.1

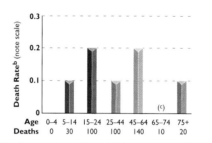

Age	0–4	5–14	15–24	25–44	45–64	65–74	75+
Deaths	0	30	100	100	140	10	20

Railroad

Includes deaths arising from railroad vehicles in motion (except involving motor vehicles), subway and elevated trains, and people boarding or alighting from standing trains. Excludes crews and people traveling in the course of employment.

	Total	Change from 2008	Death rate[a]
Deaths	400	0%	0.1

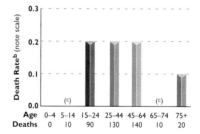

Age	0–4	5–14	15–24	25–44	45–64	65–74	75+
Deaths	0	10	90	130	140	10	20

Air transport

Includes deaths in private flying, passengers in commercial aviation, and deaths of military personnel in the United States. Excludes crews and people traveling in the course of employment.

	Total	Change from 2008	Death rate[a]
Deaths	400	0%	0.1

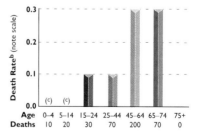

Age	0–4	5–14	15–24	25–44	45–64	65–74	75+
Deaths	10	20	30	70	200	70	0

All other public

Most important types included are mechanical suffocation; excessive natural heat or cold; firearms; fire, flames, and smoke; and machinery.

	Total	Change from 2008	Death rate[a]
Deaths	6,200	–2%	2.0

[a]Deaths per 100,000 population.
[b]Deaths per 100,000 population in each age group.
[c]Death rate less than 0.05.

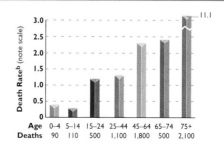

Age	0–4	5–14	15–24	25–44	45–64	65–74	75+
Deaths	90	110	500	1,100	1,800	500	2,100

HOME, 2009

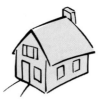

Between 1912 and 2009, unintentional home injury deaths per 100,000 population were reduced 24% to 21.3 (after adjusting for the 1948 classification change) from 28. In 1912, when there were 21 million households, an estimated 26,000 to 28,000 people were killed by unintentional home injuries. In 2009, with more than 117 million households and the population tripled, home deaths numbered 65,200. However, the number and rate of unintentional home injury deaths has been steadily increasing since 2000. This increase in deaths is largely driven by increases in both unintentional poisonings and falls.

The injury total of 21,100,000 means that 1 person out of every 14 in the United States experienced an unintentional injury in the home in 2009 that was serious enough to consult with a medical professional.

Medically consulted injuries are more numerous in the home than in public places, the workplace, and in motor vehicle crashes combined. The National Health Interview Survey estimates that about 43% of all medically consulted injuries occurred at home.

The National Safety Council adopted the U.S. Bureau of Labor Statistics' Census of Fatal Occupational Injuries count for work-related unintentional injuries beginning with 1992 data. This affected long-term historical comparisons for the Work, Home, and Public classes. Beginning with 1999 data, deaths are classified according to the 10th revision of the International Classification of Diseases. Caution should be used in comparing current data with data classified under prior revisions. See the Technical Appendix for more information.

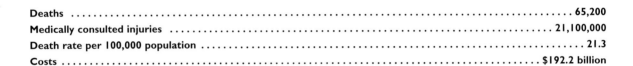

Deaths 65,200
Medically consulted injuries 21,100,000
Death rate per 100,000 population 21.3
Costs . . . . $192.2 billion

HOME DEATHS AND DEATH RATES, UNITED STATES, 1999–2009

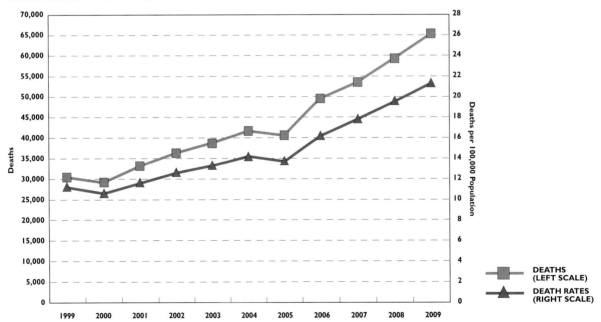

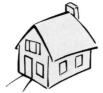

PRINCIPAL TYPES OF HOME UNINTENTIONAL INJURY DEATHS, UNITED STATES, 1987-2009

Year	Total home	Poisoning	Falls	Fire, flames, smoke[a]	Choking[b]	Mechanical suffocation	Drowning	Natural heat/cold	Firearms	Other
1987	21,400	4,100	6,300	3,900	2,500	600	700	(c)	800	2,500
1988	22,700	4,800	6,600	4,100	2,600	600	700	(c)	800	2,500
1989	22,500	5,000	6,600	3,900	2,500	600	700	(c)	800	2,400
1990	21,500	4,500	6,700	3,400	2,300	600	900	(c)	800	2,300
1991	22,100	5,000	6,900	3,400	2,200	700	900	(c)	800	2,200
1992	24,000	5,200	7,700	3,700	1,500	700	900	(c)	1,000	3,300
1993	26,100	6,500	7,900	3,700	1,700	700	900	(c)	1,100	3,600
1994	26,300	6,800	8,100	3,700	1,600	800	900	(c)	900	3,500
1995	27,200	7,000	8,400	3,500	1,500	800	900	(c)	900	4,200
1996	27,500	7,300	9,000	3,500	1,500	800	900	(c)	800	3,700
1997	27,700	7,800	9,100	3,200	1,500	800	900	(c)	700	3,500
1998	29,000	8,400	9,500	2,900	1,800	800	1,000	(c)	600	4,000
1999[d]	30,500	9,300	7,600	3,000	1,900	1,100	900	700	600	5,400
2000	29,200	9,800	7,100	2,700	2,100	1,000	1,000	400	500	4,600
2001	33,200	11,300	8,600	3,000	2,000	1,100	900	400	600	5,300
2002	36,200	13,900	9,700	2,800	1,900	1,100	900	400	500	5,000
2003	38,600	15,900	10,300	2,900	2,100	1,000	800	400	500	4,700
2004	41,500	17,500	11,300	2,900	2,200	1,200	900	400	400	4,700
2005	46,200	20,000	12,000	2,900	2,300	1,300	900	500	500	5,800
2006	49,400	23,300	12,800	2,800	2,300	1,400	1,000	600	400	4,800
2007[e]	53,500	25,800	14,200	3,000	2,100	1,400	1,000	500	400	5,100
2008[e]	59,300	30,000	15,500	2,900	2,300	1,400	1,000	500	400	5,300
2009[f]	65,200	34,300	16,900	2,900	2,300	1,500	1,100	500	400	5,300

Source: National Safety Council estimates based on data from National Center for Health Statistics and state vital statistics departments. The Council adopted the U.S. Bureau of Labor Statistics' Census of Fatal Occupational Injuries counts for work-related unintentional injuries retroactive to 1992 data. Because of the lower Work class total resulting from this change, several thousand unintentional injury deaths that were classified by the Council as work-related had to be reassigned to the Home and Public classes. For this reason, long-term historical comparisons for these three classes should be made with caution. See the Technical Appendix for an explanation of the methodological changes.
[a]Includes deaths resulting from conflagration, regardless of nature of injury.
[b]Inhalation and ingestion of food or other object that obstructs breathing.
[c]Included in Other.
[d]In 1999, a revision was made in the International Classification of Diseases. See the Technical Appendix for comparability with earlier years.
[e]Revised.
[f]Preliminary.

PRINCIPAL TYPES OF HOME UNINTENTIONAL INJURY DEATHS, UNITED STATES, 2009

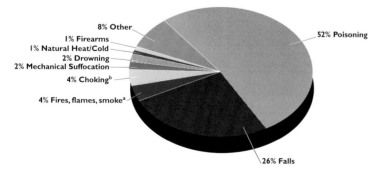

8% Other
1% Firearms
1% Natural Heat/Cold
2% Drowning
2% Mechanical Suffocation
4% Choking[b]
4% Fires, flames, smoke[a]
52% Poisoning
26% Falls

[a]Includes deaths resulting from conflagration, regardless of nature of injury.
[b]Inhalation and ingestion of food or other object that obstructs breathing.

DEATHS DUE TO UNINTENTIONAL HOME INJURIES, 2009

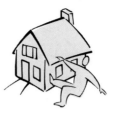

TYPE OF EVENT AND AGE OF VICTIM

All home

Includes deaths in the home and on home premises to occupants, guests, and trespassers. Also includes hired household workers, but excludes other people working on home premises.

	Total	Change from 2008	Death rate[a]
Deaths	65,200	+10%	21.3

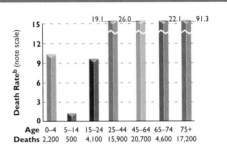

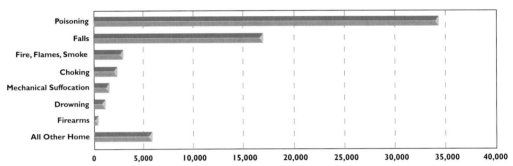

Poisoning

Includes deaths from drugs, medicines, other solid and liquid substances, and gases and vapors. Excludes poisonings from spoiled foods, salmonella, etc., which are classified as disease deaths.

	Total	Change from 2008	Death rate[a]
Deaths	34,300	+14%	11.2

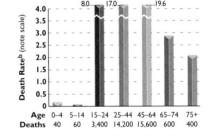

Falls

Includes deaths from falls from one level to another or on the same level in the home or on home premises.

	Total	Change from 2008	Death rate[a]
Deaths	16,900	+9%	5.5

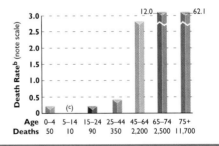

Fire, flames, and smoke

Includes deaths from fires, burns, and injuries in conflagrations in the home, such as asphyxiation, falls, and struck by falling objects. Excludes burns from hot objects or liquids.

	Total	Change from 2008	Death rate[a]
Deaths	2,900	0%	0.9

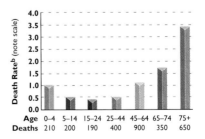

See footnotes on page 139.

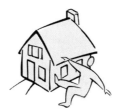

TYPE OF EVENT AND AGE OF VICTIM

Choking

Includes deaths from unintentional ingestion or inhalation of objects or food resulting in the obstruction of respiratory passages.

	Total	Change from 2008	Death rate[a]
Deaths	2,300	0%	0.7

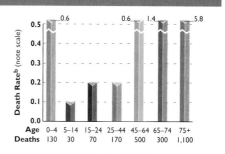

Age	0–4	5–14	15–24	25–44	45–64	65–74	75+
Deaths	130	30	70	170	500	300	1,100

Mechanical suffocation

Includes deaths from smothering by bed clothes, thin plastic materials, etc.; suffocation by cave-ins or confinement in closed spaces; and mechanical strangulation and hanging.

	Total	Change from 2008	Death rate[a]
Deaths	1,500	+7%	0.5

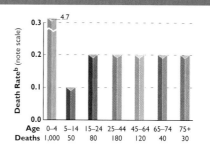

Age	0–4	5–14	15–24	25–44	45–64	65–74	75+
Deaths	1,000	50	80	180	120	40	30

Drowning

Includes drownings of people in or on home premises, such as in swimming pools and bathtubs. Excludes drowning in floods and other cataclysms.

	Total	Change from 2008	Death rate[a]
Deaths	1,100	+10%	0.4

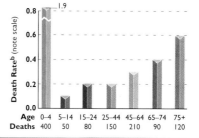

Age	0–4	5–14	15–24	25–44	45–64	65–74	75+
Deaths	400	50	80	150	210	90	120

Firearms

Includes firearms injuries in or on home premises, such as while cleaning or playing with guns. Excludes deaths from explosive materials.

	Total	Change from 2008	Death rate[a]
Deaths	400	0%	0.1

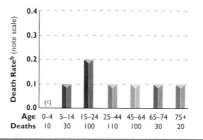

Age	0–4	5–14	15–24	25–44	45–64	65–74	75+
Deaths	10	30	100	110	100	30	20

All other home

Most important types included are natural heat and cold, struck by or against objects, machinery, and electric current.

	Total	Change from 2008	Death rate[a]
Deaths	5,800	+4%	1.9

[a]Deaths per 100,000 population.
[b]Deaths per 100,000 population in each age group.
[c]Death rate less than 0.05.

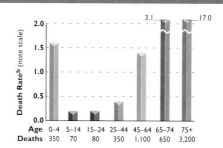

Age	0–4	5–14	15–24	25–44	45–64	65–74	75+
Deaths	350	70	80	350	1,100	650	3,200

SPORTS AND RECREATION INJURIES

In the United States in 2009, bicycle riding and basketball injuries each resulted in more than half a million emergency department visits.

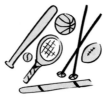

The table below shows estimates of injuries treated in hospital emergency departments and participants associated with various sports and recreational activities. Differences between the two sources in methods, coverage, classification systems, and definitions can affect comparisons among sports. Because this list of

sports is not complete, the frequency and duration of participation is not known, and the number of participants varies greatly, no inference should be made concerning the relative hazard of these sports or rank with respect to risk of injury. In particular, it is **not** appropriate to calculate injury rates from these data.

SPORTS PARTICIPATION AND INJURIES, UNITED STATES, 2009

Sport or activity	Participants	Injuries	Percent of injuries by age				
			0-4	5-14	15-24	25-64	65 & older
Archery	7,100,000	4,199	3.3	12.0	20.2	50.6	13.9
Baseball	11,500,000	165,842	3.4	46.9	27.8	21.0	0.9
Softball	11,800,000	121,175	0.5	25.8	32.5	40.1	1.0
Basketball	24,400,000	501,251	0.4	29.4	49.7	20.4	0.2
Bicycle riding[a]	38,100,000	534,928	5.3	40.8	18.2	32.1	3.7
Billiards/pool	28,200,000	5,269	1.9	20.4	24.2	51.8	1.7
Bowling	45,000,000	20,878	5.7	14.6	13.3	55.6	10.8
Boxing	[b]	18,455	0.5	9.0	53.7	36.5	0.4
Cheerleading	2,900,000[c]	31,456	0.0	49.7	49.0	1.2	0.0
Exercise	[b]	265,938[d]	2.7	12.1	18.4	53.9	12.9
Fishing	32,900,000	75,490	2.3	19.0	13.4	54.5	10.9
Football	8,900,000[e]	451,961	0.4	47.5	41.7	10.4	0.1
Golf	22,300,000	41,009[f]	4.7	20.5	7.6	42.0	25.2
Gymnastics	3,900,000	29,606[g]	4.0	70.7	21.7	3.6	0.0
Hockey, field	[b]	4,017	3.1	28.7	63.1	5.1	0.0
Horseback riding	[b]	78,499	1.8	17.4	20.1	56.9	3.8
Horseshoe pitching	[b]	2,251	3.3	3.9	17.0	56.2	19.6
Ice hockey	3,100,000	19,035	0.2	30.9	49.8	18.7	0.4
Ice skating	[b]	21,926[h]	2.7	52.0	17.4	26.5	1.4
Martial arts	[b]	28,909	0.5	24.4	25.3	49.6	0.2
Mountain biking	8,400,000	9,627	1.4	5.9	22.0	69.1	1.5
Mountain climbing	[b]	4,376	0.4	16.2	34.5	49.0	0.0
Racquetball, squash & paddleball	[b]	6,594	2.5	5.1	21.1	69.2	2.1
Roller skating	[b]	63,550[i]	1.4	50.7	14.7	32.1	1.1
Rugby	[b]	14,847	0.0	2.4	78.3	19.3	0.0
Scuba diving	[b]	1,331	1.2	6.2	34.0	52.3	6.3
Skateboarding	8,400,000	144,416	1.4	46.2	39.9	12.3	0.2
Snowboarding	6,200,000	54,188	0.0	26.1	51.1	22.5	0.2
Snowmobiling	[b]	12,154	0.6	6.3	30.4	61.0	1.7
Soccer	13,600,000	208,214	0.6	42.1	39.5	17.7	0.2
Swimming	50,200,000	175,388[j]	10.3	40.2	18.2	27.5	3.8
Tennis	10,800,000	23,611	0.6	14.5	20.2	38.4	26.3
Track & field	[b]	22,191	0.1	40.9	47.8	10.9	0.3
Volleyball	10,700,000	60,159	0.3	27.7	43.6	27.5	0.9
Water skiing	5,200,000	7,032	0.0	16.5	40.8	42.7	0.0
Weight lifting	34,500,000	86,307	3.5	8.0	34.8	50.9	2.8
Wrestling	3,000,000	41,712	0.2	36.4	57.8	5.6	0.0

Source: Participants—National Sporting Goods Association; figures include those 7 and older who participated more than once per year except for bicycle riding, swimming, and weightlifting, which include those who participated six or more times per year.
Injuries—Consumer Product Safety Commission; figures include only injuries treated in hospital emergency departments.
[a]Excludes mountain biking.
[b]Data not available.
[c]Data for 2008.
[d]Includes exercise equipment (55,578 injuries) and exercise activity (210,360 injuries).
[e]Includes participation in tackle football only.
[f]Excludes golf carts (14,629 injuries).
[g]Excludes trampolines (97,908 injuries).
[h]Excludes 6,459 injuries in skating, unspecified.
[i]Includes roller skating (45,699 injuries) and in-line skating (17,851 injuries).
[j]Includes injuries associated with swimming, swimming pools (2008 data), pool slides (2008 data), diving or diving boards, and swimming pool equipment.

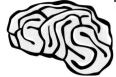

TRAUMATIC BRAIN INJURY

Each year, traumatic brain injuries contribute to a substantial number of deaths and cases of permanent disability. A TBI is caused by a bump, blow, or jolt to the head, or a penetrating head injury that disrupts the normal function of the brain. The severity of a TBI may range from "mild" (a brief change in mental status or consciousness) to "severe" (an extended period of unconsciousness or amnesia after the injury). TBI is often referred to as the "silent epidemic" because the complications from TBI, such as changes affecting thinking, sensation, language, or emotions, may not be readily apparent.

An estimated 1.7 million people sustain a TBI annually in the United States. Among them, 52,000 die, 275,000 are hospitalized, and nearly 1.4 million (about 80%) are treated and released from an emergency department. TBI is a contributing factor to one-third (30.5%) of all injury-related deaths. An unknown number of TBIs receive other types of medical care or no care.

Young children 0-4 years old, adolescents ages 15-19 years, and adults 65 and older are most likely to sustain a TBI. The most ED visits for TBI are made annually by children ages 0 to 14 years, while adults age 75 and

older have the highest rates of TBI-related hospitalization and death. By sex, TBI rates are higher for males than for females in every age group, with males 0-4 years old having the highest rates for TBI-related ED visits, hospitalizations, and deaths combined.

Falls are the leading cause of TBI, with the highest rates for children 0-4 years old and for adults age 75 and older. Falls also result in the greatest number of TBI-related ED visits (523,043) and hospitalizations (62,334). The leading cause of TBI-related deaths is motor vehicle traffic injuries, with the highest rates observed among adults 20-24 years old.

There was an increase in TBI-related ED visits (14.4%) and hospitalizations (19.5%) from 2002 to 2006. Over this same period, there was a 62% increase in ED visits for fall-related TBI among children 14 and younger. For adults age 65 and older, increases were observed from 2002 to 2006 in the number of ED visits (46%), hospitalizations (34%), and TBI-related deaths (27%).

Source: Faul, M., Xu, L., Wald, M.M., and Coronado, V.G. (2010). Traumatic Brain Injury in the United States: Emergency Department Visits, Hospitalizations and Deaths 2002-2006. Atlanta, GA: Centers for Disease Control and Prevention, National Center for Injury Prevention and Control.

ESTIMATED ANNUAL AVERAGE AND PERCENTAGE OF ALL INJURIES AND TRAUMATIC BRAIN INJURY-RELATED EMERGENCY DEPARTMENT VISITS, HOSPITALIZATIONS AND DEATHS, UNITED STATES, 2002-2006

	All injuries			TBIs		
	All visits	Number	% of all visits	Number	% of all injuries	% of all visits
ED visits[a]	96,839,411	28,697,028	29.6	1,364,797	4.8	1.4
Hospitalizations[b]	36,693,646	1,826,548	5.0	275,146	15.1	0.7
Deaths	2,432,714	169,055	6.9	51,538[c]	30.5	2.1
Total	135,965,771	30,692,631	22.6	1,691,481	5.5	1.2

[a]Persons who were hospitalized, died, or transferred to another facility were excluded.
[b]In-hospital deaths and patients who transferred from another hospital were excluded.
[c]128 mortality records (from 2002 to 2006) were omitted because of missing age information.

WEATHER

Weather-related deaths down more than 50% in 2009.

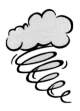

A variety of weather events resulted in 227 deaths in the United States and District of Columbia in 2009, compared with 528 deaths in 2008. Temperature extremes accounted for 21% of the deaths and ocean/lake surf accounted for an additional 18%. Primarily due to temperature extremes, June was the most deadly month with 41 weather related deaths.

Data on weather-related deaths was compiled by the National Climatic Data Center, which is part of the National Oceanic and Atmospheric Administration. NCDC data may differ from data based on death certificates that appears elsewhere in *Injury Facts*.

WEATHER-RELATED DEATHS, UNITED STATES, 2009

Event	Total	Jan.	Feb.	March	April	May	June	July	Aug.	Sept.	Oct.	Nov.	Dec.
Total	277	27	27	11	29	33	41	31	19	14	14	12	19
Tornado	22	0	9	0	7	5	0	0	0	0	1	0	0
Thunderstorm/high winds	35	0	5	1	2	10	7	2	1	0	2	2	3
Temperature extremes	59	15	5	0	0	1	16	11	3	0	2	0	6
Flood	47	4	0	4	12	9	3	1	1	6	5	1	1
Ocean/lake surf	49	0	0	2	5	4	3	8	10	4	3	7	3
Snow/ice	25	8	8	2	0	0	0	0	0	0	1	0	6
Lightning	31	0	0	1	1	2	12	9	3	3	0	0	0
Hurricane/tropical storm	1	0	0	0	0	0	0	0	1	0	0	0	0
Wild/forest fire	2	0	0	0	2	0	0	0	0	0	0	0	0
Hail	0	0	0	0	0	0	0	0	0	0	0	0	0
Precipitation	6	0	0	1	0	2	0	0	0	1	0	2	0
Drought	0	0	0	0	0	0	0	0	0	0	0	0	0
Dust storm	0	0	0	0	0	0	0	0	0	0	0	0	0
Fog	0	0	0	0	0	0	0	0	0	0	0	0	0
Funnel cloud	0	0	0	0	0	0	0	0	0	0	0	0	0
Waterspout	0	0	0	0	0	0	0	0	0	0	0	0	0

Source: National Safety Council analysis of National Climatic Data Center data.

WEATHER-RELATED FATALITIES BY MONTH, UNITED STATES, 2009

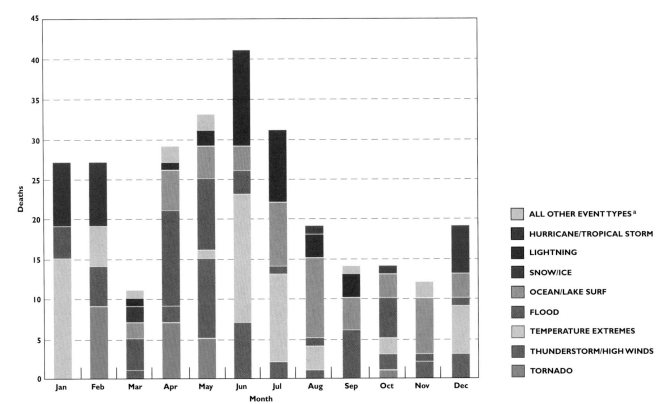

a Includes wild/forest fire, hail, and precipitation.

FIREARMS

Unintentional firearm-related deaths down nearly 5% to record low in 2007.

Firearm-related deaths from unintentional, intentional, and undetermined causes totaled 31,224 in 2007, an increase of 1% from 2006. Suicides accounted for 55.6% of firearms deaths, 40.5% were homicides, and 2.0% were unintentional deaths. Males dominated all categories of firearms deaths and accounted for 86.6% of the total.

The number of homicide deaths by firearms decreased slightly in 2007 after increasing in each of the previous two years. Unintentional firearms deaths also declined in 2007 for the second year in a row, falling to a new

record low. However, suicide deaths by firearms increased in 2007 following a decline the previous year.

Hospital emergency department surveillance data indicated an estimated 15,698 nonfatal unintentional firearm-related injuries in 2007. For assault, there was an estimated 48,676[a] nonfatal injuries, while the estimated total for intentionally self-inflicted nonfatal injuries was 4,291.[a]

Source: National Safety Council analysis of National Center for Health Statistics mortality data and National Center for Injury Prevention and Control injury surveillance data using WISQARS from www.cdc.gov/ncipc/wisqars/.
[a]Estimate for nonfatal assault-related injuries and self-inflicted nonfatal injuries do not meet standard of reliability or precision and should be used with caution.

DEATHS INVOLVING FIREARMS BY AGE AND SEX, UNITED STATES, 2007

Type & sex	All ages	Under 5 years	5-14 years	15-19 years	20-24 years	25-44 years	45-64 years	65-74 years	75+
Total firearms deaths	**31,224**	**85**	**313**	**2,669**	**4,233**	**11,422**	**8,199**	**1,938**	**2,365**
Male	27,047	51	237	2,402	3,835	9,793	6,856	1,701	2,172
Female	4,177	34	76	267	398	1,629	1,343	237	193
Unintentional	**613**	**19**	**46**	**73**	**82**	**185**	**139**	**31**	**38**
Male	537	15	41	68	79	156	122	23	33
Female	76	4	5	5	3	29	17	8	5
Suicide	**17,352**	**---**	**53**	**630**	**1,270**	**5,185**	**6,317**	**1,700**	**2,197**
Male	15,181	---	45	572	1,155	4,426	5,374	1,539	2,070
Female	2,171	---	8	58	115	759	943	161	127
Homicide	**12,632**	**63**	**201**	**1,897**	**2,772**	**5,789**	**1,605**	**185**	**120**
Male	10,767	34	141	1,696	2,503	4,969	1,243	121	60
Female	1,865	29	60	201	269	820	362	64	60
Legal intervention	**351**	**0**	**1**	**24**	**72**	**183**	**63**	**5**	**3**
Male	339	0	1	24	69	177	60	5	3
Female	12	0	0	0	3	6	3	0	0
Undetermined[a]	**276**	**3**	**12**	**45**	**37**	**80**	**75**	**17**	**7**
Male	223	2	9	42	29	65	57	13	6
Female	53	1	3	3	8	15	18	4	1

Source: The Centers for Disease Control and Prevention, WISQARS
Note: Dashes (—) indicate category not applicable.
[a]Undetermined means the intentionality of the deaths (unintentional, homicide, suicide) was not determined.

FIREARMS DEATHS BY INTENTIONALITY AND YEAR, UNITED STATES, 1998–2007

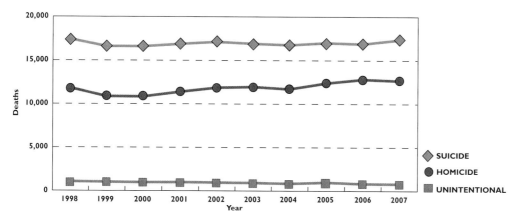

TRANSPORTATION MODE COMPARISONS

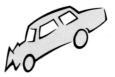

Passenger transportation incidents account for about 2 out of every 10 unintentional injury deaths. But the risk of death to the passenger, expressed on a per mile basis, varies greatly by transportation mode. Highway travel by personal vehicle presents the greatest risk; air, rail, and bus travel have much lower death rates. The tables below show the latest information on passenger transportation deaths and death rates.

The statistics for automobiles, vans, sport utility vehicles, pickups, and other light trucks shown in the tables below represent all passenger vehicle usage, both intercity and local. The bus data also include intercity

and local (transit) bus travel. Railroad includes both intercity (Amtrak) and local commuting travel. Scheduled airlines includes both large airlines and commuter airlines, but excludes on-demand air taxis and charter operations. In comparing the four modes, drivers of automobiles (except taxis), vans, SUVs, and pickup trucks are considered passengers. Bus drivers and airline or railroad crews are not considered passengers.

Other comparisons are possible based on passenger trips, vehicle miles, or vehicle trips, but passenger miles is the most commonly used basis for comparing the safety of various modes of travel.

TRANSPORTATION ACCIDENT DEATH RATES, UNITED STATES, 2006-2008

| Mode of transportation | 2008 | | | 2006-2008 average death rate |
	Passenger deaths	Passenger miles (billions)	Deaths per 100,000,000 passenger miles	
Passenger automobiles[a]	14,579	2,633.8	0.55	0.61
Vans, SUVs, pickup trucks[b]	10,765	1,817.5	0.59	0.66
Buses[c]	50	61.1	0.08	0.05
Transit buses	23	21.9	0.11	0.03
Intercity buses	11	39.2	0.03	0.03
Railroad passenger trains[d]	24	18.2	0.13	0.06
Scheduled airlines[e]	0	568.2	0.00	0.003

Source: Highway passenger deaths: Fatality Analysis Reporting System data. Railroad passenger deaths and miles: Federal Railroad Administration. Airline passenger deaths: National Transportation Safety Board. Airline passenger miles: Bureau of Transportation Statistics. Passenger miles for transit buses: American Public Transit Association. All other figures: National Safety Council estimates.
[a]Includes taxi passengers. Drivers of passenger automobiles are considered passengers.
[b]Includes two-axle, four-tire vehicles less than 10,000 pounds gross vehicle weight rating other than automobiles.
[c]Figures exclude school buses but include "other" and "unknown" bus types.
[d]Includes Amtrak and commuter rail service.
[e]Includes large airlines and scheduled commuter airlines; excludes charter, cargo, and on-demand service and suicide/sabotage.

PASSENGER DEATHS AND DEATH RATES, UNITED STATES, 1999-2008

| Year | Passenger automobiles | | Vans, SUVs, & pickup trucks | | Buses | | Railroad passenger trains | | Scheduled airlines | |
	Deaths	Rate[a]	Deaths	Rate[a]	Deaths	Rate[a]	Deaths	Rate[a]	Deaths	Rate[a]
1999	20,851	0.84	11,295	0.76	40	0.07	14	0.10	24	0.005
2000	20,689	0.81	11,545	0.76	3	0.01	4	0.03	94	0.02
2001	20,310	0.78	11,736	0.76	11	0.02	3	0.02	279	0.06
2002	20,564	0.78	12,278	0.78	36	0.06	7	0.05	0	0.00
2003	19,723	0.74	12,551	0.78	30	0.05	3	0.02	24	0.005
2004	19,183	0.71	12,678	0.75	27	0.05	3	0.02	13	0.002
2005	18,509	0.68	13,043	0.76	43	0.07	16	0.10	22	0.004
2006	17,792	0.66	12,723	0.72	15	0.02	2	0.01	52	0.01
2007	16,613	0.61	12,462	0.68	18	0.03	5	0.03	0	0.00
2008	14,579	0.55	10,765	0.59	50	0.08	24	0.13	0	0.00
10-year average	18,881	0.72	12,108	0.73	27	0.05	8	0.05	51	0.01

Source: See table above.
[a]Deaths per 100,000,000 passenger miles.

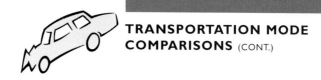

PASSENGER DEATH RATES, UNITED STATES, 2006–2008

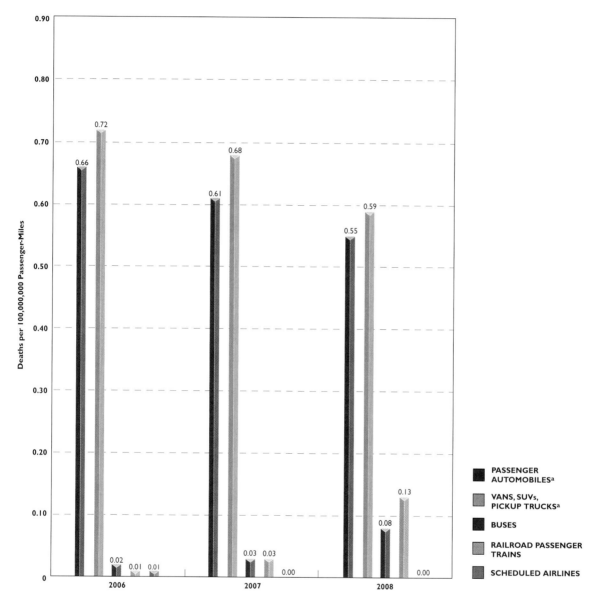

Legend
- **PASSENGER AUTOMOBILES**[a]
- **VANS, SUVs, PICKUP TRUCKS**[a]
- **BUSES**
- **RAILROAD PASSENGER TRAINS**
- **SCHEDULED AIRLINES**

Y-axis: Deaths per 100,000,000 Passenger-Miles

2006: 0.66, 0.72, 0.02, 0.01, 0.01
2007: 0.61, 0.68, 0.03, 0.03, 0.00
2008: 0.55, 0.59, 0.08, 0.13, 0.00

[a]*Drivers of these vehicles are considered passengers.*

AVIATION

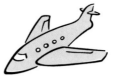

In the United States, the rate of civil aviation accidents per 100,000 flight hours has decreased since 1990 for general aviation, on-demand air taxis, and large airlines.

CIVIL AVIATION ACCIDENT RATES, UNITED STATES, 1990–2009

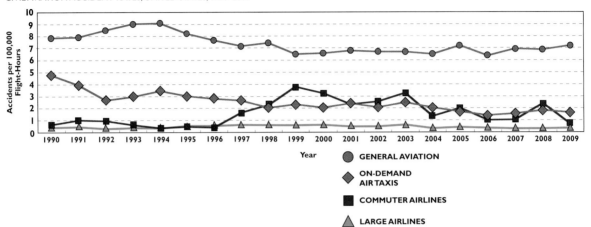

- ● GENERAL AVIATION
- ◆ ON-DEMAND AIR TAXIS
- ■ COMMUTER AIRLINES
- ▲ LARGE AIRLINES

U.S. CIVIL AVIATION ACCIDENTS, DEATHS, AND DEATH RATES, 2004-2009

| | | | | Accident rates | | | |
| | Accidents | | Total deaths[a] | Per 100,000 flight hours | | Per million aircraft miles | |
Year	Total	Fatal		Total	Fatal	Total	Fatal
Large airlines[b]							
2004	30	2	14	0.159	0.011	0.0038	0.0003
2005	40	3	22	0.206	0.015	0.0049	0.0004
2006	33	2	50	0.171	0.01	0.0041	0.0002
2007	28	1	1	0.143	0.005	0.0034	0.0001
2008	28	2	3	0.147	0.01	0.0035	0.0002
2009	30	2	52	0.167	0.011	0.004	0.0003
Commuter airlines[b]							
2004	4	0	0	1.324	0	0.0855	0
2005	6	0	0	2.002	0	0.1312	0
2006	3	1	2	0.995	0.332	0.0645	0.0215
2007	3	0	0	1.028	0	0.0651	0
2008	7	0	0	2.385	0	0.1508	0
2009	2	0	0	0.685	0	0.0432	0
On-demand air taxis[b]							
2004	66	23	64	2.04	0.71	—	—
2005	65	11	18	1.70	0.29	—	—
2006	52	10	16	1.39	0.27	—	—
2007	62	14	43	1.54	0.35	—	—
2008	58	20	69	1.81	0.62	—	—
2009	47	2	17	1.63	0.07	—	—
General aviation[b]							
2004[c]	1,617	314	559	6.49	1.26	—	—
2005[c]	1,670	321	563	7.20	1.38	—	—
2006[c]	1,523	308	706	6.35	1.28	—	—
2007[c]	1,652	288	496	6.93	1.2	—	—
2008[c]	1,566	275	494	6.86	1.21	—	—
2009[c]	1,474	272	474	7.20	1.33	—	—

Source: National Transportation Safety Board: 2009 preliminary, 2004-2008 revised; exposure data for rates from Federal Aviation Administration.
Note: Dash (—) indicates data not available.
[a]Includes passengers, crew members, and others such as persons on the ground.
[b] Civil aviation accident statistics collected by the National Transportation Safety Board are classified according to the federal air regulations under which the flights were made. The classifications are (1) large airlines operating scheduled service under Title 14, Code of Federal Regulations, part 121 (14 CFR 121); (2) commuter carriers operating scheduled service under 14 CFR 135; (3) unscheduled, "on-demand" air taxis under 14 CFR 135; and (4) "general aviation," which includes accidents involving aircraft flown under rules other than 14 CFR 121 and 14 CFR 135. Not shown in the table is nonscheduled air carrier operations under 14 CFR 121, which experienced two accidents and one fatality in 2007. Since 1997, Large Airlines includes aircraft with 10 or more seats, formerly operated as commuter carriers under 14 CFR 135.
[c] Suicide/sabotage/terrorism and stolen/unauthorized cases are included in "accident" and fatality totals but excluded from rates—General Aviation, 2004 (3/0), 2005 (2/1), 2006 (2/1), 2007 (2/2), 2008 (2/0), 2009 (2/0).

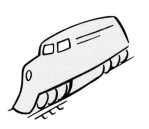

RAILROAD

Railroad deaths totaled 708 in 2009, a 12% decrease from the 2008 total of 801 and a 21% decrease from the 1999-2008 average of 898. From 2008 to 2009, there was a 15% decrease in fatalities at highway-rail crossings, while fatalities that occurred in other types of incidents decreased 10%. The latter included 431 deaths, or 93%, to trespassers. Sixteen employees were killed while on duty, a 36% decrease compared to the 2008 death toll and a 27% decrease from the 1999-2008 average of 22. Deaths to passengers on trains totaled 3, down from 24 deaths in 2008 and also down from the 10-year average of eight deaths a year.

The ratio of railroad-related deaths to nonfatal injuries and illnesses is approximately 1:11. In 2009, railroad accidents resulted in 7,679 cases of nonfatal conditions, compared with 8,905 in 2008 and the 1999-2008 average of 10,076. Nine percent of the total was attributed to highway-rail crossing incidents, which decreased by 27% from the 2008 total of 965 and by 36% from the 1999-2008 average of 1,104. Of the 4,376 nonfatal occupational railroad injuries and illnesses reported in 2009, less than 2% were attributed to highway-rail crossing incidents.

DEATHS AND NONFATAL CASES IN RAILROAD ACCIDENTS AND INCIDENTS, UNITED STATES, 1999-2009

Year	Total	Highway rail crossing incident?		Occurring in other than highway rail crossing incident		Employees on duty At highway rail crossing?		Passengers on trains[a] At highway rail crossing?	
		Yes	No	Trespassers	Others	Yes	No	Yes	No
Deaths									
1999	932	402	530	479	51	2	29	11	3
2000	937	425	512	463	49	2	22	0	4
2001	971	421	550	511	39	1	21	0	3
2002	951	357	594	540	54	1	19	0	7
2003	865	334	531	498	33	1	18	1	2
2004	891	371	520	472	48	2	23	0	3
2005	884	359	525	458	67	2	23	0	16
2006	903	369	534	511	23	4	12	0	2
2007	849	337	512	470	42	1	16	0	5
2008	801	289	512	456	56	3	22	0	24
2009	708	247	461	431	30	0	16	0	3
Nonfatal conditions									
1999	11,700	1,396	10,304	445	9,859	140	8,482	43	438
2000	11,643	1,219	10,424	414	10,010	100	8,323	10	648
2001	10,985	1,157	9,828	404	9,424	97	7,718	20	726
2002	11,103	999	10,104	395	9,709	110	6,534	26	851
2003	9,264	1,035	8,229	398	7,831	76	6,182	74	653
2004	9,194	1,094	8,100	406	7,694	116	5,906	28	675
2005	9,548	1,050	8,498	420	8,078	111	5,712	33	925
2006	8,787	1,069	7,718	480	7,238	96	5,175	95	840
2007	9,626	1,055	8,571	408	8,163	105	5,341	71	1,437
2008	8,905	965	7,940	431	7,509	73	4,873	89	1,200
2009	7,679	705	6,974	343	6,631	68	4,308	47	1,028

Source: Federal Railroad Administration
[a]Passenger cases include all circumstances, including getting on/off standing trains, stumbling aboard trains, assaults, train accidents, crossing incidents, etc.

CASUALTIES AT PUBLIC AND PRIVATE HIGHWAY-RAIL CROSSINGS, UNITED STATES, 1999-2009

Year	Deaths				Nonfatal conditions			
	Total	Motor vehicle-related	Pedestrians	Others	Total	Motor vehicle-related	Pedestrians	Others
1999	402	345	45	12	1,396	1,338	35	23
2000	425	361	51	13	1,219	1,169	34	16
2001	421	345	67	9	1,157	1,110	31	16
2002	357	310	35	12	999	939	29	31
2003	334	281	50	3	1,035	1,000	28	7
2004	371	289	73	9	1,094	1,058	30	6
2005	359	284	58	17	1,052	1,007	37	8
2006	369	305	53	11	1,071	1,037	29	5
2007	337	263	59	5	1,059	1,020	30	9
2008	289	220	64	5	968	907	50	11
2009	247	182	59	6	706	666	34	6

Source: Federal Railroad Administration

UNINTENTIONAL FATAL POISONINGS

Poisoning deaths up 8% from 2006 to 2007.

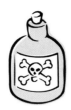

Deaths from unintentional poisoning numbered 29,846 in 2007, the latest year for which data are available. The death rate per 100,000 population was 9.9. Males are at greatest risk with a death rate of 13.2 compared to 6.7 for females. Total poisoning deaths increased 8% from 27,531 in 2006 and are 2.9 times the 1997 total. See pages 46-49 for long-term trends.

Nearly 44% of the poisoning deaths were classified in the "narcotics and psychodysleptics (hallucinogens), not elsewhere classified," catergory, which includes prescription narcotic analgesics and illegal drugs such as cocaine, heroin, cannabinol, and LSD. A recent report from the Centers for Disease Control and Prevention[a] indicated the number of fatalities involving prescription opioid analgesics in 2006 was 1.6 times the number involving cocaine and 5.88 times the number involving heroin. In addition, emergency department visits for nonmedical use of prescription and over-the-counter drugs have caught up with those for illegal drugs, with each accounting for 1.0 million ED visits in 2008.

Deaths due to alcohol poisoning nearly quadrupled from 2006 to 2007 to a total of 1,356. Although alcohol poisoning deaths for males continue to outnumber those for females by more than 3 to 1, the increase observed from 2006 to 2007 was similar for both sexes. It should be noted that alcohol also may be present in combination with other drugs.

Carbon monoxide poisoning is included in the catergory of "other gases and vapors." Additional information on human poisoning exposure cases may be found on pages 150 and 191.

[a]Unintentional Drug Poisoning in the United States, accessed July 8, 2010, at www.cdc.gov/HomeandRecreationalSafety/pdf/poison-issue-brief.pdf.

UNINTENTIONAL POISONING DEATHS BY TYPE, AGE, AND SEX, UNITED STATES, 2007

Type of poison	All ages	0-4 years	5-14 years	15-19 years	20-24 years	25-44 years	45-64 years	65 & older
Both sexes								
Total poisoning deaths	**29,846**	**53**	**81**	**838**	**2,321**	**13,275**	**12,126**	**1,152**
Deaths per 100,000 population	9.9	0.3	0.2	3.9	11.1	15.9	15.8	3.0
Total drug-related poisoning deaths	27,658	34	53	754	2,173	12,541	11,201	902
Nonopioid analgesics, antipyretics and antirheumatics (X40)[a]	290	1	1	5	13	117	110	43
Antiepileptic, sedative-hypnotic, antiparkinsonism and psychotropic drugs, n.e.c. (X41)	1,545	6	4	26	74	620	757	58
Narcotics and psychodysleptics (hallucinogens), n.e.c. (X42)	13,030	14	26	425	1,088	5,998	5,260	219
Other drugs acting on the autonomic nervous system (X43)	10	1	0	0	1	2	5	1
Other and unspecified drugs, medicaments and biological substances (X44)	12,783	12	22	298	997	5,804	5,069	581
Alcohol (X45)	1,356	1	4	48	91	499	642	71
Organic solvents and halogenated hydrocarbons and their vapors (X46)	77	1	3	9	9	32	19	4
Other gases and vapors (X47)	603	14	15	24	38	153	212	147
Pesticides (X48)	3	0	0	0	0	1	1	1
Other and unspecified chemical and noxious substances (X49)	149	3	6	3	10	49	51	27
Males								
Total poisoning deaths	**19,644**	**30**	**50**	**642**	**1,788**	**9,118**	**7,440**	**576**
Deaths per 100,000 population	13.2	0.3	0.2	5.8	16.5	21.6	19.9	3.6
Total drug-related poisoning deaths	18,029	20	33	582	1,668	8,543	6,749	434
Nonopioid analgesics, antipyretics and antirheumatics (X40)	122	1	1	2	5	54	46	13
Antiepileptic, sedative-hypnotic, antiparkinsonism and psychotropic drugs, n.e.c. (X41)	934	4	3	11	48	395	447	26
Narcotics and psychodysleptics (hallucinogens), n.e.c. (X42)	9,380	8	16	342	875	4,428	3,585	126
Other drugs acting on the autonomic nervous system (X43)	3	0	0	0	1	1	1	0
Other and unspecified drugs, medicaments and biological substances (X44)	7,590	7	13	227	739	3,665	2,670	269
Alcohol (X45)	1,033	1	3	33	74	386	483	53
Organic solvents and halogenated hydrocarbons and their vapors (X46)	64	1	3	6	8	26	17	3
Other gases and vapors (X47)	430	8	7	19	29	128	165	74
Pesticides (X48)	2	0	0	0	0	1	0	1
Other and unspecified chemical and noxious substances (X49)	86	0	4	2	9	34	26	11
Females								
Total poisoning deaths	**10,202**	**23**	**31**	**196**	**533**	**4,157**	**4,686**	**576**
Deaths per 100,000 population	6.7	0.2	0.2	1.9	5.3	10.1	11.9	2.6
Total drug-related poisoning deaths	9,629	14	20	172	505	3,998	4,452	468
Nonopioid analgesics, antipyretics and antirheumatics (X40)	168	0	0	3	8	63	64	30
Antiepileptic, sedative-hypnotic, antiparkinsonism and psychotropic drugs, n.e.c. (X41)	611	2	1	15	26	225	310	32
Narcotics and psychodysleptics (hallucinogens), n.e.c. (X42)	3,650	6	10	83	213	1,570	1,675	93
Other drugs acting on the autonomic nervous system (X43)	7	1	0	0	0	1	4	1
Other and unspecified drugs, medicaments and biological substances (X44)	5,193	5	9	71	258	2,139	2,399	312
Alcohol (X45)	323	0	1	15	17	113	159	18
Organic solvents and halogenated hydrocarbons and their vapors (X46)	13	0	0	3	1	6	2	1
Other gases and vapors (X47)	173	6	8	5	9	25	47	73
Pesticides (X48)	1	0	0	0	0	0	1	0
Other and unspecified chemical and noxious substances (X49)	63	3	2	1	1	15	25	16

Source: National Safety Council tabulations of National Center for Health Statistics mortality data.
Note: "n.e.c." means "not elsewhere classified."
[a]Numbers following titles refer to external cause of injury and poisoning classifications in ICD-10.

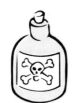

UNINTENTIONAL FATAL POISONINGS

(CONT.)

UNINTENTIONAL POISONING DEATHS, UNITED STATES, 1996–2007

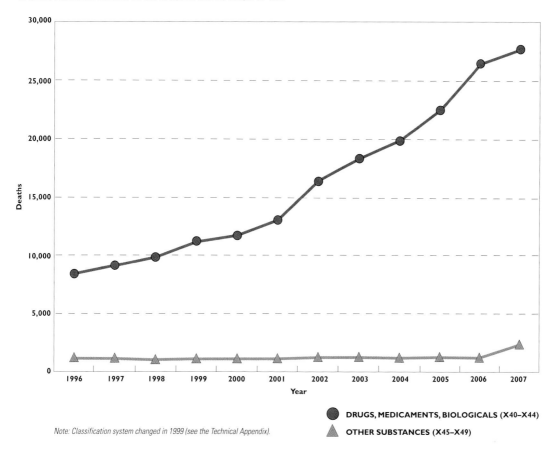

Note: Classification system changed in 1999 (see the Technical Appendix).

● DRUGS, MEDICAMENTS, BIOLOGICALS (X40–X44)

▲ OTHER SUBSTANCES (X45–X49)

ESTIMATED NUMBERS OF EMERGENCY DEPARTMENT VISITS INVOLVING LEGAL DRUGS
USED NONMEDICALLY AND ILLEGAL DRUGS, UNITED STATES, 2008

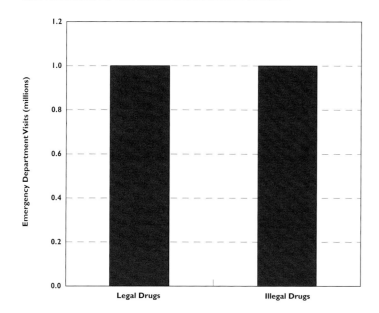

Source: Unintentional Drug Poisoning in the United States, accessed July 8, 2010,
at www.cdc.gov/HomeandRecreationalSafety/pdf/poison-issue-brief.pdf,

FATAL VS. NONFATAL UNINTENTIONAL POISONING

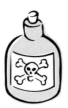

Most people think of poisoning as a childhood issue. That is true for exposure to poisons, but not for nonfatal and fatal poisonings. The pie charts below show the distribution of poisoning exposures, nonfatal poisonings, and fatal poisonings by age group. Poisoning exposure data are from the American Association of Poison Control Centers and represents calls received by poison control centers. The nonfatal data represents emergency department visits, while the fatality data are from death certificates.

Nonfatal exposures occur predominantly among young children, whereas nonfatal and fatal poisonings are overwhelmingly among adults. While more than half of the posioning exposures involve children 5 and younger, nearly 85% of the nonfatal poisonings and 99% of the fatalities occur among adults 19 and older.

POISONING EXPOSURES AND DEATHS BY AGE GROUP, UNITED STATES, SELECTED YEARS

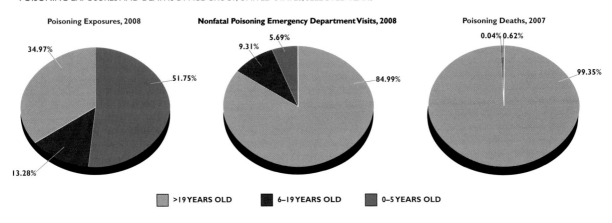

Overall, both fatal and nonfatal unintentional poisonings are on the rise. The charts below illustrate

that both categories of poisonings have increased since 2001.

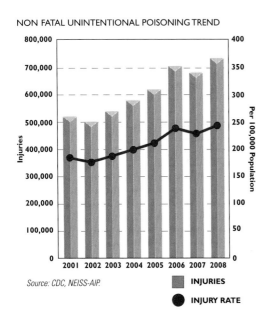

NON FATAL UNINTENTIONAL POISONING TREND

Source: CDC, NEISS-AIP.

INJURIES
INJURY RATE

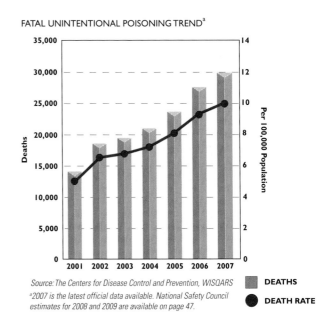

FATAL UNINTENTIONAL POISONING TREND[a]

Source: The Centers for Disease Control and Prevention, WISQARS
[a]2007 is the latest official data available. National Safety Council estimates for 2008 and 2009 are available on page 47.

DEATHS
DEATH RATE

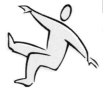

OLDER ADULT FALLS

The impact of unintentional falls on the older adult population has been highlighted in numerous editions of *Injury Facts*. In 2008 alone, 2,114,113 individuals 65 or older were treated in hospital emergency departments for nonfatal unintentional fall injuries. This compares sharply with the 55-64 age group that accounted for only 742,735 fall-related emergency department visits. The prevalence of fall-related fatalities also is strongly associated with age. As shown in the chart below, the number of fall deaths among the 65 or older age group is 4 times as much as the number of fall deaths among all other age groups. The number and rate of fall deaths among older individuals also is increasing while other ages have shown little to no increase since 1999. From 1999 to 2007, the number of unintentional fall fatalities among the 65 and older age group increased 81%, while the fatality rate per 100,000 population increased 66% over this same period.

Source: The Centers for Disease Control and Prevention, NEISS-AIP, Bureau of the Census population data, and National Safety Council analysis of National Center for Health Statistics mortality data.

FALL DEATHS AND DEATH RATES, UNITED STATES, 1999–2007

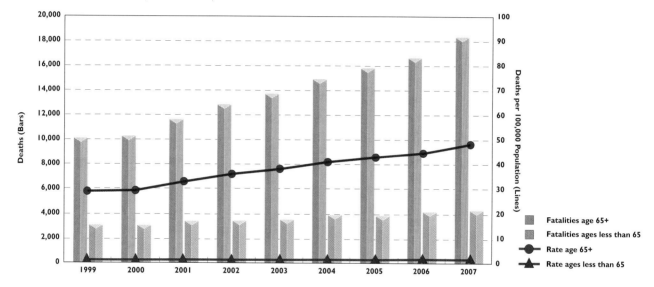

A recent study found a strong association between chronic pain and fall risk. Chronic pain measured according to number of locations, severity, or pain interference with daily activities was associated with greater risk of falls in older adults. Among people who reported severe or very severe pain, there was a 77% increased likelihood for a fall within one month compared with those who reported no pain. Even very mild pain increased the chance of a fall by 36%.

PAIN RATINGS FROM OLDER ADULTS AND PERCENT INCREASED LIKELIHOOD OF A SUBSEQUENT FALL WITHIN ONE MONTH

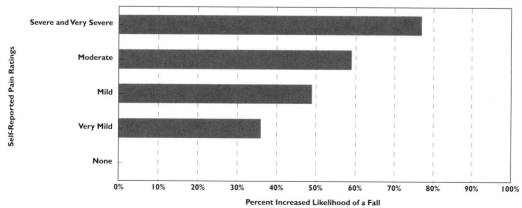

Source: Leveille, S.G., Jones, R.N., Kiely, D.K., et al. (2009). Chronic musculoskeletal pain and the occurrence of falls in an older population. Journal of the American Medical Association, 302 (20), 2214-2221.

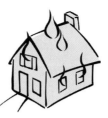

FIRES

152

A study of 34 injury specialists rated a wide range of home injury hazards and prevention strategies to determine injury prevention priorities for children 1 to 5 years of age. The study found "access to fire starting materials" to be the third most important household hazard behind "access to firearms in the home" and "direct access to a pool." In addition, the group of experts concluded that installing smoke alarms in the home was the single most important injury prevention activity.

According to the National Fire Protection Association, in 2008, an estimated 12,000 structure fires involving fire-play were reported to U.S. municipal fire departments, with associated losses of 70 civilian deaths and 840 civilian injuries. Of these structure fires, 7,600 occurred in the home, resulting in the majority of both

the deaths and injuries. While most child-play fires occur outdoors (40,600 in 2008), they accounted for relatively few deaths and injuries with no deaths and only 60 civilian fire injuries in 2008.

As shown in the graph below, fires started by 5 year olds accounted for 39% of all civilian child-play fire deaths, while fires started by 4 year olds accounted for another 27% of the deaths. While fires started by 4 and 5 year olds accounted for the most deaths, these age groups did not account for the most fire-play victims. While about 14% of the fire-play victims were 4 years old and another 16% were 5 years old, fully 34% of the victims were 3 or younger. However, fires started by these younger age groups, younger than 4, accounted for only 6% of the deaths.

CHILD PLAYING WITH FIRE, HOME FIRES BY AGES OF FIRE SETTER, 2004–2008

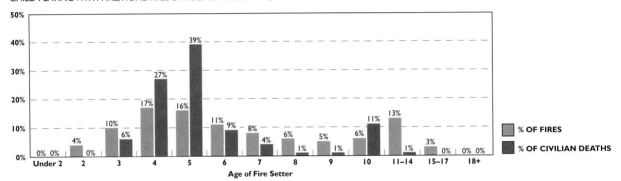

As shown in the graph below, fires involving fire-play are on the decline. Since 1980, all structure fires involving fire-play have decreased 80% and home structure fires have decreased 83%. Outside and other fires have decreased 78% since 1980. 1995 was the first full year for the child-resistant lighter standard. Since 1994, outside and other fires involving fire-play have decreased 50%, home structure fires have decreased

68%, and structure fires as a whole have decreased 59%.

Sources: Katcher, M.L., Meister, A.N., Sorkness, C.A., Staresinic, A.G., Pierce, S.E., Goodman, B.M., Peterson, N.M., Hatfield, P.M., and Schirmer, J.A. (2006). Use of the modified Delphi technique to identify and rate home injury hazard risks and prevention methods for your children. Injury Prevention. (12) 189-194.

Hall, J.R. (2010, October). Children Playing With Fires. Quincy, MA: National Fire Protection Association.

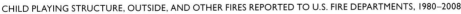

CHILD PLAYING STRUCTURE, OUTSIDE, AND OTHER FIRES REPORTED TO U.S. FIRE DEPARTMENTS, 1980–2008

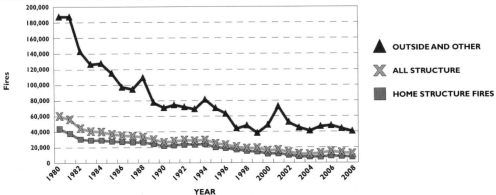

PEDALCYCLES

The estimated number of deaths from collisions between pedalcycles and motor vehicles increased from about 750 in 1940 to 1,200 in 1980, and then declined to about 800 in 2009. Nonfatal medically consulted injuries[a] were estimated at 100,000 in 2009.

In 2007, 578 pedalcyclists died in motor vehicle crashes and 242 in other accidents, according to National Center for Health Statistics mortality data. Males accounted for 89% of all pedalcycle deaths, nearly 8 times the female fatalities.

Emergency department-treated injuries associated with bicycles and bicycle accessories were estimated to total 516,261 in 2008 and 544,470 in 2009, according to the U.S. Consumer Product Safety Commission (see page 156).

A meta-analysis of bicycle helmet efficacy by Attewell, Glase, and McFadden (2001) estimated that bicycle helmets reduce the risk of all head injuries by 60% and brain injury by 58%. In 2009, 21 states, the District of Columbia, and at least 201 localities had bicycle helmet-use laws, according to the Bicycle Helmet Safety Institute.

Source: National Safety Council estimates and tabulations of National Center for Health Statistics mortality data obtained via WISQARS at www.cdc.gov/injury/wisqars/index.html. Population data for rates are from the U.S. Census Bureau. Data from Bicycle Helmet Safety Institute retrieved 9/29/10 from www.bhsi.org.
Attewell, R.G., Glase, K., and McFadden, M. (2001). Bicycle helmet efficacy: a meta-analysis. Accident Analysis & Prevention, 33 (3). 345-352.
[a]Nonfatal medically consulted injuries are not comparable to estimates provided in earlier editions that used the definition of disabling injury. Please see the Technical Appendix for more information regarding medically consulted injuries.

PEDALCYCLE DEATHS AND DEATH RATES BY SEX AND AGE GROUP, UNITED STATES, 2007

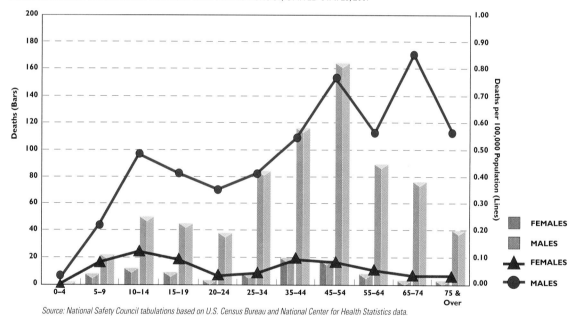

Source: National Safety Council tabulations based on U.S. Census Bureau and National Center for Health Statistics data.

PEDALCYCLE FATALITIES BY MONTH, UNITED STATES, 2007

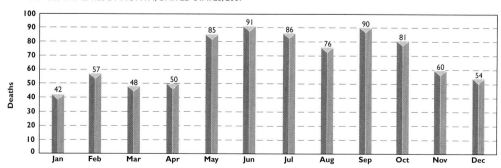

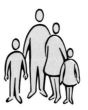

154

The leading risks for unintentional injury vary with age and are different for deaths and for nonfatal injuries. The tables here and on the next page list, for eight age groups, the five leading causes of UI death and the five leading causes of hospital emergency department visits, which is one measure of nonfatal injuries.

For all ages, the five leading causes account for 84% of all UI deaths and 75% of UI ED visits. Only motor vehicle crashes and falls are common to both lists. Motor vehicle crashes rank first for UI deaths and fourth for UI ED visits. Falls rank third for UI deaths and first for ED UI visits.

The five leading causes of UI deaths account for

between 80% and 93% of such deaths depending on the age group. The leading causes of UI ED visits account for between 73% and 88% of such hospital visits.

For deaths, motor vehicle crashes; poisoning; falls; fire, flames, and smoke; and drowning are most often among the top five with choking, firearms, and mechanical suffocation sometimes included. For ED visits, falls, struck by or against, overexertion, motor vehicle occupant injuries, and cut or pierce injuries are most often in the top five. In the younger age groups, bites and stings (except dog bites), foreign body injuries, and struck by or against are among the leading risks.

LEADING UNINTENTIONAL INJURY RISKS, ALL AGES, UNITED STATES, 2007

Rank	Unintentional injury deaths				Emergency department UI visits			
	Event	Number	Percent	Rate[a]	Event	Number	Percent	Rate[a]
—	Total	123,706	100.0%	41.1	Total	27,731,818	100.0%	9,204
1	Motor vehicle crashes	43,945	35.5%	14.6	Falls	8,035,635	29.0%	2,667
2	Poisoning	29,846	24.1%	9.9	Struck by/against	4,554,023	16.4%	1,512
3	Falls	22,631	18.3%	7.5	Overexertion	3,542,728	12.8%	1,176
4	Choking[b]	4,344	3.5%	1.4	Motor vehicle occupant	2,655,425	9.6%	881
5	Drowning	3,443	2.8%	1.1	Cut or pierce	2,123,862	7.7%	705

LEADING UNINTENTIONAL INJURY RISKS, YOUNG CHILDREN (AGES 0-4), UNITED STATES, 2007

Rank	Unintentional injury deaths				Emergency department UI visits			
	Event	Number	Percent	Rate[a]	Event	Number	Percent	Rate[a]
—	Total	2,873	100.0%	13.9	Total	2,201,699	100.0%	10,621
1	Mechanical suffocation	961	33.4%	4.6	Falls	949,089	43.1%	4,578
2	Motor vehicle crashes	675	23.5%	3.3	Struck by or against	403,451	18.3%	1,946
3	Drowning	515	17.9%	2.5	Bite or sting (except dog)	146,427	6.7%	706
4	Fires, flames, and smoke	239	8.3%	1.2	Foreign body	136,507	6.2%	658
5	Choking[b]	147	5.1%	0.7	Overexertion	89,111	4.0%	430

LEADING UNINTENTIONAL INJURY RISKS, CHILDREN AND YOUNG ADOLESCENTS (AGES 5-14), UNITED STATES, 2007

Rank	Unintentional injury deaths				Emergency department UI visits			
	Event	Number	Percent	Rate[a]	Event	Number	Percent	Rate[a]
—	Total	2,194	100.0%	5.5	Total	3,858,134	100.0%	9,614
1	Motor vehicle crashes	1,285	58.6%	3.2	Falls	1,209,433	31.3%	3,014
2	Drowning	224	10.2%	0.6	Struck by or against	979,498	25.4%	2,441
3	Fires, flames, and smoke	211	9.6%	0.5	Overexertion	364,989	9.5%	910
4	Poisoning	81	3.7%	0.2	Cut or pierce	248,849	6.4%	620
5	Mechanical suffocation	72	3.3%	0.2	Pedalcyclist	210,735	5.5%	525

LEADING UNINTENTIONAL INJURY RISKS, TEENS (AGES 15-19), UNITED STATES, 2007

Rank	Unintentional injury deaths				Emergency department UI visits			
	Event	Number	Percent	Rate[a]	Event	Number	Percent	Rate[a]
—	Total	6,493	100.0%	30.3	Total	2,784,818	100.0%	12,985
1	Motor vehicle crashes	4,723	72.7%	22.0	Struck by or against	610,705	21.9%	2,848
2	Poisoning	838	12.9%	3.9	Falls	476,366	17.1%	2,221
3	Drowning	317	4.9%	1.5	Overexertion	416,783	15.0%	1,943
4	Falls	86	1.3%	0.4	Motor vehicle occupant	387,574	13.9%	1,807
4	Fires, flames, and smoke	86	1.3%	0.4	Cut or pierce	208,722	7.5%	973

See source and footnotes on page 155.

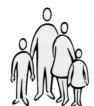

LEADING UNINTENTIONAL INJURY RISKS, YOUNG ADULTS (AGES 20-24), UNITED STATES, 2007

Rank	Unintentional injury deaths				Emergency department UI visits			
	Event	Number	Percent	Rate[a]	Event	Number	Percent	Rate[a]
—	Total	9,404	100.0%	44.9	Total	2,559,020	100.0%	12,208
1	Motor vehicle crashes	5,845	62.2%	27.9	Struck by or against	438,310	17.1%	2,091
2	Poisoning	2,321	24.7%	11.1	Falls	418,889	16.4%	1,998
3	Drowning	313	3.3%	1.5	Motor vehicle occupant	394,080	15.4%	1,880
4	Falls	147	1.6%	0.7	Overexertion	385,893	15.1%	1,841
5	Fires, flames, and smoke	108	1.1%	0.5	Cut or pierce	255,524	10.0%	1,219

LEADING UNINTENTIONAL INJURY RISKS, ADULTS (AGES 25-44), UNITED STATES, 2007

Rank	Unintentional injury deaths				Emergency department UI visits			
	Event	Number	Percent	Rate[a]	Event	Number	Percent	Rate[a]
—	Total	31,908	100.0%	38.2	Total	7,962,994	100.0%	9,538
1	Motor vehicle crashes	13,457	42.2%	16.1	Falls	1,536,502	19.3%	1,840
2	Poisoning	13,275	41.6%	15.9	Overexertion	1,365,774	17.2%	1,636
3	Falls	927	2.9%	1.1	Struck by or against	1,235,085	15.5%	1,479
4	Drowning	798	2.5%	1.0	Motor vehicle occupant	985,102	12.4%	1,180
5	Fires, flames, and smoke	529	1.7%	0.6	Cut or pierce	767,008	9.6%	919

LEADING UNINTENTIONAL INJURY RISKS, ADULTS (AGES 45-64), UNITED STATES, 2007

Rank	Unintentional injury deaths				Emergency department UI visits			
	Event	Number	Percent	Rate[a]	Event	Number	Percent	Rate[a]
—	Total	32,508	100.0%	42.4	Total	5,252,852	100.0%	6,858
1	Poisoning	12,126	37.3%	15.8	Falls	1,517,161	28.9%	1,981
2	Motor vehicle crashes	10,889	33.5%	14.2	Overexertion	725,557	13.8%	947
3	Falls	3,043	9.4%	4.0	Struck by or against	653,421	12.4%	853
4	Fires, flames, and smoke	980	3.0%	1.3	Motor vehicle occupant	537,051	10.2%	701
5	Drowning	805	2.5%	1.1	Cut or pierce	431,803	8.2%	564

LEADING UNINTENTIONAL INJURY RISKS, OLDER ADULTS (AGES 65-74), UNITED STATES, 2007

Rank	Unintentional injury deaths				Emergency department UI visits			
	Event	Number	Percent	Rate[a]	Event	Number	Percent	Rate[a]
—	Total	8,753	100.0%	45.2	Total	1,190,552	100.0%	6,146
1	Motor vehicle crashes	2,940	33.6%	15.2	Falls	566,773	47.6%	2,926
2	Falls	2,594	29.6%	13.4	Struck by or against	115,580	9.7%	597
3	Poisoning	602	6.9%	3.1	Overexertion	106,770	9.0%	551
4	Choking[b]	561	6.4%	2.9	Motor vehicle occupant	94,830	8.0%	490
5	Fires, flames, and smoke	421	4.8%	2.2	Cut or pierce	75,370	6.3%	389

LEADING UNINTENTIONAL INJURY RISKS, ELDERLY (AGE 75 AND OLDER), UNITED STATES, 2007

Rank	Unintentional injury deaths				Emergency department UI visits			
	Event	Number	Percent	Rate[a]	Event	Number	Percent	Rate[a]
—	Total	29,539	100.0%	159.0	Total	1,917,631	100.0%	10,325
1	Falls	15,740	53.3%	84.7	Falls	1,360,994	71.0%	7,328
2	Motor vehicle	4,122	14.0%	22.2	Struck by or against	117,523	6.1%	633
3	Choking[b]	2,529	8.6%	13.6	Overexertion	87,787	4.6%	473
4	Fires, flames, and smoke	708	2.4%	3.8	Motor vehicle occupant	77,578	4.0%	418
5	Poisoning	547	1.9%	2.9	Cut or pierce	47,887	2.5%	258

Source: National Safety Council analysis of NCHS mortality data and CDC, NCIPC, NEISS-AIP data.
[a]*Deaths or emergency department visits per 100,000 population.*
[b]*Inhalation and ingestion of food or other objects.*

INJURIES ASSOCIATED WITH CONSUMER PRODUCTS

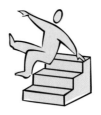

More than 2 million injury-related emergency department visits each year are associated with stairs, steps, floors, and flooring materials.

The following list of items found in and around the home was selected from the U.S. Consumer Product Safety Commission's National Electronic Injury Surveillance System for 2009. NEISS estimates are calculated from a statistically representative sample of hospitals in the United States. Injury totals represent estimates of the number of hospital emergency department-treated cases nationwide associated with various products. However, product involvement may or may not be the cause of the injury.

CONSUMER PRODUCT-RELATED INJURIES TREATED IN HOSPITAL EMERGENCY DEPARTMENTS, 2009
(excluding most sports or sports equipment; see page 140)

Description	Injuries
Home workshop equipment	
Saws (hand or power)	86,617
Hammers	32,933
Tools (not specified)	24,264
Packaging and containers, household	
Household containers and packaging	224,227
Bottles and jars	75,340
Bags	41,215
Paper products	24,864
Housewares	
Knives	409,590
Tableware and flatware (excl. knives)	97,389
Drinking glasses	81,552
Waste containers, trash baskets, etc.	37,750
Cookware, bowls, and canisters	31,294
Scissors	29,121
Manual cleaning equipment (excludes buckets)	23,839
Other kitchen gadgets	20,864
Home furnishing, fixtures, and accessories	
Beds	613,870
Chairs	352,691
Tables, n.e.c.[a]	344,036
Household cabinets, racks, and shelves	289,311
Bathtubs and showers	274,109
Ladders	188,492
Sofas, couches, davenports, divans, etc.	175,972
Rugs and carpets	142,515
Other furniture[b]	125,669
Toilets	86,450
Stools	58,326
Misc. decorating items	41,827
Benches	33,976
Sinks	27,377
Mirrors or mirror glass	25,156
Home structures and construction materials	
Floors or flooring materials	1,334,455
Stairs or steps	1,266,319
Ceilings and walls	341,956
Other doors[c]	322,951
Porches, balconies, open-side floors	145,345
Nails, screws, tacks or bolts	132,385
Windows	115,561
Fences or fence posts	112,445
Door sills or frames	57,850
Counters or countertops	53,134
Handrails, railings or banisters	47,281
Poles	43,937
Glass doors	28,173
House repair and construction materials	23,925
Cabinet or door hardware	20,947

Description	Injuries
General household appliances	
Refrigerators	40,536
Ranges or ovens (not specified)	29,655
Heating, cooling, and ventilating equipment	
Pipes (excluding smoking pipes)	31,343
Home Communication and Entertainment Equipment	
Televisions	68,486
Computers (equipment and electronic games)	32,434
Personal use items	
Footwear	169,208
Wheelchairs	129,001
Crutches, canes, walkers	108,751
Jewelry	83,535
Daywear	60,274
First aid equipment	42,567
Razors and shavers	40,742
Other clothing[d]	38,056
Desk supplies	34,105
Coins	33,934
Hair grooming equipment and accessories	23,866
Luggage	23,808
Yard and garden equipment	
Lawn mowers	86,272
Pruning, trimming and edging equipment	41,880
Other unpowered garden tools[e]	28,969
Chainsaws	26,593
Manual snow or ice removal tools	26,518
Sports and recreation	
Bicycles	544,470
Skateboards	144,416
Toys, n.e.c.	101,394
Trampolines	97,908
Monkey bars or other playground climbing equipment	78,024
Minibikes or trailbikes	74,913
Swings or swing sets	66,018
Scooters (unpowered)	59,429
Dancing	52,911
Aquariums and other pet supplies	51,008
Slides or sliding boards	49,693
Other playground equipment[f]	36,369
Sleds	29,058
Bleachers	21,309
Amusement park attractions (including rides)	20,301
Miscellaneous products	
Carts	48,423
Hot water	40,741
Elevators, escalators, moving walks	21,876

Source: U.S. Consumer Product Safety Commission, National Electronic Injury Surveillance System, Product Summary Report, All Products, CY2009.
Note: Products are listed above if the estimate was greater than 20,000 cases.
n.e.c. = not elsewhere classified.
[a]Excludes baby-changing tables (4,666 injuries) and television tables or stands (12,616 injuries).
[b]Excludes cabinets, racks, shelves, desks, bureaus, chests, buffets, etc. (289,311 injuries).

[c]Excludes glass doors (28,173 injuries) and garage doors (17,719 injuries).
[d]Excludes costumes, masks, daywear, footwear (169,208 injuries), nightwear (4,755 injuries), and outerwear (15,646 injuries).
[e]Includes cultivators, hoes, pitchforks, rakes, shovels, spades, and trowels.
[f]Excludes monkey bars (78,024 injuries), seesaws (3,658 injuries), slides (49,693 injuries), and swings (66,018 injuries).

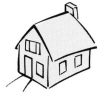
PRINCIPAL TYPES OF HOME AND COMMUNITY UNINTENTIONAL INJURY DEATHS, UNITED STATES, 1987-2009

Year	Total home and community[a]	Falls	Drowning	Poisoning	Choking[b]	Fire, flames, smoke	Firearms	Mechanical suffocation	Air transport	Water transport	Rail transport[c]	Other
1987	39,800	10,300	3,900	4,900	3,600	4,400	1,400	(d)	900	800	400	9,200
1988	41,100	10,700	3,800	5,700	3,700	4,600	1,400	(d)	700	800	400	9,300
1989	40,700	10,800	3,700	5,900	3,500	4,400	1,400	(d)	800	700	400	9,100
1990	38,900	11,000	3,700	5,400	3,300	3,800	1,300	(d)	700	800	400	8,500
1991	39,700	11,400	3,700	6,000	3,100	3,800	1,400	(d)	700	700	500	8,400
1992	43,000	12,100	3,400	6,900	3,100	3,900	1,400	(d)	700	700	600	10,200
1993	45,800	12,500	3,700	8,400	3,200	3,900	1,500	(d)	600	700	600	10,700
1994	45,900	12,800	3,300	8,900	3,100	3,900	1,300	(d)	600	600	600	10,800
1995	47,300	13,400	3,700	9,000	3,100	3,700	1,200	(d)	600	700	500	11,400
1996	48,500	14,300	3,400	9,400	3,200	3,700	1,100	(d)	700	600	500	11,600
1997	49,400	14,700	3,500	10,100	3,200	3,400	1,000	(d)	500	600	400	12,000
1998	51,600	15,500	3,900	10,700	3,500	3,100	900	(d)	500	600	500	12,400
1999[e]	52,700	12,400	3,500	12,100	3,900	3,200	900	1,600	500	600	400	13,600
2000	51,900	12,600	3,400	12,700	4,300	2,900	800	1,300	500	500	400	12,500
2001	55,000	14,200	3,300	14,000	4,100	3,200	800	1,400	700	500	400	12,400
2002	58,700	15,600	3,400	17,500	4,100	3,100	700	1,400	500	500	400	11,500
2003	61,800	16,600	3,200	19,300	4,300	3,200	700	1,300	600	500	400	11,700
2004	64,200	18,000	3,300	20,900	4,400	3,100	600	1,400	400	500	400	11,200
2005	69,600	18,800	3,500	23,500	4,400	3,100	(d)	1,500	400	500	400	13,500
2006	73,300	20,000	3,500	27,400	4,400	3,000	(d)	1,600	400	400	400	12,200
2007[f]	77,200	21,800	3,400	29,700	4,300	3,200	(d)	1,600	400	400	400	12,000
2008[f]	83,700	23,600	3,400	34,200	4,500	3,100	(d)	1,600	400	400	400	12,100
2009[g]	90,300	25,500	3,500	38,800	4,500	3,100	(d)	1,700	400	400	400	12,000

Source: National Safety Council estimates based on data from National Center for Health Statistics and state vital statistics departments. The Council adopted the Bureau of Labor Statistics Census of Fatal Occupational Injuries counts for work-related unintentional injuries retroactive to 1992 data. Because of the lower Work class total resulting from this change, several thousand unintentional injury deaths that had been classified by the Council as work-related had to be reassigned to the Home and Public classes. For this reason, long-term historical comparisons for these three classes should be made with caution. See the Technical Appendix for an explanation of the methodological changes.
[a]Includes some deaths not shown separately.
[b]Inhalation and ingestion of food or other object that obstructs breathing.
[c]Includes subways and elevated trains.
[d]Estimates for both home and public are not available.
[e]In 1999, a revision was made in the International Classification of Diseases. See the Technical Appendix for comparability with earlier years.
[f]Revised.
[g]Preliminary.

OVERVIEW OF INTENTIONAL INJURY DEATHS, UNITED STATES, 2007

Total Injury Deaths: 182,479

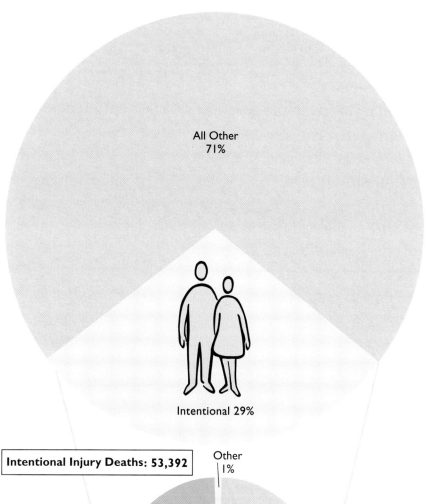

All Other
71%

Intentional 29%

Intentional Injury Deaths: 53,392

Other
1%

Homicide
34%

Suicide
65%

Age Distribution of Homicides

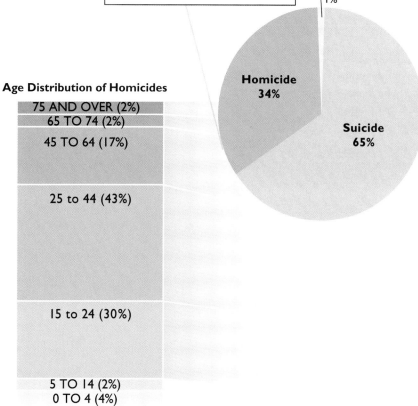

75 AND OVER (2%)
65 TO 74 (2%)
45 TO 64 (17%)
25 to 44 (43%)
15 to 24 (30%)
5 TO 14 (2%)
0 TO 4 (4%)

Age Distribution of SUICIDE

75 AND OVER (9%)
65 TO 74 (7%)
45 to 64 (37%)
25 TO 44 (35%)
15 to 24 (12%)

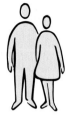

Injuries may be divided into three broad groups— unintentional, intentional, and undetermined intent. Most of *Injury Facts* presents data on unintentional (accidental) injuries. This section presents data on intentional injuries.

Under the World Health Organization's Safe Communities initiative, for which the National Safety Council is the affiliate support center in the United States, injury prevention is not limited to unintentional injuries. Data on intentional injuries is presented here to support Safe Communities and complement the unintentional injury data shown in other sections of *Injury Facts*.

Intentional injuries may be divided into four subgroups: intentional self-harm (suicide), assault (homicide), legal intervention, and operations of war. The diagram below illustrates the injury groupings and shows the death totals for 2007.

INJURY DEATHS BY INTENT, UNITED STATES, 2007

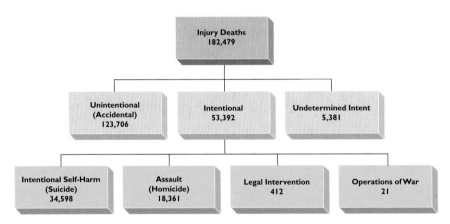

Intentional self-harm includes suicide and attempted suicide by purposely self-inflicted poisoning or injury. The most common methods of intentional self-harm that result in death are firearms; hanging, strangulation, and suffocation; and poisoning.

Assault includes homicide and injuries inflicted by another person with intent to injure or kill (excluding legal intervention and operations of war). The most common means of homicide are firearms; sharp objects; and hanging, strangulation, and suffocation.

Legal intervention includes legal execution. Operations of war include injuries to military personnel and civilians caused by war and civil insurrection. The death must have occurred in the United States. In the vital statistics system, war deaths (and other deaths) occurring outside the United States are counted by the country in which they occurred.

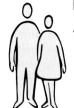

Each of the three broad groups of injuries was among the 15 leading causes of deaths in the United States in 2007. Unintentional (accidental) injuries ranked 5th, intentional self-harm (suicide) ranked 11th, and assault (homicide) ranked 15th.

Intentional self-harm ranked as high as second (after unintentional injuries) for people ages 13 and from 28 to 34, and ranked third for those ages 12, 13, and 15-27. Suicide deaths were highest at ages 44 and 48

(825) and ranked fourth at these ages after cancer, heart disease, and unintentional injuries. Assault ranked as high as second (after unintentional injuries) for people ages 2 and 15-27. It ranked third among people ages 1, 3, 4, 6, 13, 14, and 29 to 31. Homicide deaths were highest at age 19 (683). For people ages 15-31, accidents, homicide, and suicide were the three leading causes of death. The graph below shows the number of deaths due to injuries by single year of age from 0 to 100.

INJURY DEATHS BY AGE, UNITED STATES, 2007

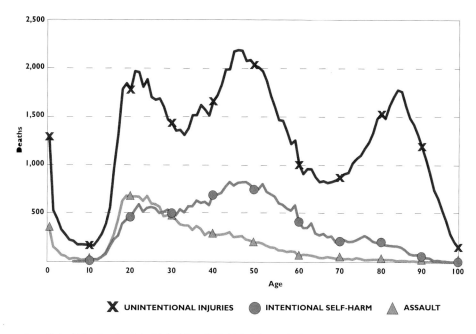

Source: National Safety Council analysis of National Center for Health Statistics mortality data.

Males have higher death rates than females for injuries of all intents. Males also have higher nonfatal injury rates than females for unintentional injuries and assault.

Females, however, have a higher injury rate than males for intentional self-harm.

DEATH AND NONFATAL INJURY RATES BY INTENT AND SEX, UNITED STATES, 2007

Sex	Deaths per 100,000 population			Nonfatal Injuries per 100,000 population		
	Unintentional	Homicide	Suicide	Unintentional	Assault	Self-harm
Both sexes	41.1	6.1	11.5	9,204	514	131
Males	53.8	9.8	18.4	10,208	638	109
Females	28.7	2.5	4.8	8,226	394	152
Ratio of male to female	1.9	3.9	3.8	1.2	1.6	0.7

Source: The Centers for Disease Control and Prevention, the National Center for Injury Prevention and Contol, and Web-based Injury Statistics Query and Reporting System.

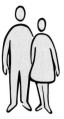

TRENDS

162

The graph below shows the trends from 1992 to the present in injury deaths and death rates. Unintentional injury deaths and death rates have increased by 47.4% and 26.5%, respectively. Suicide deaths increased 13.5%, but the death rate declined 2.4%. Homicide deaths and death rates decreased 27.0% and 37.8%, respectively, over the 1992-2007 period. Age-adjusted death rates, which remove the effects of the changing age distribution of the population, increased 20.1% for unintentional injuries and decreased 5.8% for suicide and 35.3% for homicide.

INJURY DEATHS AND DEATH RATES, UNITED STATES, 1992–2007

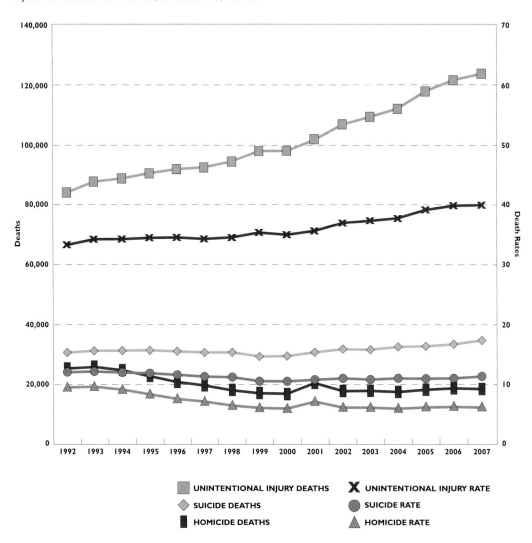

Source: National Safety Council analysis of National Center for Health Statistics mortality data.

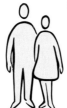

Several national surveys provide information on the amount of medical care provided for injuries. The National Electronic Injury Surveillance System All Injuries Program (NEISS-AIP) provides estimates of the number of injury episodes treated in hospital emergency departments. The most recent estimates (2008) are 27.9 million cases involving unintentional injuries, 1.6 million involving assault, and 0.4 million involving self harm.[a]

The National Hospital Ambulatory Medical Care Survey (NHAMCS) is another survey of emergency department visits with results that are similar to the NEISS-AIP. The latest NHAMCS estimates (2007) are 26.0 million unintentional injury visits, 1.5 million assault visits, and 0.5 million self-harm visits. Another 0.3 million visits were for injuries of undetermined intent.[b]

The NHAMCS also provides estimates of the number of hospital outpatient department visits for injuries or poisonings. In 2007, about 7.3 million visits were for unintentional injuries or poisonings and 457,000 were for intentional injuries or poisonings. An additional 2.3 million visits were for injuries or poisonings of undetermined intent.[c]

The National Ambulatory Medical Care Survey (NAMCS) gives estimates of the number of physician office visits for injuries. In 2007, more than 68.8 million office visits were for unintentional injuries or poisoning and about 1.7 million visits were for intentional injuries or poisoning. An additional 27.2 million visits were for injuries or poisoning episodes of unknown intent.[d]

According to the National Hospital Discharge Survey, about 1.9 million people were hospitalized for intentional and unintentional injuries in 2007.[e]

Apart from surveys of medical care utilization for intentional injuries, there are estimates of the general incidence of self-harm and violent behavior within the population. Overall, there is one suicide for every 25 attempts. For youth between 15 and 24 years old, the ratio is 1 suicide for every 100-200 attempts. For adults age 65 and older, there is one suicide for every four attempts.[f]

The National Crime Victimization Survey for 2008 reported a total of 21.3 million victimizations (involving either a person or household as the victim), of which 5.0 million were personal crimes and 16.3 million were property crimes. Of the personal crimes, 4.9 million were crimes of violence, which include rape and sexual assault (0.2 million), robbery (0.6 million), and assault (4.1 million). Personal theft accounted for more than 0.1 million victimizations. A weapon was present in 20% of violent crime incidents.[g]

[a]The Centers for Disease Control and Prevention, the National Center for Injury Prevention and Contol, and Web-based Injury Statistics Query and Reporting System. Retrieved Sept. 24, 2010, from http://webappa.cdc.gov/sasweb/ncipc/nfirates2001.html.
[b]Pitts, S.R., Niska, R.W., Xu, J., and Burt, C.W. (2008). National hospital ambulatory medical care survey: 2007 emergency department summary. National Health Statistics Report, No. 7. Hyattsville, MD: National Center for Health Statistics.
[c]Hing, E., Hall, M.J., and Xu, J. (2010). National hospital ambulatory medical care survey: 2007 outpatient department summary. National Health Statistics Report, No. 4. Hyattsville, MD: National Center for Health Statistics.
[d]Cherry, D.K., Hing, E., Woodwell, D.A., and Rechtsteiner, E.A. (2010). National ambulatory medical care survey: 2007 summary. National Health Statistics Report, No. 3. Hyattsville, MD: National Center for Health Statistics.
[e]DeFrances, C.J., Lucas, C.A., Buie, V.C., and Golosinskiy, A. (2010). National hospital discharge survey: 2007 summary. National Health Statistics Report, No. 5. Hyattsville, MD: National Center for Health Statistics.
[f]Goldsmith, S.K., Pellmar, T.C., Kleinman, A.M., and Bunney, W.E. (Eds.). (2002). Reducing Suicide: A National Imperative. Washington, DC: National Academy Press.
[g]Rand, M.R. (2009). Criminal Victimization, 2007. NCJ 224390. Washington, DC: U.S. Department of Justice, Bureau of Justice Statistics.

ASSAULT/HOMICIDE

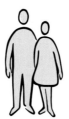

Assault includes homicide and injuries inflicted by another person with intent to injure or kill (excluding legal intervention and operations of war). The four leading forms of fatal assault injuries account for 84% of the total—firearms (69%), sharp objects (11%), hanging, strangulation, and suffocation (3%), and smoke, fire, and flames (1%).

ASSAULT/HOMICIDE DEATHS AND DEATH RATES BY AGE GROUP, UNITED STATES, 2007

	Total	0–4	5–14	15–24	25–44	45–64	65–74	75+
Total	**18,361**	**750**	**346**	**5,551**	**7,810**	**3,120**	**411**	**373**
Rate^a	6.1	3.6	0.9	13.1	9.4	4.1	2.1	2.0
Firearms	12,632	63	201	4,669	5,789	1,605	185	120
Rate^a	4.2	0.3	0.5	11.0	6.9	2.1	1.0	0.6
Sharp objects	1,981	9	35	444	875	496	66	56
Rate^a	0.7	(^b)	0.1	1.0	1.0	0.6	0.3	0.3
Hanging, strangulation, and suffocation	637	62	26	108	226	161	23	31
Rate^a	0.2	0.3	0.1	0.3	0.3	0.2	0.1	0.2
Smoke, fire, and flames	139	18	20	15	41	32	8	5
Rate^a	(^b)	0.1	(^b)	(^b)	(^b)	(^b)	(^b)	(^b)
Other means	2,963	598	64	315	879	826	129	161
Rate^a	1.0	2.9	0.2	0.7	1.1	1.1	0.7	0.9

^aDeaths per 100,000 population in each age group.
^bLess than 0.05.

HOMICIDE DEATH RATES BY AGE GROUP, UNITED STATES, 1994–2007

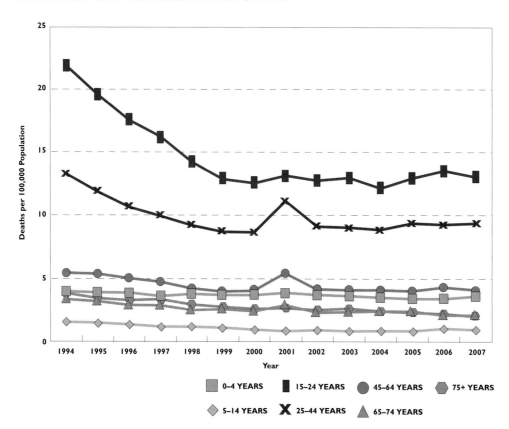

Source: National Safety Council analysis of National Center for Health Statistics mortality data.

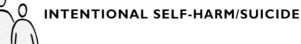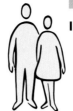

INTENTIONAL SELF-HARM/SUICIDE

Intentional self-harm includes suicide and attempted suicide by purposely self-inflicted poisoning or injury. The four leading forms of fatal self-harm injuries account for 92% of the total—firearms (50%), hanging, strangulation, and suffocation (24%), self-poisoning by drugs and medicines (14%), and self-poisoning by other chemicals and noxious substances (4%). It is generally accepted that children younger than 5 cannot commit suicide.

INTENTIONAL SELF-HARM/SUICIDE DEATHS AND DEATH RATES BY AGE GROUP, UNITED STATES, 2007

	Total	0–4	5–14	15–24	25–44	45–64	65–74	75+
Total	34,598	—	184	4,140	12,000	12,847	2,444	2,983
Rate^a	11.5	—	0.5	9.8	14.4	16.8	12.6	16.1
Firearms	17,352	—	53	1,900	5,185	6,317	1,700	2,197
Rate^a	5.8	—	0.1	4.5	6.2	8.2	8.8	11.8
Hanging, strangulation, and suffocation	8,161	—	122	1,533	3,609	2,314	275	308
Rate^a	2.7	—	0.3	3.6	4.3	3.0	1.4	1.7
Poisoning by drugs and medicines	4,772	—	7	273	1,644	2,408	249	191
Rate^a	1.6	—	(^b)	0.6	2.0	3.1	1.3	1.0
Poisoning by other substances	1,586	—	0	89	577	754	71	95
Rate^a	0.5	—	(^b)	0.2	0.7	1.0	0.4	0.5
Other means	2,727	—	2	345	985	1,054	149	192
Rate^a	0.9	—	(^b)	0.8	1.2	1.4	0.8	1.0

Note: Dashes (—) indicate not applicable.
^aDeaths per 100,000 population in each age group.
^bLess than 0.05.

SUICIDE DEATH RATES BY AGE GROUP, UNITED STATES, 1994–2007

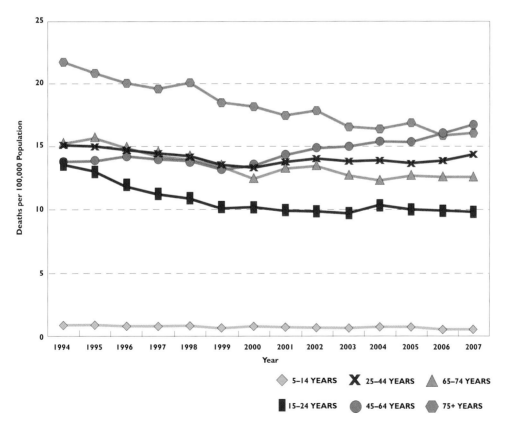

Source: National Safety Council analysis of National Center for Health Statistics mortality data.

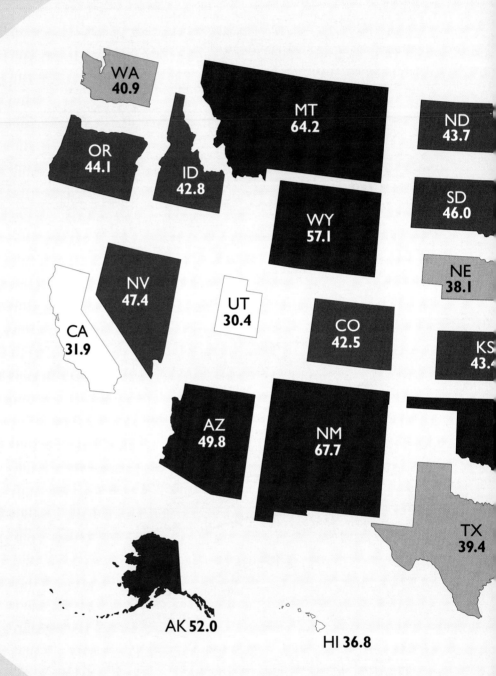

WA
40.9

MT
64.2

ND
43.7

OR
44.1

ID
42.8

SD
46.0

WY
57.1

NE
38.1

NV
47.4

UT
30.4

CO
42.5

KS
43.4

CA
31.9

AZ
49.8

NM
67.7

TX
39.4

AK 52.0

HI 36.8

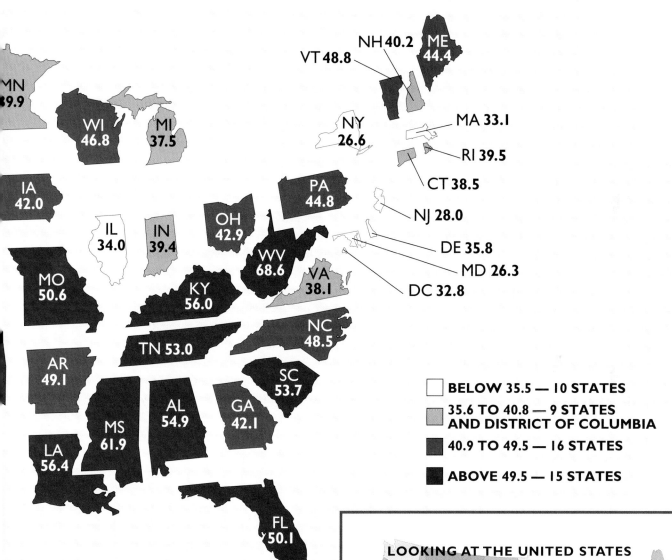

MN
39.9

WI
46.8

MI
37.5

VT 48.8

NH 40.2

ME
44.4

NY
26.6

MA 33.1

RI 39.5

CT 38.5

NJ 28.0

IA
42.0

IL
34.0

IN
39.4

OH
42.9

PA
44.8

DE 35.8

MD 26.3

MO
50.6

WV
68.6

VA
38.1

DC 32.8

KY
56.0

NC
48.5

AR
49.1

TN 53.0

SC
53.7

MS
61.9

AL
54.9

GA
42.1

LA
56.4

FL
50.1

☐ BELOW 35.5 — 10 STATES

⬜ 35.6 TO 40.8 — 9 STATES
AND DISTRICT OF COLUMBIA

⬛ 40.9 TO 49.5 — 16 STATES

■ ABOVE 49.5 — 15 STATES

LOOKING AT THE UNITED STATES IN A NEW WAY

The map illustrated on these two pages scales the 50 states and the District of Columbia in proportion to unintentional injury death rates per 100,000 population. With this scaling, states with below average unintentional injury death rates appear smaller than normal, while states with above average rates appear larger than normal. For comparison, the small map provided in this callout box reflects the traditional view of the United States.

Motor vehicle crashes are the leading cause of unintentional injury deaths in 39 states and the District of Columbia.

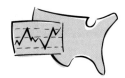

This section on state-level data includes data for occupational and motor vehicle injuries, as well as general injury mortality.

Death rates by state of residence for unintentional injuries can vary greatly from one type of injury to the next, as well as from state to state. The graph on the next page shows the death rates (per 100,000 population) for total UI deaths in each state and the four leading types of UI deaths nationally: motor vehicle crashes, poisonings, falls, and choking (inhalation or ingestion of food or other object that obstructs breathing).

The map on page 170 shows graphically the overall UI death rates by state of residence. Rates by region were lowest in the Middle Atlantic and highest in the East South Central states.

The charts on pages 171-173 show (a) total UI deaths by state of residence and where UIs rank as a cause of death in each state, and (b) the five leading causes of UI deaths in each state.

UIs as a whole are the fifth leading cause of death in the United States, in 22 states and in the District of Columbia. UIs are the third leading cause of death in 11 states, the fourth leading cause in 16 states, and the sixth leading cause in Washington.

In 2007, motor vehicle crashes were the leading cause of UI deaths in 39 states and the District of Columbia. Poisoning was the leading cause in seven states. Falls were the leading cause in Minnesota, Rhode Island, Vermont, and Wisconsin.

The second leading cause of UI deaths was poisoning in 29 states and the District of Columbia, while falls was the second leading cause in 15 states. Motor vehicle crashes were second in seven states.

The most common third leading causes of UI deaths were falls in 31 states and the District of Columbia, while poisoning was the third leading cause in 13 states. Motor vehicle crashes ranked third in Massachusetts, New Hampshire, Rhode Island, and Washington. Drowning was the third leading cause in Alaska, while fire, flames, and smoke was the third leading cause in Maryland.

Choking was the fourth leading cause of UI deaths in 32 states, while the fourth ranking cause was drowning in 11 states, and fires, flames, and smoke in five states and the District of Columbia. Natural heat and cold ranked fourth in Alaska and South Dakota, and poisoning was fourth in Maryland. (Poisoning and drowning were tied as the fourth leading cause in Maryland and were included in both counts.)

Fires, flames, and smoke was the fifth leading UI cause of death in 22 states. Drowning ranked fifth in 13 states and choking was fifth in 11 states and the District of Columbia. The fifth ranking cause was natural heat and cold in New Mexico and North Dakota, while mechanical suffocation was the fifth leading cause in Minnesota and Missouri. Air transportation was the fifth leading cause of UI death in Wyoming. (States with ties for fifth leading causes were included in multiple counts.)

The table on pages 174 and 175 shows the number of UI deaths by state of occurrence for the 15 most common types of injury events. State populations are also shown to facilitate computation of detailed death rates.

The table on page 176 consists of a four-year state-by-state comparison of UI deaths by state of residence and death rates for 2004 through 2007.

Page 177 shows fatal occupational injuries by state and number of deaths for some of the principal types of events: transportation accidents, assaults and violent acts, contacts with objects and equipment, falls, exposure to harmful substances or environments, and fires and explosions.

Nonfatal occupational injury and illness incidence rates for most states are shown in the table on page 178 and graphically in the map on page 179. States not shown do not have state occupational safety and health plans.

Pages 180 and 181 show motor vehicle-related deaths and death rates by state in both tables and maps. The maps show death rates based on population, vehicle miles traveled, and registered vehicles.

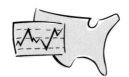

STATE DATA (CONT.)

UNINTENTIONAL INJURY DEATH RATES BY STATE, UNITED STATES, 2007

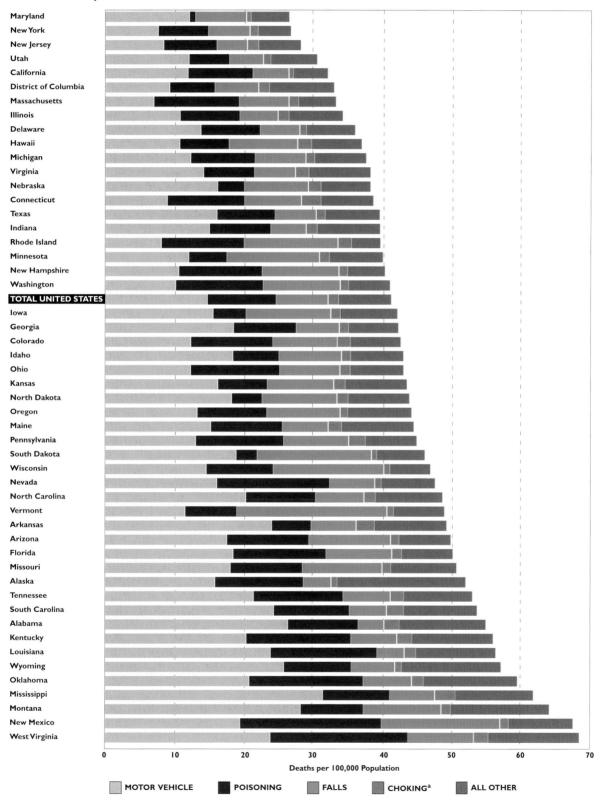

Deaths per 100,000 Population

MOTOR VEHICLE   POISONING   FALLS   CHOKING[a]   ALL OTHER

[a]Suffocation by ingestion or inhalation of food or other object.

STATE DATA

NATIONAL SAFETY COUNCIL® INJURY FACTS® 2011 EDITION

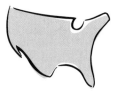

UNINTENTIONAL INJURY DEATH RATES BY STATE

170

UNINTENTIONAL INJURY DEATHS PER 100,000 POPULATION BY STATE, UNITED STATES 2007

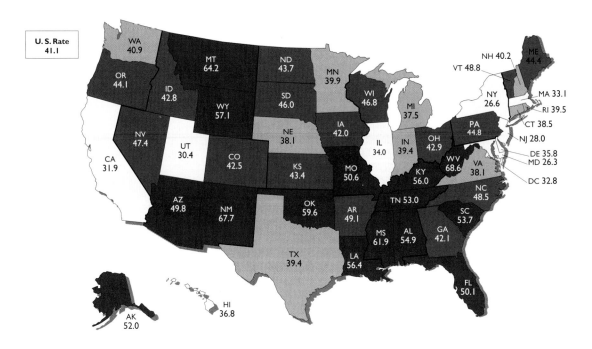

U.S. Rate
41.1

WA 40.9
MT 64.2
ND 43.7
MN 39.9
NH 40.2
VT 48.8
ME 44.4
OR 44.1
ID 42.8
WY 57.1
SD 46.0
WI 46.8
NY 26.6
MA 33.1
RI 39.5
CT 38.5
NV 47.4
UT 30.4
CO 42.5
NE 38.1
IA 42.0
IL 34.0
IN 39.4
OH 42.9
PA 44.8
NJ 28.0
DE 35.8
MD 26.3
DC 32.8
CA 31.9
MI 37.5
WV 68.6
VA 38.1
AZ 49.8
NM 67.7
KS 43.4
MO 50.6
KY 56.0
NC 48.5
OK 59.6
AR 49.1
TN 53.0
SC 53.7
TX 39.4
MS 61.9
AL 54.9
GA 42.1
LA 56.4
FL 50.1
AK 52.0
HI 36.8

REGIONAL RATES

NEW ENGLAND (CT, ME, MA, NH, RI, VT)	37.3
MIDDLE ATLANTIC (NJ, NY, PA)	32.5
EAST NORTH CENTRAL (IL, IN, MI, OH, WI)	39.3
WEST NORTH CENTRAL (IA, KS, MN, MO, NE, ND, SD)	44.0
SOUTH ATLANTIC (DE, DC, FL, GA, MD, NC, SC, VA, WV)	45.1
EAST SOUTH CENTRAL (AL, KY, MS, TN)	55.6
WEST SOUTH CENTRAL (AR, LA, OK, TX)	44.4
MOUNTAIN (AZ, CO, ID, MT, NV, NM, UT, WY)	47.4
PACIFIC (AK, CA, HI, OR, WA)	34.5

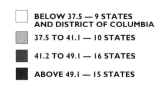

BELOW 37.5 — 9 STATES
AND DISTRICT OF COLUMBIA

37.5 TO 41.1 — 10 STATES

41.2 TO 49.1 — 16 STATES

ABOVE 49.1 — 15 STATES

Source: National Center for Health Statistics and U.S. Census Bureau.

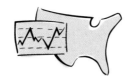

UNINTENTIONAL INJURY DEATHS BY STATE

The following series of charts is a state-by-state ranking of the five leading causes of deaths due to unintentional injuries based on 2007 data. The data are classified by state of residence. The first line of each section gives the rank of UI deaths among all causes of death, the total number of UI deaths, and the rate of UI deaths per 100,000 population in the state. The following lines list the five leading types of UI deaths in the state along with the number and rate for each type.

UNINTENTIONAL INJURY DEATHS BY STATE OF RESIDENCE, UNITED STATES, 2007

TOTAL UNITED STATES

Rank	Cause	Deaths	Rate
5	All UI	123,706	41.1
1	Motor vehicle	43,945	14.6
2	Poisoning[a]	29,846	9.9
3	Falls	22,631	7.5
4	Choking[b]	4,344	1.4
5	Drowning[c]	3,443	1.1

ALABAMA

Rank	Cause	Deaths	Rate
4	All UI	2,542	54.9
1	Motor vehicle	1,212	26.2
2	Poisoning[a]	471	10.2
3	Falls	170	3.7
4	Choking[b]	106	2.3
5	Fires, flames, smoke	88	1.9

ALASKA

Rank	Cause	Deaths	Rate
3	All UI	354	52.0
1	Motor vehicle	107	15.7
2	Poisoning[a]	87	12.8
3	Falls	27	4.0
3	Drowning[c]	27	4.0
4	Natural heat or cold	19	2.8

ARIZONA

Rank	Cause	Deaths	Rate
3	All UI	3,161	49.8
1	Motor vehicle	1,104	17.4
2	Poisoning[a]	757	11.9
3	Falls	742	11.7
4	Drowning	93	1.5
5	Choking[b]	82	1.3

ARKANSAS

Rank	Cause	Deaths	Rate
5	All UI	1,391	49.1
1	Motor vehicle	675	23.8
2	Falls	184	6.5
3	Poisoning[a]	162	5.7
4	Choking[b]	75	2.6
5	Fires, flames, smoke	66	2.3

CALIFORNIA

Rank	Cause	Deaths	Rate
5	All UI	11,614	31.9
1	Motor vehicle	4,306	11.8
2	Poisoning[a]	3,372	9.3
3	Falls	1,892	5.2
4	Drowning[c]	372	1.0
5	Choking[b]	237	0.7

COLORADO

Rank	Cause	Deaths	Rate
3	All UI	2,056	42.5
1	Motor vehicle	593	12.2
2	Poisoning[a]	567	11.7
3	Falls	448	9.3
4	Choking[b]	94	1.9
5	Drowning[c]	63	1.3

CONNECTICUT

Rank	Cause	Deaths	Rate
5	All UI	1,343	38.5
1	Poisoning[a]	386	11.1
2	Motor vehicle	309	8.9
3	Falls	287	8.2
4	Choking[b]	99	2.8
5	Drowning[c]	36	1.0

DELAWARE

Rank	Cause	Deaths	Rate
5	All UI	309	35.8
1	Motor vehicle	118	13.7
2	Poisoning[a]	73	8.5
3	Falls	49	5.7
4	Fires, flames, smoke	11	1.3
5	Choking[b]	9	1.0

DISTRICT OF COLUMBIA

Rank	Cause	Deaths	Rate
5	All UI	193	32.8
1	Motor vehicle	54	9.2
2	Poisoning[a]	38	6.5
3	Falls	37	6.3
4	Fires, flames, smoke	12	2.0
5	Choking[b]	9	1.5

FLORIDA

Rank	Cause	Deaths	Rate
4	All UI	9,113	50.1
1	Motor vehicle	3,329	18.3
2	Poisoning[a]	2,446	13.4
3	Falls	1,722	9.5
4	Drowning[c]	390	2.1
5	Choking[b]	254	1.4

GEORGIA

Rank	Cause	Deaths	Rate
3	All UI	4,012	42.1
1	Motor vehicle	1,745	18.3
2	Poisoning[a]	857	9.0
3	Falls	595	6.2
4	Choking[b]	126	1.3
5	Drowning[c]	125	1.3
5	Fire, flames, smoke	125	1.3

HAWAII

Rank	Cause	Deaths	Rate
4	All UI	470	36.8
1	Motor vehicle	136	10.6
2	Falls	126	9.9
3	Poisoning[a]	90	7.0
4	Drowning[c]	40	3.1
5	Choking[b]	26	2.0

IDAHO

Rank	Cause	Deaths	Rate
4	All UI	641	42.8
1	Motor vehicle	273	18.2
2	Falls	135	9.0
3	Poisoning[a]	99	6.6
4	Drowning[c]	23	1.5
5	Choking[b]	20	1.3

ILLINOIS

Rank	Cause	Deaths	Rate
5	All UI	4,367	34.0
1	Motor vehicle	1,375	10.7
2	Poisoning[a]	1,094	8.5
3	Falls	699	5.4
4	Choking[b]	204	1.6
5	Fires, flames, smoke	137	1.1

INDIANA

Rank	Cause	Deaths	Rate
5	All UI	2,499	39.4
1	Motor vehicle	942	14.9
2	Poisoning[a]	560	8.8
3	Falls	325	5.1
4	Choking[b]	100	1.6
5	Fires, flames, smoke	86	1.4

IOWA

Rank	Cause	Deaths	Rate
5	All UI	1,252	42.0
1	Motor vehicle	459	15.4
2	Falls	366	12.3
3	Poisoning[a]	141	4.7
4	Choking[b]	42	1.4
5	Drowning[c]	29	1.0

KANSAS

Rank	Cause	Deaths	Rate
5	All UI	1,205	43.4
1	Motor vehicle	447	16.1
2	Falls	266	9.6
3	Poisoning[a]	197	7.1
4	Choking[b]	47	1.7
5	Drowning[c]	38	1.4

See source and footnotes on page 173.

NATIONAL SAFETY COUNCIL® INJURY FACTS® 2011 EDITION

171

UNINTENTIONAL INJURY DEATHS
BY STATE (CONT.)

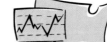

UNINTENTIONAL INJURY DEATHS BY STATE OF RESIDENCE, UNITED STATES, 2007 (Cont.)

KENTUCKY

Rank	Cause	Deaths	Rate
4	All UI	2,372	56.0
1	Motor vehicle	853	20.1
2	Poisoning[a]	640	15.1
3	Falls	283	6.7
4	Choking[b]	97	2.3
5	Fires, flames, smoke	79	1.9

LOUISIANA

Rank	Cause	Deaths	Rate
3	All UI	2,466	56.4
1	Motor vehicle	1,036	23.7
2	Poisoning[a]	672	15.4
3	Falls	174	4.0
4	Fires, flames, smoke	86	2.0
5	Choking[b]	77	1.8

MAINE

Rank	Cause	Deaths	Rate
5	All UI	584	44.4
1	Motor vehicle	198	15.1
2	Poisoning[a]	136	10.3
3	Falls	87	6.6
4	Choking[b]	25	1.9
5	Drowning[c]	16	1.2

MARYLAND

Rank	Cause	Deaths	Rate
5	All UI	1,480	26.3
1	Motor vehicle	675	12.0
2	Falls	410	7.3
3	Fires, flames, smoke	85	1.5
4	Poisoning[a]	49	0.9
5	Drowning[c]	47	0.8

MASSACHUSETTS

Rank	Cause	Deaths	Rate
5	All UI	2,139	33.1
1	Poisoning[a]	789	12.2
2	Falls	463	7.2
3	Motor vehicle	450	7.0
4	Choking[b]	89	1.4
5	Drowning[c]	52	0.8

MICHIGAN

Rank	Cause	Deaths	Rate
5	All UI	3,764	37.5
1	Motor vehicle	1,229	12.2
2	Poisoning[a]	922	9.2
3	Falls	741	7.4
4	Choking[b]	124	1.2
5	Fires, flames, smoke	123	1.2

MINNESOTA

Rank	Cause	Deaths	Rate
4	All UI	2,066	39.9
1	Falls	692	13.4
2	Motor vehicle	618	11.9
3	Poisoning[a]	283	5.5
4	Choking[b]	75	1.4
5	Mechanical suffocation	52	1.0

MISSISSIPPI

Rank	Cause	Deaths	Rate
3	All UI	1,808	61.9
1	Motor vehicle	914	31.3
2	Poisoning[a]	281	9.6
3	Falls	192	6.6
4	Choking[b]	86	2.9
5	Fires, flames, smoke	85	2.9

MISSOURI

Rank	Cause	Deaths	Rate
5	All UI	2,975	50.6
1	Motor vehicle	1,054	17.9
2	Falls	679	11.6
3	Poisoning[a]	609	10.4
4	Fires, flames, smoke	99	1.7
5	Drowning[c]	78	1.3
5	Mechanical suffocation	78	1.3

MONTANA

Rank	Cause	Deaths	Rate
3	All UI	614	64.2
1	Motor vehicle	268	28.0
2	Falls	108	11.3
3	Poisoning[a]	87	9.1
4	Drowning[c]	17	1.8
5	Choking[b]	13	1.4

NEBRASKA

Rank	Cause	Deaths	Rate
5	All UI	674	38.1
1	Motor vehicle	284	16.0
2	Falls	163	9.2
3	Poisoning[a]	68	3.8
4	Choking[b]	33	1.9
5	Fires, flames, smoke	16	0.9

NEVADA

Rank	Cause	Deaths	Rate
3	All UI	1,212	47.4
1	Poisoning[a]	417	16.3
2	Motor vehicle	407	15.9
3	Falls	164	6.4
4	Drowning[c]	38	1.5
5	Fires, flames, smoke	32	1.3

NEW HAMPSHIRE

Rank	Cause	Deaths	Rate
4	All UI	527	40.2
1	Poisoning[a]	157	12.0
2	Falls	145	11.0
3	Motor vehicle	138	10.5
4	Choking[b]	16	1.2
5	Fires, flames, smoke	10	0.8

NEW JERSEY

Rank	Cause	Deaths	Rate
5	All UI	2,425	28.0
1	Motor vehicle	719	8.3
2	Poisoning[a]	662	7.7
3	Falls	375	4.3
4	Choking[b]	136	1.6
5	Fires, flames, smoke	66	0.8

NEW MEXICO

Rank	Cause	Deaths	Rate
3	All UI	1,329	67.7
1	Poisoning[a]	401	20.4
2	Motor vehicle	379	19.3
3	Falls	340	17.3
4	Choking[b]	25	1.3
5	Natural heat or cold	24	1.2

NEW YORK

Rank	Cause	Deaths	Rate
5	All UI	5,160	26.6
1	Motor vehicle	1,478	7.6
2	Poisoning[a]	1,379	7.1
3	Falls	1,158	6.0
4	Choking[b]	217	1.1
5	Fires, flames, smoke	179	0.9

NORTH CAROLINA

Rank	Cause	Deaths	Rate
4	All UI	4,389	48.5
1	Motor vehicle	1,818	20.1
2	Poisoning[a]	914	10.1
3	Falls	627	6.9
4	Choking[b]	150	1.7
5	Fires, flames, smoke	144	1.6

NORTH DAKOTA

Rank	Cause	Deaths	Rate
5	All UI	279	43.7
1	Motor vehicle	115	18.0
2	Falls	69	10.8
3	Poisoning[a]	28	4.4
4	Choking[b]	10	1.6
5	Natural heat or cold	9	1.4

See source and footnotes on page 173.

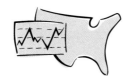

UNINTENTIONAL INJURY DEATHS BY STATE OF RESIDENCE, UNITED STATES, 2007 (Cont.)

OHIO

Rank	Cause	Deaths	Rate
5	All UI	4,922	42.9
1	Poisoning[a]	1,473	12.8
2	Motor vehicle	1,399	12.2
3	Falls	995	8.7
4	Choking[b]	165	1.4
5	Fires, flames, smoke	124	1.1

OKLAHOMA

Rank	Cause	Deaths	Rate
4	All UI	2,149	59.6
1	Motor vehicle	743	20.6
2	Poisoning[a]	596	16.5
3	Falls	254	7.0
4	Fires, flames, smoke	79	2.2
5	Choking[b]	62	1.7

OREGON

Rank	Cause	Deaths	Rate
5	All UI	1,646	44.1
1	Motor vehicle	490	13.1
2	Falls	396	10.6
3	Poisoning[a]	373	10.0
4	Drowning[c]	61	1.6
5	Choking[b]	39	1.0

PENNSYLVANIA

Rank	Cause	Deaths	Rate
5	All UI	5,568	44.8
1	Motor vehicle	1,604	12.9
2	Poisoning[a]	1,566	12.6
3	Falls	1,166	9.4
4	Choking[b]	302	2.4
5	Fires, flames, smoke	181	1.5

RHODE ISLAND

Rank	Cause	Deaths	Rate
5	All UI	416	39.5
1	Falls	143	13.6
2	Poisoning[a]	124	11.8
3	Motor vehicle	85	8.1
4	Choking[b]	20	1.9
5	Drowning[c]	6	0.6

SOUTH CAROLINA

Rank	Cause	Deaths	Rate
4	All UI	2,364	53.7
1	Motor vehicle	1,062	24.1
2	Poisoning[a]	481	10.9
3	Falls	239	5.4
4	Choking[b]	110	2.5
5	Fires, flames, smoke	89	2.0

SOUTH DAKOTA

Rank	Cause	Deaths	Rate
5	All UI	366	46.0
1	Motor vehicle	149	18.7
2	Falls	131	16.5
3	Poisoning[a]	24	3.0
4	Natural heat or cold	9	1.1
5	Fires, flames, smoke	8	1.0

TENNESSEE

Rank	Cause	Deaths	Rate
4	All UI	3,257	53.0
1	Motor vehicle	1,303	21.2
2	Poisoning[a]	798	13.0
3	Falls	418	6.8
4	Choking[b]	124	2.0
5	Fires, flames, smoke	114	1.9

TEXAS

Rank	Cause	Deaths	Rate
4	All UI	9,392	39.4
1	Motor vehicle	3,800	15.9
2	Poisoning[a]	1,999	8.4
3	Falls	1,416	5.9
4	Choking[b]	316	1.3
5	Drowning[c]	300	1.3

UTAH

Rank	Cause	Deaths	Rate
3	All UI	811	30.4
1	Motor vehicle	320	12.0
2	Poisoning[a]	154	5.8
3	Falls	130	4.9
4	Choking[b]	29	1.1
5	Drowning[c]	18	0.7

VERMONT

Rank	Cause	Deaths	Rate
4	All UI	303	48.8
1	Falls	134	21.6
2	Motor vehicle	71	11.4
3	Poisoning[a]	46	7.4
4	Drowning[c]	8	1.3
5	Fires, flames, smoke	7	1.1

VIRGINIA

Rank	Cause	Deaths	Rate
4	All UI	2,931	38.1
1	Motor vehicle	1,081	14.0
2	Poisoning[a]	562	7.3
3	Falls	454	5.9
4	Choking[b]	151	2.0
5	Fires, flames, smoke	102	1.3

WASHINGTON

Rank	Cause	Deaths	Rate
6	All UI	2,637	40.9
1	Poisoning[a]	810	12.6
2	Falls	715	11.1
3	Motor vehicle	649	10.1
4	Choking[b]	78	1.2
5	Drowning[c]	72	1.1

WEST VIRGINIA

Rank	Cause	Deaths	Rate
4	All UI	1,241	68.6
1	Motor vehicle	429	23.7
2	Poisoning[a]	360	19.9
3	Falls	173	9.6
4	Choking[b]	39	2.2
5	Fires, flames, smoke	36	2.0

WISCONSIN

Rank	Cause	Deaths	Rate
4	All UI	2,619	46.8
1	Falls	894	16.0
2	Motor vehicle	809	14.4
3	Poisoning[a]	538	9.6
4	Fires, flames, smoke	61	1.1
5	Choking[b]	48	0.9

WYOMING

Rank	Cause	Deaths	Rate
3	All UI	299	57.1
1	Motor vehicle	134	25.6
2	Poisoning[a]	51	9.7
3	Falls	33	6.3
4	Drowning[c]	9	1.7
5	Air transportation	7	1.3

Source: National Safety Council tabulations of National Center for Health Statistics mortality data.
[a]Solid, liquid, gas, and vapor poisoning.
[b]Inhalation or ingestion of food or other objects.
[c]Excludes water transport drownings.

UNINTENTIONAL INJURY DEATHS BY STATE AND EVENT

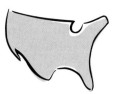

UNINTENTIONAL INJURY DEATHS BY STATE OF OCCURRENCE AND TYPE OF EVENT, UNITED STATES, 2007

State	Population (000)	Total[a]	Motor vehicle[b]	Poisoning	Falls	Choking[c]	Drowning[d]	Fires flames, smoke	Mechanical suffocation
Total U.S.	301,290	123,706	43,945	29,846	22,631	4,344	3,433	3,286	1,653
Alabama	4,627	2,548	1,226	459	165	106	82	91	33
Alaska	681	373	107	88	26	6	33	14	13
Arizona	6,353	3,207	1,122	763	755	82	98	33	44
Arkansas	2,831	1,306	632	148	171	74	41	63	11
California	36,378	11,501	4,190	3,405	1,879	228	374	229	103
Colorado	4,843	2,137	628	583	460	94	61	26	23
Connecticut	3,490	1,332	301	381	287	102	31	29	7
Delaware	862	323	127	73	49	9	9	9	—
Dist. of Columbia	588	257	66	45	59	8	—	19	3
Florida	18,200	9,287	3,371	2,511	1,729	252	464	133	132
Georgia	9,523	3,977	1,719	842	597	120	109	146	50
Hawaii	1,277	502	139	92	129	27	59	4	3
Idaho	1,496	644	279	94	141	19	20	12	12
Illinois	12,826	4,147	1,280	1,082	648	204	95	133	80
Indiana	6,336	2,498	938	549	333	102	60	82	61
Iowa	2,983	1,237	458	142	353	43	26	24	9
Kansas	2,777	1,152	432	200	237	44	31	36	18
Kentucky	4,236	2,297	844	629	254	95	50	75	28
Louisiana	4,373	2,513	1,042	686	182	76	74	89	31
Maine	1,315	588	205	131	87	26	20	5	6
Maryland	5,619	1,417	673	22	399	35	41	82	17
Massachusetts	6,468	2,132	447	793	465	87	45	36	18
Michigan	10,050	3,645	1,163	903	729	124	96	122	82
Minnesota	5,182	2,039	593	292	683	71	41	32	53
Mississippi	2,921	1,754	897	275	183	83	40	80	42
Missouri	5,878	3,120	1,099	614	735	75	88	108	80
Montana	957	626	288	81	106	14	21	8	8
Nebraska	1,769	687	286	68	171	35	13	17	12
Nevada	2,554	1,303	458	430	180	34	38	32	21
New Hampshire	1,312	525	128	153	153	17	9	8	4
New Jersey	8,653	2,297	701	622	343	132	48	56	25
New Mexico	1,964	1,338	414	406	320	22	18	16	15
New York	19,429	4,974	1,365	1,372	1,133	213	93	181	54
North Carolina	9,042	4,459	1,834	913	658	153	108	151	43
North Dakota	638	328	135	32	88	14	10	3	—
Ohio	11,478	4,836	1,349	1,470	976	164	95	119	84
Oklahoma	3,608	2,134	749	591	239	58	67	81	16
Oregon	3,736	1,664	498	382	402	40	57	33	21
Pennsylvania	12,420	5,625	1,611	1,590	1,188	308	83	196	47
Rhode Island	1,053	433	86	122	151	23	8	4	—
South Carolina	4,405	2,366	1,099	482	220	108	66	65	43
South Dakota	796	388	169	20	141	5	6	8	5
Tennessee	6,149	3,568	1,467	808	471	135	83	121	49
Texas	23,843	9,391	3,796	1,994	1,437	322	292	216	104
Utah	2,669	843	335	153	128	30	21	19	16
Vermont	621	293	66	51	129	6	7	7	—
Virginia	7,699	2,890	1,079	554	446	151	67	100	28
Washington	6,450	2,603	618	811	720	77	64	37	30
West Virginia	1,810	1,297	470	362	188	41	23	33	14
Wisconsin	5,599	2,600	810	532	880	46	46	59	44
Wyoming	523	305	156	45	28	4	10	4	4

See source and footnotes on page 175.

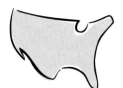

UNINTENTIONAL INJURY DEATHS BY STATE OF OCCURRENCE AND TYPE OF EVENT, UNITED STATES, 2007 (Cont.)

State	Natural heat or cold	Struck by/against object	Machinery	Firearms	Electric current	Water trans.	Air trans.	Rail trans.	All other accidents
Total U.S.	1,020	812	659	613	369	486	550	437	9,612
Alabama	18	16	13	28	10	—	15	5	280
Alaska	20	2	—	—	4	9	28	—	22
Arizona	57	13	—	15	11	6	16	12	179
Arkansas	14	19	8	21	5	11	5	7	76
California	76	55	41	45	29	35	59	72	681
Colorado	17	18	15	4	—	7	11	—	189
Connecticut	17	6	—	3	4	—	3	8	150
Delaware	—	—	—	—	—	—	3	—	35
Dist. of Columbia	3	—	—	—	—	—	—	—	47
Florida	15	50	28	13	26	55	45	28	435
Georgia	20	45	26	23	8	21	22	16	213
Hawaii	—	—	—	—	—	—	5	—	35
Idaho	9	—	6	8	—	10	5	—	26
Illinois	46	24	22	16	24	15	13	34	431
Indiana	22	10	16	16	5	5	9	15	275
Iowa	15	21	22	3	3	8	9	5	96
Kansas	9	7	21	3	4	4	—	—	103
Kentucky	22	19	11	28	5	9	7	5	216
Louisiana	5	10	17	34	11	26	6	10	214
Maine	9	—	—	—	—	16	—	—	74
Maryland	23	11	3	4	4	4	7	9	83
Massachusetts	19	7	—	—	8	—	10	7	186
Michigan	40	20	26	12	7	18	4	4	295
Minnesota	15	9	12	—	3	8	10	6	209
Mississippi	11	22	9	26	5	14	—	4	62
Missouri	43	20	16	25	11	5	12	—	187
Montana	10	—	3	—	—	—	13	3	66
Nebraska	4	8	5	4	—	—	3	—	58
Nevada	14	11	—	3	4	3	13	—	58
New Hampshire	6	4	5	—	—	5	—	—	30
New Jersey	19	10	3	3	7	11	—	14	301
New Mexico	25	7	9	7	5	—	17	7	50
New York	55	28	28	8	9	19	12	21	383
North Carolina	34	18	32	35	4	18	13	15	430
North Dakota	11	—	4	—	—	—	—	—	22
Ohio	27	26	28	13	14	3	18	23	427
Oklahoma	34	10	12	7	13	4	14	4	235
Oregon	13	11	5	6	—	10	16	6	163
Pennsylvania	34	46	33	23	10	6	8	20	422
Rhode Island	4	—	—	—	—	—	—	—	27
South Carolina	20	11	9	14	6	11	6	7	199
South Dakota	7	—	3	—	—	—	—	—	19
Tennessee	19	23	24	30	5	12	11	3	307
Texas	39	85	57	81	64	27	21	29	827
Utah	10	10	7	—	3	3	17	—	89
Vermont	3	3	—	—	—	—	—	—	17
Virginia	26	33	15	10	11	14	9	4	343
Washington	23	18	23	3	—	21	27	9	120
West Virginia	12	16	7	14	5	5	4	4	99
Wisconsin	18	17	20	8	6	10	11	5	88
Wyoming	5	—	3	—	—	3	5	—	33

Source: National Safety Council analysis of National Center for Health Statistics mortality data. Dashes (—) indicate data that do not meet publication guidelines.
[a]*Deaths are by place of occurrence and exclude nonresident aliens.*
[b]*See page 180 for motor vehicle deaths by place of residence.*
[c]*Suffocation by inhalation or ingestion of food or object obstructing breathing.*
[d]*Excludes water transport drownings.*

UNINTENTIONAL INJURY TRENDS BY STATE

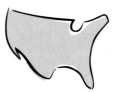

Nationwide, unintentional injury deaths increased 10% from 2004-2007 and the death rate increased 8%. By state, the greatest decrease in the number of UI deaths and death rates occurred in South Dakota (-12% and -15%, respectively). The greatest increase in UI deaths and death rates occurred in Rhode Island (+40% and +43%, respectively). Although somewhat larger, the

increases in UI deaths and death rates for Massachusetts were largely due to a classification change in 2005 that resulted in the reclassification of most poisonings from undetermined to unintentional.

The table below shows the trend in UI deaths and death rates by state over the most recent four years for which data are available.

UNINTENTIONAL INJURY DEATHS BY STATE OF RESISDENCE, UNITED STATES, 2004-2007

State	Deaths[a]				Deaths per 100,000 population			
	2007[b]	2006	2005	2004	2007[b]	2006	2005	2004
Total U.S.	123,706	121,599	117,809	112,012	41.1	40.8	39.7	38.1
Alabama	2,542	2,506	2,395	2,403	54.9	54.6	52.7	53.2
Alaska	354	316	313	326	52.0	46.7	47.2	49.6
Arizona	3,161	3,352	3,150	2,770	49.8	54.3	52.9	48.2
Arkansas	1,391	1,415	1,329	1,406	49.1	50.5	47.9	51.2
California	11,614	11,375	11,129	10,633	31.9	31.5	30.8	29.7
Colorado	2,056	1,917	1,947	1,810	42.5	40.3	41.8	39.4
Connecticut	1,343	1,302	1,134	1,261	38.5	37.3	32.4	36.1
Delaware	309	329	293	294	35.8	38.7	34.8	35.5
Dist. of Columbia	193	224	207	219	32.8	38.3	35.6	37.8
Florida	9,113	8,917	8,868	8,229	50.1	49.5	49.9	47.4
Georgia	4,012	3,879	3,762	3,667	42.1	41.6	41.2	41.0
Hawaii	470	441	436	390	36.8	34.6	34.2	31.0
Idaho	641	682	606	593	42.8	46.7	42.4	42.5
Illinois	4,367	4,451	4,182	4,133	34.0	34.9	32.8	32.5
Indiana	2,499	2,480	2,480	2,395	39.4	39.4	39.6	38.5
Iowa	1,252	1,188	1,202	1,108	42.0	40.0	40.5	37.5
Kansas	1,205	1,198	1,149	1,144	43.4	43.5	41.8	41.8
Kentucky	2,372	2,446	2,405	2,260	56.0	58.2	57.6	54.6
Louisiana	2,466	2,422	3,072	2,300	56.4	57.1	68.2	51.2
Maine	584	572	579	480	44.4	43.6	43.9	36.5
Maryland	1,480	1,456	1,376	1,412	26.3	26.0	24.6	25.4
Massachusetts[c]	2,139	2,214	1,907	1,366	33.1	34.4	29.6	21.2
Michigan	3,764	3,590	3,451	3,312	37.5	35.6	34.2	32.8
Minnesota	2,066	1,919	1,922	1,867	39.9	37.3	37.5	36.6
Mississippi	1,808	1,856	1,936	1,703	61.9	64.1	66.6	58.9
Missouri	2,975	3,009	2,848	2,728	50.6	51.6	49.1	47.4
Montana	614	558	524	535	64.2	59.0	56.1	57.8
Nebraska	674	683	704	743	38.1	38.8	40.0	42.5
Nevada	1,212	1,091	1,104	1,021	47.4	43.9	45.8	43.8
New Hampshire	527	460	477	445	40.2	35.1	36.5	34.3
New Jersey	2,425	2,590	2,561	2,324	28.0	30.0	29.4	26.8
New Mexico	1,329	1,297	1,267	1,223	67.7	66.9	65.8	64.3
New York	5,160	5,235	4,645	4,530	26.6	27.0	24.0	23.5
North Carolina	4,389	4,156	4,123	4,019	48.5	47.0	47.5	47.1
North Dakota	279	275	287	274	43.7	43.2	45.2	43.1
Ohio	4,922	4,821	4,438	4,234	42.9	42.1	38.7	36.9
Oklahoma	2,149	2,039	2,005	1,947	59.6	57.1	56.6	55.3
Oregon	1,646	1,586	1,469	1,444	44.1	43.1	40.4	40.2
Pennsylvania	5,568	5,299	5,446	5,200	44.8	42.8	43.9	42.0
Rhode Island	416	434	334	298	39.5	41.0	31.1	27.6
South Carolina	2,364	2,315	2,272	2,094	53.7	53.5	53.5	49.9
South Dakota	366	452	402	416	46.0	57.4	51.9	54.0
Tennessee	3,257	3,307	3,147	3,156	53.0	54.5	52.8	53.6
Texas	9,392	9,140	8,598	8,323	39.4	39.1	37.5	37.0
Utah	811	715	743	697	30.4	27.7	29.8	28.8
Vermont	303	301	272	253	48.8	48.5	43.7	40.8
Virginia	2,931	2,703	2,638	2,630	38.1	35.4	34.9	35.2
Washington	2,637	2,679	2,543	2,341	40.9	42.1	40.4	37.7
West Virginia	1,241	1,177	940	1,110	68.6	65.1	51.8	61.3
Wisconsin	2,619	2,524	2,490	2,303	46.8	45.3	45.0	41.9
Wyoming	299	306	302	243	57.1	59.7	59.4	48.1

Source: Deaths are from the National Center for Health Statistics. Rates are National Safety Council estimates based on data from the National Center for Health Statistics and the U.S. Census Bureau. See Technical Appendix for comparability.
[a]Deaths for each state are by state of residence and exclude nonresident aliens.
[b]Latest official figures.
[c]Starting in 2005, Massachusetts changed the classification of most poisonings from undetermined to unintentional.

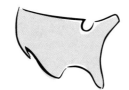

FATAL OCCUPATIONAL INJURIES BY STATE

In general, the states with the largest number of people employed have the largest number of work-related fatalities. The four largest states—California, Florida, New York, and Texas—accounted for about 28% of the total 2009 fatalities in the United States. Each state's industry mix, geographic features, age of population, and other characteristics of the workforce must be considered when evaluating state fatality profiles. Overall, the six leading events or exposures account for all but 16 of the 4,340 total occupational fatalities in 2009.

FATAL OCCUPATIONAL INJURIES BY STATE AND EVENT OR EXPOSURE, UNITED STATES, 2008-2009

State	2008 total[a]	2009						
		Total[b]	Transpor-tation[c]	Assualts & violent acts[d]	Contacts with objects & equipment	Falls	Exposure to harmful substances or environments	Fires & explosions
Total	5,214	4,340	1,682	788	734	617	390	113
Alabama	107	70	33	14	12	5	5	—
Alaska	33	17	9	—	4	—	—	—
Arizona	100	50	23	6	10	5	6	—
Arkansas	85	75	35	10	12	7	8	—
California	465	301	95	79	41	54	24	6
Colorado	105	80	34	16	9	13	6	—
Connecticut	28	34	9	13	3	7	—	—
Delaware	11	7	3	—	—	—	—	—
District of Columbia	9	10	3	6	—	—	—	—
Florida	291	243	90	35	31	36	47	—
Georgia	182	96	47	14	11	11	10	3
Hawaii	19	13	8	—	3	—	—	—
Idaho	36	26	14	—	7	—	—	—
Illinois	193	158	46	36	32	26	16	—
Indiana	143	123	47	20	25	20	9	—
Iowa	93	78	47	3	15	7	4	—
Kansas	73	76	33	8	16	11	5	3
Kentucky	106	97	37	15	21	10	12	—
Louisiana	135	138	60	13	30	15	16	3
Maine	24	16	10	—	—	—	—	—
Maryland	60	65	23	17	9	10	4	—
Massachusetts	68	59	20	9	12	11	7	—
Michigan	123	93	27	23	22	11	9	—
Minnesota	65	60	22	10	14	9	4	—
Mississippi	80	64	33	12	4	6	4	5
Missouri	148	142	59	24	27	20	10	—
Montana	40	50	22	13	7	—	3	—
Nebraska	53	57	26	4	9	13	4	—
Nevada	41	24	13	3	3	3	—	—
New Hampshire	7	6	3	—	—	—	—	—
New Jersey	92	99	33	23	12	23	5	3
New Mexico	31	42	20	7	6	5	4	—
New York	213	184	63	47	29	24	12	8
North Carolina	161	125	47	25	17	18	9	9
North Dakota	28	25	11	—	4	6	3	—
Ohio	168	132	39	26	22	28	10	4
Oklahoma	102	77	43	6	14	4	8	—
Oregon	55	66	34	10	14	4	3	—
Pennsylvania	241	166	55	37	25	31	13	5
Rhode Island	6	7	—	—	4	—	—	—
South Carolina	87	73	29	12	11	10	9	—
South Dakota	30	24	10	—	10	—	—	—
Tennessee	135	105	42	18	24	12	6	3
Texas	463	480	163	93	65	82	61	15
Utah	64	48	27	—	7	4	—	6
Vermont	10	12	7	—	—	—	—	—
Virginia	156	118	42	31	21	16	8	—
Washington	84	75	23	22	19	5	3	—
West Virginia	53	41	19	—	12	—	3	4
Wisconsin	77	94	32	18	21	14	7	—
Wyoming	33	19	11	—	—	4	—	—

Source: U.S. Department of Labor, Bureau of Labor Statistics
Note: Dashes (—) indicate no data or data that do not meet publication criteria.
[a]Data for 2008 revised and total includes two deaths for which state of occurrence could not be determined.
[b]Data for 2009 preliminary and total includes zero deaths for which state of occurrence could not be determined.
[c]Includes highway, nonhighway, air, water, and rail fatalities, and fatalities resulting from being struck by a vehicle.
[d]Includes violence by persons, self-inflicted injury, and attacks by animals.

NONFATAL OCCUPATIONAL INCIDENCE RATES BY STATE

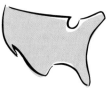

NONFATAL OCCUPATIONAL INJURY AND ILLNESS INCIDENCE RATES[a] BY STATE, PRIVATE INDUSTRY, 2008

State	Total recordable cases	Cases with days away from work[b]	Cases with job transfer or restriction	Other recordable cases
Private industry[c]	**3.9**	**1.1**	**0.9**	**1.9**
Alabama	4.1	1.0	1.0	2.1
Alaska	5.1	2.0	0.7	2.4
Arizona	3.7	1.0	0.8	1.9
Arkansas	4.5	0.9	0.9	2.7
California	3.9	1.1	1.1	1.6
Colorado	—	—	—	—
Connecticut	4.6	1.5	1.0	2.0
Delaware	3.3	1.2	0.5	1.5
District of Columbia	1.9	0.8	0.1	1.0
Florida	3.8	1.1	0.9	1.9
Georgia	3.3	0.9	0.8	1.6
Hawaii	4.3	2.3	0.4	1.6
Idaho	—	—	—	—
Illinois	3.6	1.1	0.8	1.7
Indiana	4.7	1.1	1.2	2.4
Iowa	5.0	1.2	1.2	2.5
Kansas	4.5	1.0	1.1	2.4
Kentucky	4.7	1.4	1.2	2.2
Louisiana	2.8	0.9	0.4	1.4
Maine	6.0	1.6	1.8	2.7
Maryland	3.3	1.2	0.5	1.6
Massachusetts	3.6	1.5	0.5	1.7
Michigan	4.4	1.1	1.1	2.2
Minnesota	4.2	1.0	0.9	2.3
Mississippi	—	—	—	—
Missouri	3.6	0.8	0.9	1.9
Montana	6.4	2.1	0.8	3.5
Nebraska	4.4	1.2	0.9	2.3
Nevada	4.5	1.2	1.3	2.1
New Hampshire	—	—	—	—
New Jersey	3.2	1.2	0.6	1.4
New Mexico	3.8	1.2	0.7	1.9
New York	2.8	1.4	0.2	1.3
North Carolina	3.4	0.8	0.8	1.7
North Dakota	—	—	—	—
Ohio	—	—	—	—
Oklahoma	4.5	1.2	0.9	2.4
Oregon	4.6	1.5	1.1	2.1
Pennsylvania	—	—	—	—
Rhode Island	—	—	—	—
South Carolina	3.1	0.9	0.7	1.4
South Dakota	—	—	—	—
Tennessee	4.2	1.0	1.1	2.1
Texas	3.1	0.8	0.9	1.3
Utah	4.7	1.0	1.0	2.6
Vermont	5.5	1.6	0.9	2.9
Virginia	3.1	1.0	1.6	1.5
Washington	5.6	1.8	0.9	2.9
West Virginia	4.7	2.1	0.4	2.1
Wisconsin	4.9	1.4	1.1	2.4
Wyoming	4.6	1.6	0.5	2.4

Source: Bureau of Labor Statistics, U.S. Department of Labor
Note: Because of rounding, components may not add to totals. Dashes (—) indicate data not available.
[a]Incidence rates represent the number of injuries and illnesses per 100 full-time workers using 200,000 hours as the equivalent.
[b]Days-away-from-work cases include those that result in days away from work with or without job transfer or restriction.
[c]Data cover all 50 states.

NONFATAL OCCUPATIONAL INJURY AND ILLNESS INCIDENCE RATES FOR TOTAL RECORABLE CASES BY STATE, PRIVATE INDUSTRY, 2008

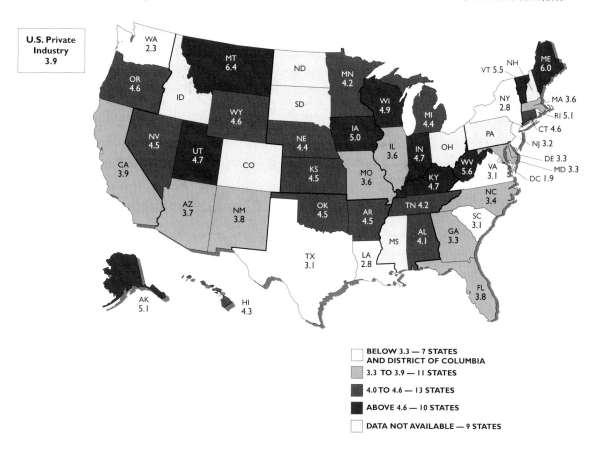

U.S. Private Industry 3.9

☐ BELOW 3.3 — 7 STATES
AND DISTRICT OF COLUMBIA

▨ 3.3 TO 3.9 — 11 STATES

▨ 4.0 TO 4.6 — 13 STATES

■ ABOVE 4.6 — 10 STATES

☐ DATA NOT AVAILABLE — 9 STATES

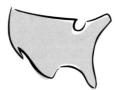

MOTOR VEHICLE DEATHS BY STATE, UNITED STATES, 2006-2009

State	Motor vehicle traffic deaths (place of accident)				Total motor vehicle deaths[a] (place of residence)			
	Number		Mileage rate[b]		Number		Population rate[b]	
	2009	2008	2009	2008	2007[c]	2006	2007	2006
Total U.S.[a]	35,900	39,700	1.2	1.3	43,945	45,316	14.6	15.2
Alabama	848	968	1.4	1.6	1,212	1,224	26.2	26.7
Alaska	64	62	1.3	1.2	107	85	15.7	12.6
Arizona	806	937	1.3	1.5	1,104	1,323	17.4	21.4
Arkansas	592	600	1.8	1.9	675	729	23.8	26.0
California	3,063	3,396	0.9	1.1	4,306	4,464	11.8	12.4
Colorado	465	548	1.0	1.2	593	591	12.2	12.4
Connecticut	227	304	0.7	1.0	309	363	8.9	10.4
Delaware	118	122	1.3	1.3	118	140	13.7	16.5
District of Columbia	33	39	0.9	1.1	54	40	9.2	6.8
Florida	2,575	2,983	1.3	1.5	3,329	3,466	18.3	19.2
Georgia	1,289	1,507	1.2	1.4	1,745	1,751	18.3	18.8
Hawaii	109	107	1.1	1.1	136	157	10.6	12.3
Idaho	226	232	1.5	1.5	273	298	18.2	20.4
Illinois	911	1,043	0.9	1.0	1,375	1,416	10.7	11.1
Indiana	693	814	1.0	1.2	942	954	14.9	15.2
Iowa	372	412	1.2	1.4	459	457	15.4	15.4
Kansas	386	385	1.3	1.3	447	491	16.1	17.8
Kentucky	791	826	1.7	1.8	853	932	20.1	22.2
Louisiana	824	915	1.8	2.1	1,036	1,017	23.7	24.0
Maine	161	157	1.1	1.1	198	193	15.1	14.7
Maryland	549	588	1.0	1.1	675	727	12.0	13.0
Massachusetts	348	363	0.6	0.7	450	487	7.0	7.6
Michigan	871	980	0.9	1.0	1,229	1,176	12.2	11.7
Minnesota	415	455	0.7	0.8	618	610	11.9	11.9
Mississippi	700	783	1.6	1.9	914	968	31.3	33.4
Missouri	878	960	1.3	1.4	1,054	1,111	17.9	19.0
Montana	220	229	2.0	2.1	268	264	28.0	27.9
Nebraska	223	208	1.2	1.1	284	270	16.0	15.3
Nevada	343	324	1.2	1.5	407	442	15.9	17.8
New Hampshire	110	140	0.8	1.1	138	129	10.5	9.9
New Jersey	586	589	0.8	0.8	719	774	8.3	9.0
New Mexico	361	366	1.4	1.4	379	469	19.3	24.2
New York	1,089	1,224	0.8	0.9	1,478	1,599	7.6	8.3
North Carolina	1,317	1,442	1.3	1.4	1,818	1,704	20.1	19.3
North Dakota	140	104	1.8	1.4	115	114	18.0	17.9
Ohio	1,022	1,192	0.9	1.1	1,399	1,367	12.2	11.9
Oklahoma	718	749	1.5	1.6	743	787	20.6	22.1
Oregon	377	416	1.1	1.2	490	510	13.1	13.9
Pennsylvania	1,256	1,464	1.2	1.4	1,604	1,625	12.9	13.1
Rhode Island	83	65	1.0	0.8	85	89	8.1	8.4
South Carolina	894	920	1.8	1.9	1,062	1,044	24.1	24.1
South Dakota	131	121	1.5	1.4	149	193	18.7	24.5
Tennessee	989	1,035	1.4	1.5	1,303	1,379	21.2	22.7
Texas	2,948	3,408	1.2	1.5	3,800	3,907	15.9	16.7
Utah	244	275	0.9	1.1	320	342	12.0	13.2
Vermont	74	73	1.0	1.0	71	91	11.4	14.7
Virginia	757	821	0.9	1.0	1,081	962	14.0	12.6
Washington	491	521	0.9	0.9	649	743	10.1	11.7
West Virginia	357	378	1.7	1.9	429	420	23.7	23.2
Wisconsin	542	587	0.9	1.0	809	769	14.4	13.8
Wyoming	134	159	1.4	1.8	134	153	25.6	29.8

Source: Motor Vehicle Traffic Deaths are provisional counts from state traffic authorities; Total Motor Vehicle Deaths are from the National Center for Health Statistics (see also page 174).
[a]*Includes both traffic and nontraffic motor vehicle deaths. See definitions of motor vehicle traffic and nontraffic accidents on page 207.*
[b]*The mileage death rate is deaths per 100,000,000 vehicle miles; the population death rate is deaths per 100,000 population. Death rates are National Safety Council estimates.*
[c]*Latest year available. See Technical Appendix for comparability.*

MILEAGE DEATH RATES, 2009
MOTOR VEHICLE TRAFFIC DEATHS PER 100,000,000 VEHICLE MILES

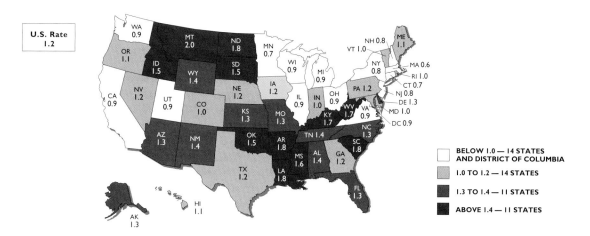

U.S. Rate
1.2

BELOW 1.0 — 14 STATES
AND DISTRICT OF COLUMBIA

1.0 TO 1.2 — 14 STATES

1.3 TO 1.4 — 11 STATES

ABOVE 1.4 — 11 STATES

REGISTRATION DEATH RATES, 2009
MOTOR VEHICLE TRAFFIC DEATHS PER 10,000 MOTOR VEHICLES

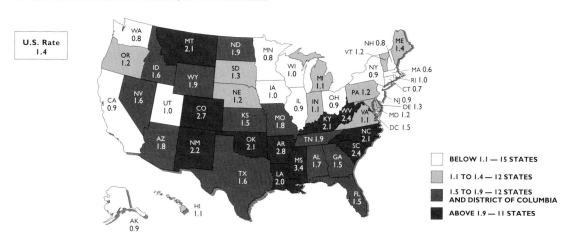

U.S. Rate
1.4

BELOW 1.1 — 15 STATES

1.1 TO 1.4 — 12 STATES

1.5 TO 1.9 — 12 STATES
AND DISTRICT OF COLUMBIA

ABOVE 1.9 — 11 STATES

POPULATION DEATH RATES, 2009
MOTOR VEHICLE TRAFFIC DEATHS PER 100,000 POPULATION

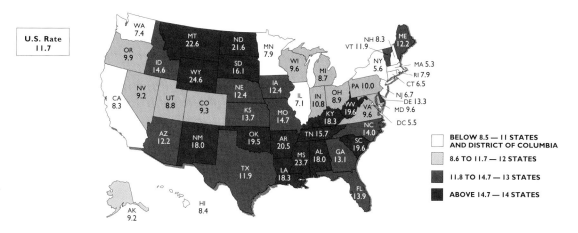

U.S. Rate
11.7

BELOW 8.5 — 11 STATES
AND DISTRICT OF COLUMBIA

8.6 TO 11.7 — 12 STATES

11.8 TO 14.7 — 13 STATES

ABOVE 14.7 — 14 STATES

Source: Rates estimated by National Safety Council based on data from state traffic authorities, the National Center for Health Statistics, the Federal Highway Administration, and the U.S. Census Bureau.

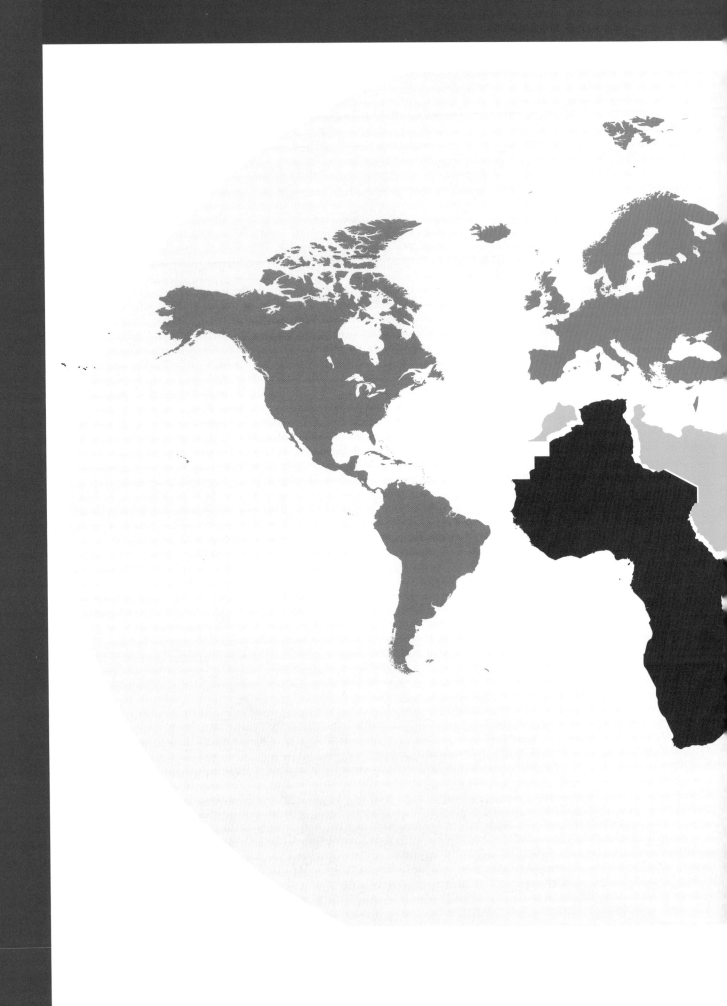

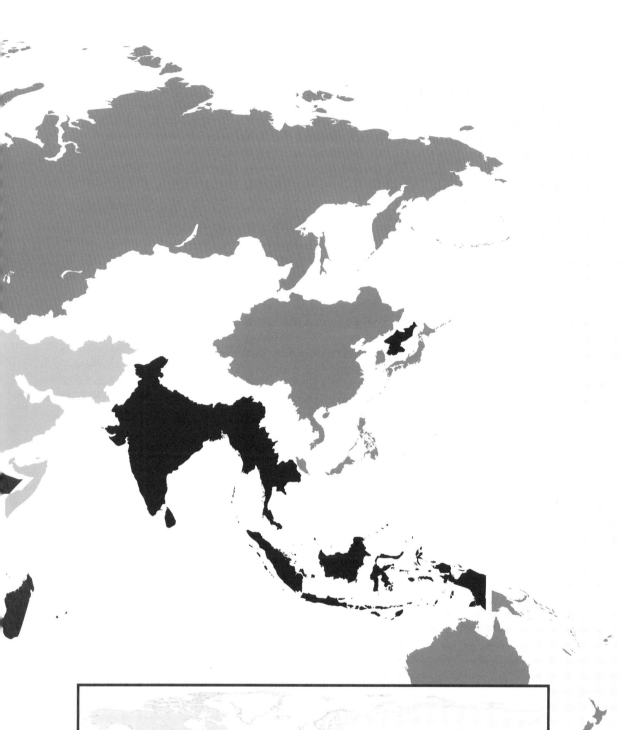

LOOKING AT THE WORLD IN A NEW WAY

The six regions of the world illustrated on these two pages are scaled to reflect the relative impact of unintentional fatal injuries. Impact is measured using total unintentional fatality rates, which are further explored in the body of this section. For comparison, the small map provided in this call out box reflects the traditional view of the world.

INTERNATIONAL DATA

Unintentional injuries account for 9% of years of life lost.

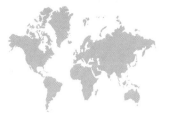

This section on international injury and fatalities includes data for occupational and motor vehicle injuries, as well as general unintentional injury and mortality. The two primary data sources used in this section are the World Health Organization and International Labor Organization.

WHO estimates that 9% of the years of life lost are caused by unintentional injuries. The charts on pages 185-188 show graphically the unintentional injury death rates in 2008 for the world overall, as well as six geographic regions. As measured in deaths per 100,000 population, the South East Asian Region has the highest average unintentional fatality rate with 68. This contrasts sharply with the Region of the Americas, which has the lowest average unintentional fatality rate of 38. Overall, the world has an average unintentional fatality rate of 59. The relative differences in fatality rates across the six regions of the world also are illustrated using the world map provided at the start of this section. Unlike traditional maps, this map is scaled in proportion to each region's average fatality rate. Because of this scaling, the Region of the Americas is depicted to be relatively small compared with other regions with substantially higher fatality rates, such as the South East Asian and African Regions.

Looking at specific causes, road traffic accidents are the leading cause of unintentional fatalities for each region in the world. The overall fatality rate for road traffic accidents is 21. Unintentional fatality rates tend to be high for the youngest children, ages 0 to 4, decrease for older children ages 5 to 14, and then increase steadily with age.

WHO highlights the importance of road traffic safety in its report, *Global status report on road safety: Time for action.* The report confirms previous research that road traffic fatality rates are much higher in low- and middle-income countries than in higher-income countries. It

highlights that while developing countries represent more than 90% of road traffic deaths, they account for less than half of the world's registered vehicles. In addition, almost half of those killed in road traffic crashes are pedestrians, cyclists, and motorcyclists. This proportion is highest in the poorest countries of the world.

The charts on pages 189-193 provide the unintentional injury deaths and death rates for 53 countries. The most current year of mortality data available is reported for motor vehicle, poisonings, falls, drowning, and overall unintentional injury deaths. Looking at overall age trends across the world, the 65 and older age group has the highest rate of unintentional injury deaths per 100,000 population, while the 5- to 14-year-old age group has the lowest. Death rates for all causes except poisonings peak for the 65 and older age group. The poisoning death rate peaks for the 45 to 64 age group. Because of differences in recordkeeping, comparisons among countries are not recommended.

The charts on pages 194 and 195 detail the occupational deaths and death rates by country for the past five years. Because of the wide range of recordkeeping standards used in the world, countries with similar recordkeeping practices are grouped together. Although comparison among countries is not recommended even within these recordkeeping groupings, trends over the years are evident.

Of the 46 countries listed on page 195, 26 show improvement in the occupational death rate. Fourteen of these improving countries have decreased work-related deaths by at least one worker per units measured. Six of the 14 countries that show an increased death rate are up by at least one worker per units measured over the years reported.

Source: World Health Organization. (2009). Global status report on road safety: Time for action. *Downloaded from* www.who.int/violence_injury_prevention/road_safety_status/ *on Aug. 6, 2010.*

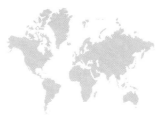

INTERNATIONAL UNINTENTIONAL INJURY DEATHS

As part of the Global Burden of Disease project, the World Health Organization makes mortality and burden of disease projections based on 2004 mortality estimates. Those projections are used in this section to compare the impact unintentional injuries have in six regions of the world and overall.

In the 2010 edition of *Injury Facts*, WHO's burden of disease measure that quantifies the overall impact of diseases and injuries at the individual or societal level was spotlighted. WHO measures the burden of disease using an estimate of disability-adjusted life years, which is the sum of the years of life lost due to premature mortality and the years lost due to disability. This edition of *Injury Facts* is focused on exploring WHO's regional mortality estimates.

WHO mortality estimates are developed using a set of statistical models to project trends based on economic and social development, and using the historically observed relationships of these with cause-specific mortality rates.

This section presents unintentional injury fatality rates (per 100,000 population) projections representing 2008 for the world overall and for six regions: Africa, Americas, Mediterranean, European, South East Asian, and Western Pacific.

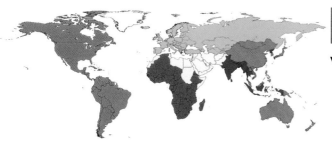

WORLD

WHO estimates that in 2008 nearly 4 million unintentional injury deaths occurred worldwide. As illustrated in the chart below, the unintentional injury rate in the world per 100,000 population is greatest among the 80 and older age group. The 80 and older age group has a total unintentional fatality rate of 299 compared to

an average rate of 59 across all age groups. Looking at causes, road traffic accidents has the highest fatality rate of 21. Road traffic accidents are the leading unintentional fatality cause for all age groups younger than 70. Starting with the 70-79 age group, falls represent the leading cause of death, accounting for 33% of all fatalities.

WORLD: UNINTENTIONAL DEATH RATE BY AGE GROUP, 2008

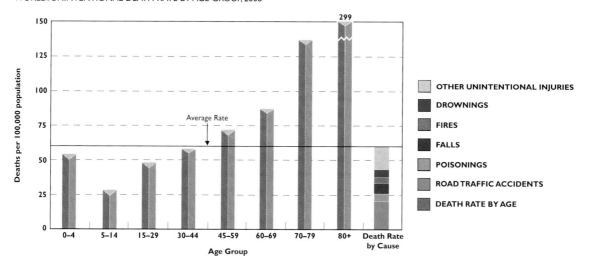

Source: National Safety Council analysis of World Health Organization Burden of Disease Project data.

INTERNATIONAL UNINTENTIONAL INJURY DEATHS: AFRICAN REGION

The African Region represented by 46 countries has the second highest average unintentional death rate in the world after the South East Asian Region with 68 per 100,000 population. Although road traffic accidents are the most prevalent cause overall, falls are the leading cause for individuals 80 and older.

AFRICAN REGION: UNINTENTIONAL DEATH RATE BY AGE GROUP, 2008

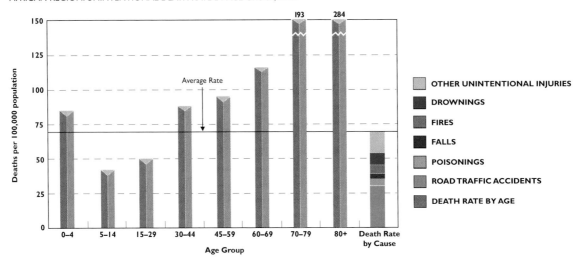

REGION OF THE AMERICAS

The Americas, represented by 35 countries, has the lowest average unintentional death rate in the world with 38 per 100,000 population. As in the rest of the world, unintentional death rates spike for the 80 and older age group, driven largely by fall deaths. For all but the 80 and older age group, road traffic accidents are the leading cause of unintentional death.

REGION OF THE AMERICAS: UNINTENTIONAL DEATH RATE BY AGE GROUP, 2008

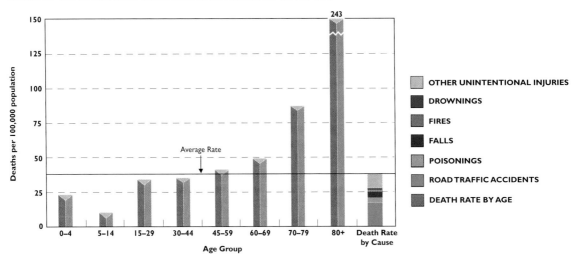

Source: National Safety Council analysis of World Health Organization Burden of Disease Project data.

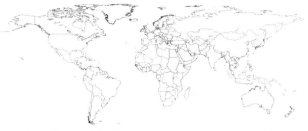

The Eastern Mediterranean Region, represented by 21 countries, has the third highest unintentional fatality rate with 62 per 100,000 population. Road traffic accidents are the leading cause among all age groups.

Falls represent the second leading cause for all age groups except for the 30-44 group. Among the 30-44 age group, fire is the second leading cause of death.

EASTERN MEDITERRANEAN REGION: UNINTENTIONAL DEATH RATE BY AGE GROUP, 2008

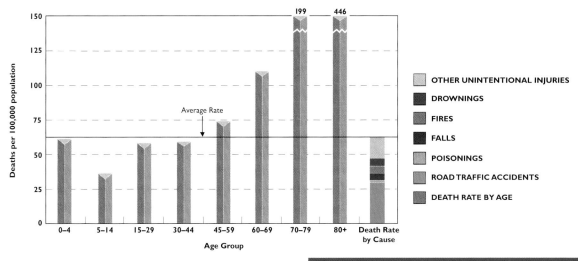

EUROPEAN REGION

The European Region, represented by 52 countries, has an average unintentional fatality rate of 57 per 100,000 population. Looking at the age groups, there is no one dominate cause. Drowning is the leading cause among

children younger than 5, road traffic accidents are the leading cause among 5-44 year olds and 60-69 year olds, poisoning is the leading cause for 45-59 year olds, and falls are the leading cause for the 70 and older age groups.

EUROPEAN REGION: UNINTENTIONAL DEATH RATE BY AGE GROUP, 2008

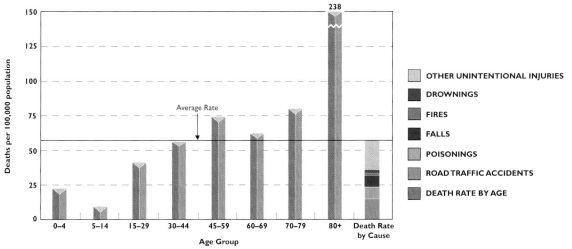

Source: National Safety Council analysis of World Health Organization Burden of Disease Project data.

INTERNATIONAL UNINTENTIONAL INJURY DEATHS: SOUTH EAST ASIAN REGION

The South East Asian Region is represented by 11 countries including India and has the highest average unintentional fatality rate with 79 per 100,000 population. Although road traffic accidents are the most prevalent cause overall, falls represent the top cause for the 70 and older age groups while fire is the lead cause among children younger than five.

SOUTH EAST ASIAN REGION: UNINTENTIONAL DEATH RATE BY AGE GROUP, 2008

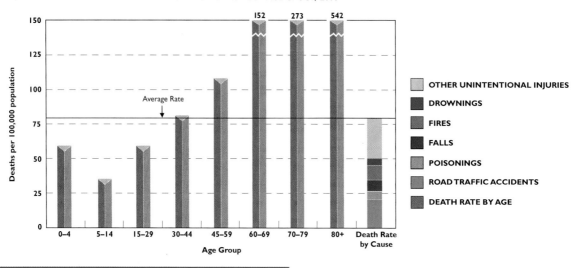

WESTERN PACIFIC REGION

The Western Pacific Region is represented by 27 countries including China and has the second lowest unintentional fatality rate behind the Americas Region with 47 per 100,000 population. Although road traffic accidents are the most prevalent cause overall, drowning represent the top cause for the 0–14 age group, while falls are the leading cause for individuals 80 and older.

WESTERN PACIFIC REGION: UNINTENTIONAL DEATH RATE BY AGE GROUP, 2008

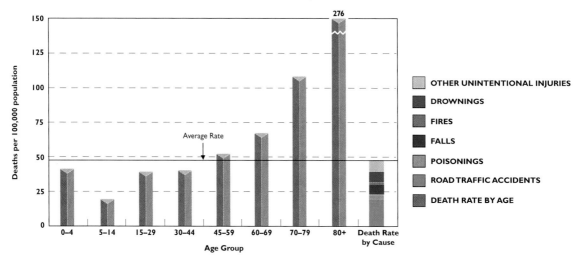

Source: National Safety Council analysis of World Health Organization Burden of Disease Project data.

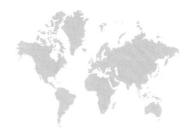

The term "Accidents and Adverse Effects" used in the International Classification of Diseases system refers to all causes of unintentional injury deaths, including transportation accidents, unintentional poisonings, falls, fires, burns, natural and environmental factors, drowning, suffocation, medical and surgical complications and misadventures, and other causes such as those involving machinery, firearms, or electric

current. The data presented in the table below are identified by codes V01–X59, Y85–Y86 of the tenth ICD revision (except where noted).

The tables on pages 189-193 show the number of injury deaths and the unadjusted death rates for 53 countries for which mortality data and population estimates were obtained.

UNINTENTIONAL INJURY DEATHS AND DEATH RATES BY AGE GROUP, LATEST YEAR AVAILABLE

Country	Year	Deaths		Deaths per 100,000 population[a]						
		Total	% male	All ages	0-4	5-14	15-24	25-44	45-64	65+
Argentina	2006	10,957	72%	27.7	18.5	8.9	25.9	26.4	31.8	64.3
Australia	2006	5,120	64%	25.1	7.3	3.2	21.8	20.9	18.6	81.6
Austria	2008	2,581	61%	31.0	5.8	2.1	19.1	12.3	20.6	111.1
Brazil	2005	58,299	80%	30.8	13.0	10.2	32.0	34.1	38.3	80.5
Canada	2004	8,986	60%	28.0	5.3	4.1	21.7	18.3	21.2	96.7
Chile	2005	4,772	77%	29.8	10.7	5.4	21.5	28.6	38.2	101.9
Colombia	2006	11,229	78%	26.7	23.2	9.5	23.7	28.0	30.8	85.7
Costa Rica	2006	1,333	77%	31.2	5.8	8.9	24.1	28.5	41.1	155.3
Croatia	2008	2,110	62%	47.6	5.7	4.2	32.7	30.5	36.2	141.9
Cuba	2006	4,229	59%	37.2	9.0	6.3	15.1	19.1	24.5	209.9
Cyprus	2007	275	71%	32.7	7.1	7.4	35.5	20.8	21.3	122.5
Czech Republic	2008	4,170	64%	40.0	5.3	2.7	22.4	23.5	41.8	121.5
Denmark	2006	1,812	55%	33.3	2.8	3.5	19.8	15.1	20.8	135.6
Ecuador	2006	5,157	77%	37.1	23.1	13.2	30.6	39.8	52.9	120.1
El Salvador	2006	2,513	80%	42.1	9.8	10.8	27.4	55.7	72.7	151.3
Estonia	2008	924	77%	68.9	17.8	6.3	42.5	60.4	107.6	99.1
Finland	2008	3,014	68%	56.7	3.8	2.2	21.4	30.4	69.9	155.4
France	2007	24,049	55%	38.8	5.0	2.9	18.8	17.3	25.0	149.2
Germany	2006	18,755	57%	22.8	4.1	2.2	14.5	10.7	15.2	69.9
Hong Kong, SAR	2007	873	70%	12.6	1.4	1.8	4.1	8.7	12.0	44.6
Hungary	2005	5,061	64%	50.2	6.7	4.1	21.9	29.4	53.0	151.5
Iceland	2008	63	65%	19.7	0.0	0.0	10.6	8.5	15.9	103.4
Ireland	2007	1,013	67%	23.3	4.5	2.4	23.0	19.6	22.7	74.0
Israel	2006	1,231	62%	17.5	7.6	3.8	13.9	10.7	13.1	85.0
Italy	2007	19,893	57%	33.5	3.3	2.7	22.1	17.0	15.6	108.5
Japan	2008	39,861	60%	31.6	5.9	2.2	8.2	7.8	18.7	104.0
Kazakhstan[b]	2008	19,693	78%	125.6	42.5	23.1	99.5	180.7	175.3	152.6
Kyrgyzstan	2006	2,571	77%	49.8	44.4	12.2	21.7	66.8	105.3	82.0
Latvia	2007	2,141	75%	94.1	15.8	16.3	39.9	87.2	156.8	125.0
Lithuania	2008	2,997	76%	89.2	18.6	10.7	35.5	77.1	166.4	116.3
Mexico	2006	36,180	77%	33.7	25.5	9.1	29.9	33.5	45.4	118.0
Netherlands	2008	3,735	50%	22.6	3.4	1.8	8.5	8.0	10.4	102.6
Nicaragua	2005	1,184	81%	21.6	10.6	7.2	22.8	25.8	31.0	105.1
Norway	2007	1,867	55%	39.6	3.4	2.4	18.5	22.0	24.8	165.9
Panama	2006	1,064	76%	33.2	25.7	7.8	27.7	31.0	41.3	129.9
Paraguay	2006	1,534	78%	25.5	12.9	6.9	31.1	28.9	31.7	73.7
Poland	2007	15,870	73%	41.6	6.4	5.5	27.0	32.7	54.6	93.8
Republic of Korea	2006	15,633	69%	32.0	9.9	5.4	12.0	17.6	41.6	144.6
Romania	2008	9,759	77%	45.4	20.6	13.3	30.0	34.0	67.2	78.2
Russian Federation[b]	2006	282,785	78%	198.5	35.3	21.2	120.1	244.1	283.5	226.6
Serbia	2008	1,910	78%	26.0	4.1	4.8	21.7	20.4	27.1	55.2
Slovakia	2005	2,085	78%	38.7	11.5	4.7	20.9	31.6	63.4	73.3
Slovenia	2008	1,007	63%	49.4	3.1	2.7	26.4	23.9	42.2	166.1
South Africa	2006	10,974	67%	22.9	31.0	8.6	15.3	28.8	25.9	57.3
Spain	2005	12,515	69%	28.8	5.3	3.6	24.0	21.8	22.5	76.4
Sweden	2007	3,117	60%	34.1	1.7	1.7	15.2	12.6	23.2	128.5
Switzerland[b]	2007	3,782	61%	50.1	4.6	3.2	28.7	28.8	41.2	163.4
Thailand	2006	20,847	79%	32.0	19.1	18.0	40.8	33.2	34.5	39.9
Ukraine[b]	2006	64,556	79%	138.5	34.8	16.7	71.6	158.1	224.8	137.9
United Kingdom	2007	14,569	58%	23.9	4.1	2.4	16.5	15.7	15.7	80.1
United States of America	2005	117,809	65%	39.7	13.5	6.0	37.4	36.8	40.1	100.0
Uzbekistan	2005	6,342	75%	24.2	36.6	11.2	13.7	31.7	34.5	41.2
Venezuela	2005	8,518	77%	33.7	29.0	11.2	31.5	40.2	40.8	92.2

Source: National Safety Council tabulations of World Health Organization data.
[a]*Population estimates based on data from WHO and the U.S. Census Bureau (International Data Base)*
[b]*Data include deaths due to all external causes, including self-harm and assault.*

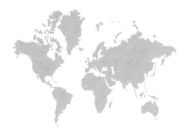

The International Classification of Diseases system identifies motor vehicle traffic accidents by codes V02–V04, V09, V12–V14, V19–V79, V86–V89 of the 10th ICD revision. A motor vehicle is a mechanically or electrically powered device used in the transportation of people or property on a land highway. A motor vehicle traffic accident involves a motor vehicle in transport (i.e., in motion or on a roadway) on a public highway.

MOTOR VEHICLE DEATHS AND DEATH RATES BY AGE GROUP, LATEST YEAR AVAILABLE

Country	Year	Deaths		Deaths per 100,000 population[a]						
		Total	% male	All ages	0-4	5-14	15-24	25-44	45-64	65+
Argentina	2006	3,799	75%	9.6	3.0	3.4	11.5	11.5	12.7	11.8
Australia	2006	1,395	75%	6.8	1.7	1.5	13.4	7.9	5.5	8.0
Austria	2008	346	79%	4.2	0.5	0.6	7.6	3.5	3.8	6.5
Brazil	2005	25,977	82%	13.7	2.0	3.0	19.0	18.2	16.2	18.3
Canada	2004	2,834	71%	8.8	1.2	2.3	16.2	8.8	7.9	12.1
Chile	2005	1,118	81%	7.0	1.8	1.2	7.4	9.2	9.1	10.3
Colombia	2006	5,168	79%	12.3	2.9	3.2	13.4	16.3	14.7	28.7
Costa Rica	2006	512	83%	12.0	1.7	2.9	10.8	13.8	18.8	32.4
Croatia	2008	578	80%	13.0	1.9	1.9	22.4	15.4	12.5	13.2
Cuba	2006	973	80%	8.6	2.5	2.2	8.1	9.8	9.9	14.1
Cyprus	2007	103	82%	12.2	4.7	4.2	25.6	9.9	9.4	19.4
Czech Republic	2008	779	75%	7.5	1.5	1.5	11.5	7.9	7.2	9.3
Denmark	2006	300	72%	5.5	1.2	1.2	12.9	4.5	4.5	8.9
Ecuador	2006	954	76%	6.9	1.6	2.2	7.8	9.7	9.7	10.6
El Salvador	2006	1,628	80%	27.3	5.8	6.7	19.5	38.2	45.4	88.5
Estonia	2008	142	73%	10.6	2.7	2.4	17.5	8.6	12.6	11.7
Finland	2008	317	75%	6.0	0.7	1.2	10.8	5.4	4.9	10.1
France	2007	4,407	76%	7.1	1.3	1.4	13.5	8.5	5.8	8.3
Germany	2006	4,250	73%	5.2	1.0	1.0	10.2	5.2	4.4	6.1
Hong Kong, SAR	2007	153	65%	2.2	0.9	1.0	1.7	1.7	2.0	5.9
Hungary	2005	1,275	76%	12.6	2.1	2.4	14.2	14.6	14.4	15.0
Iceland	2008	14	79%	4.4	0.0	0.0	6.4	3.2	4.0	13.6
Ireland	2007	248	74%	5.7	2.2	1.2	12.1	4.8	4.3	10.4
Israel	2006	312	74%	4.4	1.5	1.2	9.5	4.6	4.5	4.4
Italy	2007	5,337	80%	9.0	1.1	1.6	16.8	10.4	6.8	10.9
Japan	2008	6,830	68%	5.4	1.0	1.0	5.1	3.0	4.6	12.2
Kazakhstan[b]	2008	3,694	74%	23.6	5.6	7.7	25.1	34.8	26.3	22.4
Kyrgyzstan	2006	534	77%	10.3	2.5	3.1	7.0	15.9	17.9	17.0
Latvia	2007	432	74%	19.0	2.8	3.8	19.1	21.5	24.0	20.0
Lithuania	2008	525	72%	15.6	2.6	4.5	20.6	17.6	17.2	15.9
Mexico	2006	11,261	78%	10.5	3.7	3.1	13.3	13.2	13.7	17.1
Netherlands	2008	647	74%	3.9	0.5	1.0	6.7	3.8	3.2	6.7
Nicaragua	2005	439	82%	8.0	2.7	2.3	8.4	11.7	12.7	24.2
Norway	2007	232	72%	4.9	0.7	1.1	7.4	5.1	4.7	8.1
Panama	2006	472	78%	14.7	3.7	3.0	16.2	19.5	21.5	26.0
Paraguay	2006	715	80%	11.9	1.5	2.3	18.6	16.3	14.3	19.0
Poland	2007	5,385	76%	14.1	2.4	2.8	17.8	14.5	15.4	19.7
Republic of Korea	2006	7,609	73%	15.6	4.3	3.2	9.1	10.6	22.0	52.6
Romania	2008	2,804	75%	13.0	2.7	3.9	14.3	12.6	16.6	16.7
Russian Federation[b]	2006	38,241	73%	26.8	4.2	6.5	31.5	34.4	26.7	28.0
Serbia	2008	778	81%	10.6	1.7	2.1	12.3	9.7	11.7	16.7
Slovakia	2005	625	77%	11.6	2.3	2.4	12.7	12.5	14.5	14.5
Slovenia	2008	222	84%	10.9	3.1	1.1	19.2	11.5	10.7	11.5
South Africa	2006	5,641	72%	11.8	4.5	4.8	9.8	18.9	15.0	15.0
Spain	2005	4,617	79%	10.6	1.5	2.1	17.0	11.0	10.1	13.6
Sweden	2007	435	71%	4.8	0.2	0.8	8.7	4.3	4.7	6.6
Switzerland[b]	2007	415	78%	5.5	1.6	1.2	8.7	4.4	4.9	10.1
Thailand	2006	8,668	81%	13.3	2.5	4.4	23.4	15.6	12.9	10.5
Ukraine[b]	2006	9,885	76%	21.2	3.6	4.9	26.2	26.8	23.0	18.5
United Kingdom	2007	3,122	76%	5.1	0.9	1.2	10.1	5.6	3.9	6.5
United States of America	2005	45,343	70%	15.3	3.8	3.6	25.9	16.7	14.9	20.1
Uzbekistan	2005	2,247	79%	8.6	3.2	3.8	5.1	13.3	13.7	18.3
Venezuela	2005	3,185	79%	12.6	3.7	3.6	13.5	17.4	17.4	25.8

Source: National Safety Council tabulations of World Health Organization data.
[a]Population estimates based on data from WHO and the U.S. Census Bureau (International Data Base).
[b]Data include deaths due to all transportation-related causes, ICD-10 codes V01–V99.

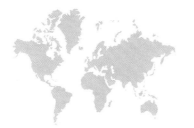

INTERNATIONAL POISONING DEATHS AND DEATH RATES

The International Classification of Diseases system identifies unintentional poisonings by codes X40–X49, which include cases of accidental poisoning by drugs, medicaments, biological substances, alcohol, solvents, gases, vapors, and pesticides. Other accidental poisonings by unspecified chemicals and noxious substances also are included.

UNINTENTIONAL POISONING DEATHS AND DEATH RATES BY AGE GROUP, LATEST YEAR AVAILABLE

Country	Year	Deaths		Deaths per 100,000 population[a]						
		Total	% male	All ages	0-4	5-14	15-24	25-44	45-64	65+
Argentina	2006	250	72%	0.6	0.9	0.1	0.3	0.5	1.0	1.3
Australia	2006	675	69%	3.3	0.2	0.1	2.2	5.3	4.3	3.0
Austria	2008	20	75%	0.2	0.0	0.0	0.3	0.2	0.2	0.6
Brazil	2005	231	71%	0.1	0.2	0.0	0.1	0.1	0.1	0.2
Canada	2004	954	71%	3.0	0.1	0.1	1.6	4.6	4.3	2.1
Chile	2005	109	71%	0.7	0.3	0.2	0.4	0.8	0.8	2.0
Colombia	2006	123	80%	0.3	0.4	0.1	0.3	0.3	0.5	0.4
Costa Rica	2006	55	91%	1.3	0.0	0.0	0.8	1.7	2.4	3.8
Croatia	2008	141	84%	3.2	0.0	0.4	3.1	6.2	2.1	2.7
Cuba	2006	79	87%	0.7	0.3	0.1	0.2	0.6	1.4	1.2
Cyprus	2007	8	88%	1.0	0.0	0.0	1.7	1.7	0.0	1.0
Czech Republic	2008	308	73%	3.0	0.2	0.1	1.3	2.4	5.9	2.7
Denmark	2006	188	77%	3.5	0.0	0.1	4.3	5.8	4.1	1.4
Ecuador	2006	211	85%	1.5	0.3	0.1	1.2	1.6	3.7	4.2
El Salvador	2006	259	91%	4.3	0.2	0.2	0.9	6.6	14.0	8.2
Estonia	2008	204	82%	15.2	0.0	0.0	8.5	22.4	24.7	8.7
Finland	2008	873	75%	16.4	0.0	0.0	7.3	16.0	33.6	10.9
France	2007	1,182	57%	1.9	0.2	0.1	0.8	1.8	1.9	4.8
Germany	2006	758	75%	0.9	0.1	0.0	0.7	1.6	1.0	0.6
Hong Kong, SAR	2007	246	83%	3.6	0.0	0.1	0.6	5.4	5.4	1.5
Hungary	2005	154	69%	1.5	0.2	0.0	1.7	1.7	2.1	1.6
Iceland	2008	8	50%	2.5	0.0	0.0	0.0	2.1	2.6	10.9
Ireland	2007	235	68%	5.4	0.0	0.0	5.4	8.6	6.7	3.6
Israel	2006	2	100%	0.1	0.0	0.0	0.0	0.1	0.2	0.0
Italy	2007	520	77%	0.9	0.1	0.1	0.5	1.6	0.6	0.8
Japan	2008	895	66%	0.7	0.1	0.0	0.5	1.0	0.8	0.8
Kazakhstan	2008	2,666	76%	17.0	3.0	1.6	6.5	25.9	30.1	22.7
Kyrgyzstan	2006	648	78%	12.5	2.5	0.4	2.7	17.1	39.2	24.0
Latvia	2007	347	75%	15.2	0.0	1.9	4.5	17.4	29.2	12.3
Lithuania	2008	720	78%	21.4	3.2	1.1	3.2	23.4	45.6	17.0
Mexico	2006	1,537	84%	1.4	0.6	0.2	0.8	1.7	2.7	4.2
Netherlands	2008	152	76%	0.9	0.0	0.0	0.6	1.7	1.0	0.7
Nicaragua	2005	17	71%	0.3	0.3	0.0	0.5	0.5	0.0	0.6
Norway	2007	341	74%	7.2	0.0	0.0	7.1	12.3	9.2	3.8
Panama	2006	110	62%	3.4	3.4	0.0	0.3	0.7	4.3	33.3
Paraguay	2006	20	75%	0.3	0.7	0.1	0.3	0.4	0.3	0.0
Poland	2007	1,754	84%	4.6	0.1	0.2	0.7	4.9	9.5	4.0
Republic of Korea	2006	296	66%	0.6	0.0	0.1	0.1	0.3	0.7	3.3
Romania	2008	1,066	72%	5.0	2.1	0.7	1.5	3.2	8.9	9.2
Russian Federation	2006	55,303	78%	38.8	3.8	1.2	14.4	51.9	65.0	32.7
Serbia	2008	99	86%	1.3	0.6	0.1	1.4	2.4	0.8	1.5
Slovakia	2005	162	80%	3.0	0.0	0.0	1.2	3.6	6.2	1.3
Slovenia	2008	70	87%	3.4	0.0	0.0	2.8	4.4	5.0	2.4
South Africa	2006	1,234	54%	2.6	15.3	0.4	0.5	1.6	1.8	2.8
Spain	2005	885	78%	2.0	0.0	0.1	1.4	3.8	1.4	1.5
Sweden	2007	351	81%	3.8	0.2	0.1	2.9	4.8	6.4	2.9
Switzerland	2007	208	73%	2.8	0.3	0.0	2.6	5.8	2.3	0.7
Thailand	2006	51	65%	0.1	0.1	0.0	0.0	0.1	0.1	0.2
Ukraine	2006	12,175	79%	26.1	3.4	0.8	4.5	28.7	55.7	18.2
United Kingdom	2007	1,533	74%	2.5	0.0	0.1	1.6	4.7	3.1	1.2
United States of America	2005	23,618	67%	8.0	0.2	0.1	5.9	13.2	12.3	2.5
Uzbekistan	2005	426	77%	1.6	0.9	0.3	0.8	2.9	2.9	2.6
Venezuela	2005	82	70%	0.3	0.9	0.2	0.3	0.2	0.3	0.8

Source: National Safety Council tabulations of World Health Organization data.
[a]Population estimates based on data from WHO and the U.S. Census Bureau (International Data Base).

INTERNATIONAL FALL-RELATED DEATHS AND DEATH RATES

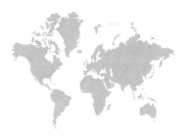

"Accidental falls" are identified by codes W00–W19 in the 10th revision of the International Classification of Diseases system.

UNINTENTIONAL FALL DEATHS AND DEATH RATES BY AGE GROUP, LATEST YEAR AVAILABLE

Country	Year	Deaths		Deaths per 100,000 population[a]						
		Total	% male	All ages	0-4	5-14	15-24	25-44	45-64	65+
Argentina	2006	346	68%	0.9	0.3	0.2	0.3	0.5	1.0	4.0
Australia	2006	1,160	48%	5.7	0.2	0.0	0.6	0.6	1.9	38.1
Austria	2008	863	57%	10.4	1.0	0.2	1.0	2.2	6.2	45.9
Brazil	2005	6,876	69%	3.6	0.8	0.5	0.8	2.2	5.1	29.9
Canada	2004	2,229	48%	6.9	0.4	0.2	0.4	0.8	3.0	41.9
Chile	2005	725	56%	4.5	0.3	0.0	0.6	1.8	4.2	37.5
Colombia	2006	1,178	79%	2.8	1.0	0.4	1.1	2.0	4.0	21.4
Costa Rica	2006	89	83%	2.1	0.0	0.1	0.5	1.8	4.6	11.8
Croatia	2008	842	42%	19.0	0.5	0.0	0.7	1.6	8.9	92.7
Cuba	2006	1,643	45%	14.5	0.4	0.3	0.9	1.4	4.2	123.6
Cyprus	2007	29	69%	3.4	0.0	0.0	2.5	2.7	1.6	15.3
Czech Republic	2008	1,035	53%	9.9	0.6	0.0	1.0	2.8	7.2	47.1
Denmark	2006	312	49%	5.7	0.0	0.0	0.2	0.7	3.2	30.5
Ecuador	2006	494	75%	3.5	1.5	0.8	2.4	2.9	5.3	20.4
El Salvador	2006	260	67%	4.4	0.8	0.6	0.7	2.6	6.9	41.8
Estonia	2008	124	75%	9.2	0.0	0.0	0.5	5.1	13.5	25.2
Finland	2008	1,154	54%	21.7	0.7	0.2	0.9	2.1	12.3	105.0
France	2007	5,409	48%	8.7	0.3	0.3	0.7	1.2	4.7	42.5
Germany	2006	8,381	45%	10.2	0.5	0.1	0.5	1.0	4.3	44.5
Hong Kong, SAR	2007	183	67%	2.6	0.5	0.0	1.1	0.6	1.8	14.2
Hungary	2005	2,102	49%	20.8	0.0	0.2	0.4	2.7	14.1	103.0
Iceland	2008	22	59%	6.9	0.0	0.0	0.0	0.0	1.3	57.2
Ireland	2007	242	53%	5.6	1.0	0.0	0.3	2.1	5.2	33.6
Israel	2006	80	56%	1.1	0.6	0.2	0.1	0.3	0.5	8.6
Italy	2007	2,958	55%	5.0	0.3	0.2	0.6	1.1	2.6	19.4
Japan	2008	7,170	59%	5.7	0.4	0.1	0.6	1.0	3.0	20.3
Kazakhstan	2008	527	76%	3.4	2.9	0.5	2.2	4.6	4.0	6.0
Kyrgyzstan	2006	87	83%	1.7	1.4	1.4	0.7	2.2	2.5	2.1
Latvia	2007	288	71%	12.7	0.9	0.5	1.7	6.7	19.5	32.0
Lithuania	2008	504	75%	15.0	0.0	0.6	2.3	7.3	27.5	35.7
Mexico	2006	2,287	77%	2.1	0.9	0.3	0.9	1.4	3.8	14.4
Netherlands	2008	1,372	42%	8.3	0.3	0.1	0.2	0.9	2.9	45.8
Nicaragua	2005	84	76%	1.5	0.5	0.2	0.8	1.3	3.3	18.3
Norway	2007	348	54%	7.4	0.0	0.2	1.0	0.5	3.5	42.5
Panama	2006	98	73%	3.1	0.9	0.5	0.5	1.8	3.5	26.5
Paraguay	2006	70	74%	1.2	1.3	0.4	0.6	1.1	1.5	5.8
Poland	2007	3,867	57%	10.1	0.3	0.2	1.3	3.3	9.3	48.3
Republic of Korea	2006	3,419	60%	7.0	1.4	0.4	0.6	2.1	7.5	47.1
Romania	2008	1,433	81%	6.7	1.6	0.4	1.7	3.4	11.1	16.9
Russian Federation	2006	11,394	74%	8.0	1.7	0.6	3.6	7.7	11.3	15.4
Serbia	2008	304	74%	4.1	0.3	0.0	0.8	1.1	4.1	15.0
Slovakia	2005	472	74%	8.8	0.8	0.3	1.2	3.6	14.3	32.2
Slovenia	2008	550	47%	27.0	0.0	0.0	0.4	2.4	14.8	136.5
South Africa	2006	129	70%	0.3	0.1	0.1	0.1	0.2	0.3	2.1
Spain	2005	1,763	58%	4.1	0.4	0.1	1.0	1.5	2.5	16.8
Sweden	2007	795	55%	8.7	0.0	0.1	0.4	0.5	4.5	42.0
Switzerland	2007	1,308	46%	17.3	0.3	0.2	1.9	1.8	5.3	92.7
Thailand	2006	842	78%	1.3	0.2	0.1	0.4	1.0	2.4	4.4
Ukraine	2006	3,106	80%	6.7	1.3	0.5	2.1	6.0	11.2	10.4
United Kingdom	2007	4,088	48%	6.7	0.1	0.1	0.5	1.2	3.5	33.7
United States of America	2005	19,656	52%	6.6	0.2	0.1	0.6	1.1	3.6	43.0
Uzbekistan	2005	444	79%	1.7	1.9	1.1	1.2	1.9	2.4	3.3
Venezuela	2005	702	63%	2.8	0.8	0.4	0.7	1.5	3.0	32.1

Source: National Safety Council tabulations of World Health Organization data.
[a]Population estimates based on data from WHO and the U.S. Census Bureau (International Data Base).

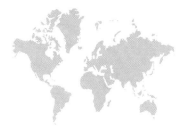

UNINTENTIONAL DROWNING DEATHS AND DEATH RATES

The International Classification of Diseases system identifies drowning by codes W65–W74, which include cases of unintentional drowning and submersion while in or following a fall in a bathtub, swimming pool, or natural body of water. Other specified and unspecified cases of drowning and submersion also are included.

UNINTENTIONAL DROWNING DEATHS AND DEATH RATES BY AGE GROUP, LATEST YEAR AVAILABLE

Country	Year	Deaths Total	Deaths % male	Deaths per 100,000 population[a] All ages	0-4	5-14	15-24	25-44	45-64	65+
Argentina	2006	576	82%	1.5	4.1	1.3	1.7	1.1	1.0	1.0
Australia	2006	178	74%	0.9	2.4	0.2	0.7	0.9	0.8	1.1
Austria	2008	68	74%	0.8	2.0	0.3	0.8	0.5	0.5	1.9
Brazil	2005	6,171	86%	3.3	2.8	2.9	4.6	3.1	2.8	2.9
Canada	2004	251	80%	0.8	1.3	0.5	0.9	0.7	0.7	1.0
Chile	2005	488	88%	3.1	3.0	1.2	3.5	2.9	3.4	5.7
Colombia	2006	1,077	80%	2.6	5.5	2.3	2.8	1.9	1.5	4.2
Costa Rica	2006	132	83%	3.1	1.9	3.0	4.3	2.7	3.8	1.3
Croatia	2008	93	82%	2.1	1.0	0.8	0.9	1.5	2.6	4.2
Cuba	2006	253	90%	2.2	2.8	2.2	2.1	2.3	1.9	2.5
Cyprus	2007	31	71%	3.7	0.0	3.2	3.3	2.7	2.1	12.2
Czech Republic	2008	170	78%	1.6	0.8	0.0	0.7	1.2	2.5	3.0
Denmark	2006	46	89%	0.8	0.0	0.9	0.7	0.4	1.4	1.1
Ecuador	2006	521	81%	3.7	5.6	2.6	4.2	3.8	3.2	4.4
El Salvador	2006	238	86%	4.0	2.0	2.6	5.0	5.4	4.0	3.5
Estonia	2008	77	73%	5.7	6.8	0.8	3.0	4.3	9.1	7.8
Finland	2008	118	86%	2.2	1.4	0.2	0.9	1.5	2.9	4.9
France	2007	970	70%	1.6	1.1	0.3	0.7	1.0	1.9	3.7
Germany	2006	418	71%	0.5	0.7	0.4	0.2	0.3	0.6	0.9
Hong Kong, SAR	2007	43	65%	0.6	0.0	0.3	0.4	0.3	0.9	1.6
Hungary	2005	192	82%	1.9	1.3	0.7	1.5	2.0	2.5	2.1
Iceland	2008	1	100%	0.6	0.0	0.0	4.1	0.0	0.0	0.0
Ireland	2007	51	90%	1.2	0.3	0.2	1.7	1.2	1.4	1.7
Israel	2006	45	78%	0.6	0.8	0.5	0.6	0.7	0.5	0.9
Italy	2007	387	82%	0.7	0.3	0.2	0.8	0.6	0.6	1.1
Japan	2008	6,464	53%	5.1	1.0	0.4	0.8	0.8	2.6	18.1
Kazakhstan	2008	1,106	83%	7.1	6.2	4.4	7.2	9.4	6.8	4.6
Kyrgyzstan	2006	270	74%	5.2	16.4	2.5	1.8	5.6	6.2	3.9
Latvia	2007	237	81%	10.4	7.5	6.2	5.1	10.8	14.6	11.5
Lithuania	2008	322	84%	9.6	4.5	3.1	4.7	9.3	18.0	7.7
Mexico	2006	2,310	83%	2.1	3.1	1.3	2.9	1.8	1.9	3.5
Netherlands	2008	77	73%	0.5	1.2	0.2	0.2	0.2	0.7	0.8
Nicaragua	2005	196	87%	3.6	1.2	2.1	5.3	4.1	4.1	6.5
Norway	2007	52	73%	1.1	0.7	0.2	1.2	0.6	1.0	3.2
Panama	2006	120	88%	3.7	4.6	1.7	5.4	3.2	3.9	6.4
Paraguay	2006	125	90%	2.1	3.3	1.0	3.4	1.3	2.0	3.4
Poland	2007	958	85%	2.5	1.2	0.9	2.3	2.3	3.7	2.5
Republic of Korea	2006	757	78%	1.5	0.6	0.9	1.2	1.1	2.1	3.9
Romania	2008	941	82%	4.4	2.1	4.2	3.7	3.6	5.6	5.7
Russian Federation	2006	12,212	84%	8.6	3.7	4.9	6.9	10.8	10.2	7.3
Serbia	2008	89	80%	1.2	0.0	1.0	1.4	0.7	1.5	1.9
Slovakia	2005	138	80%	2.6	3.1	0.8	1.8	2.1	4.4	2.4
Slovenia	2008	27	70%	1.3	0.0	0.0	0.8	1.1	2.1	1.8
South Africa	2006	207	70%	0.4	1.7	1.0	0.1	0.1	0.0	0.1
Spain	2005	494	82%	1.1	1.1	0.2	0.8	0.8	1.2	2.4
Sweden	2007	108	83%	1.2	0.4	0.1	0.9	0.6	1.5	2.7
Switzerland	2007	51	71%	0.7	1.1	0.4	0.8	0.4	0.6	1.2
Thailand	2006	4,666	76%	7.2	11.9	9.7	4.0	5.8	7.6	9.3
Ukraine	2006	3,881	84%	8.3	4.3	4.7	6.2	10.4	10.7	6.4
United Kingdom	2007	224	81%	0.4	0.4	0.2	0.5	0.4	0.4	0.4
United States of America	2005	3,582	79%	1.2	2.7	0.6	1.5	1.0	1.0	1.3
Uzbekistan	2005	1,042	67%	4.0	15.5	3.3	1.7	2.9	2.7	3.2
Venezuela	2005	590	83%	2.3	3.8	2.0	3.5	1.8	1.7	1.7

Source: National Safety Council tabulations of World Health Organization data.
[a]Population estimates based on data from WHO and the U.S. Census Bureau (International Data Base).

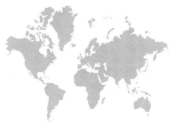

Counts and rates of fatal work-related injuries are shown on this page and the next. Comparisons between countries should be made with caution, and should take into account the differences in sources, coverage, and types of cases included.

OCCUPATIONAL DEATHS BY COUNTRY, 2004-2008

Country	Deaths					Source of data	Maximum period[a]	Coverage		
	2004	2005	2006	2007	2008			Worker types[b]	% of total employment[c]	Activities excluded
Injuries only—Compensated cases										
France	626	474	537	622	—	IR	varies	E	75	P
Injuries only—Reported cases										
Austria	132	124	107	108	115	IR	none	E, SE	71	none
Azerbaijan	72	54	81	128	72	LR	—	E	—	—
Belarus	248	235	228	214	185	C	same year	E	—	none
Czech Republic	185	163	152	188	174	AR	none	E,SE	95	AF, Pol
Hungary	160	125	123	118	—	LR	90 days	E,SE	98	none
Ireland	50	74	51	67	57	LR	none	E,SE	100	none
Japan	1,620	1,514	1,472	1,357	1,268	LR	—	E	—	C
Latvia	61	56	53	58	—	S	none	E	—	none
Norway	38	48	31	38	51	LR	none	E	100	none
Poland	490	468	493	479	523	LR	6 months	E,SE	76	Agr
Portugal	306	300	253	276	—	IR	one year	E,SE	67	PA, AF
Singapore	51	44	62	63	67	LR	none	E	33	none
Slovakia	79	76	95	97	80	C	none	IE	98	none
Spain	695	662	682	572	530	IR	1 month	I	85	PA, AF
Sweden	57	67	68	75	—	IR	none	E,SE	97	none
Trinidad and Tobago	3	18	11	—	—	LR	—	E,SE	100	none
Ukraine	1,068	989	972	1,069	927	LR	4 months	E	71	AF
United Kingdom	179	173	203	—	—	LR	1 year	E,SE	92	SF, AT
United States	5,764	5,734	5,840	5,657	—	C	none	E,SE	100	none
Injuries and commuting accidents—Compensated cases										
Croatia	38	62	76	74	79	IR	immediate	E, SE	84	none
Germany	949	863	941	812	765	IR	none	E, SE	100	none
Italy	930	918	987	847	744	IR	none	I	76	none
Injuries and commuting accidents—Reported cases										
Cyprus	14	13	18	15	12	LR	none	E	74	none
Hong Kong, China	187	187	187	172	—	LR	none	E	77	none
Lithuania	94	118	108	101	77	LR	none	E,SE	64	AF
Macau, China	2	15	6	14	14	LR	none	E	56	P
Romania	432	531	423	485	419	LR	same year	E,SE	61	AF, P
Russian Federation	3,290	3,090	2,900	2,990	2,550	S	none	E	5	Low rates
Slovenia	21	21	32	43	—	LR	1 month	I	85	none
Injuries and diseases—Compensated cases										
Australia[d]	178	182	192	193	207	IR	3 years	E	83	AF
Canada	458	491	442	392	465	IR	none	E, SE	85	AF
Malta	12	6	8	7	3	IR	—	E,SE	—	none
Switzerland	67	45	51	59	—	IR	same year	IE	88	none
Injuries and diseases—Reported cases										
Iceland	2	3	6	—	—	AR	—	E	—	none
Kazakhstan	345	357	414	341	341	LR	varies	E,SE	54	none
Sri Lanka	42	52	84	77	49	LR	1 year	E	35	M, E, TSC, C
Turkey	843	1,096	1,601	—	—	IR	—	IE	25	none
Injuries, diseases, and commuting accidents—Compensated cases										
Estonia	34	24	28	21	21	IR	1 year	I	100	AF, Pol
Israel	88	82	84	76	89	IR	same year	E,SE	100	none
Korea, Republic of[e]	1,417	1,288	1,238	1,267	1,332	IR	—	I	45	none
Thailand	861	1,444	808	741	—	IR	—	I	16	none
Injuries, diseases, and commuting accidents—Reported cases										
Bahrain	13	29	25	22	23	IR	none	E,SE	100	none
Bulgaria	130	130	169	179	—	AR	—	E,SE	35	none
Jordan	52	63	87	—	—	IR	none	E	—	AF
Kyrgyzstan	41	24	22	—	—	LR	none	E	33	none
Mauritius	7	4	1	1	3	IR	30 days	E	75	P
Mexico	1,364	1,367	1,328	1,279	1,412	IR	none	IE	32	none
New Zealand	82	109	98	84	77	IR	1 year	E,SE	100	none

Source: International Labour Organization, ILO Department of Statistics, accessed Sept. 22, 2010, from http://laborsta.ilo.org.
Note: Dash (—) means data not available. See footnotes on page 195.

Source of data	Worker types	Economic activities		
AR=Administrative reports	E=Employees	AF=Armed forces	E=Electricity, gas, and water	PA=Public administration
C=Census	I=Insured persons	Agr=Agriculture	Low=Activities with low rates of injuries	Pol=Police
IR=Insurance records	IE=Insured employees	AT=Air transport	M=Manufacturing	SF=Sea fishing
LR=Labor inspectorate records	SE=Self-employed	C=Construction	P=Public sector	TSC=Transport, storage, and communications
S=Survey				

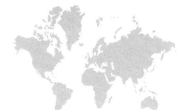

OCCUPATIONAL DEATH RATES

The International Labour Organization estimates about 2.3 million people die from work-related accidents and disease each year, including close to 360,000 fatal accidents and an estimated 1.95 million fatal work-related diseases. The total equates to about 5,500 worker deaths per day due to an accident or disease from their work.

Source: International Labor Organization (2009). World Day for Safety and Health at Work 2009—Facts On Safety and Health at Work. Accessed Sept. 23, 2010, at www.ilo.org/wcmsp5/groups/public/---dgreports/---dcomm/documents/publications/wcms_105146.pdf.

OCCUPATIONAL DEATH RATES BY COUNTRY, 2004-2008

Country	Coverage[e]	2004	2005	2006	2007	2008
Deaths per 100,000 employed persons						
Injuries only						
Belarus	RC	6.4	6.1	5.8	5.4	5.1
Hungary	RC	4.1	3.2	3.13	3.01	2.99
Ireland	RC	2.5	3.3	2.2	2.8	2.5
Moldova, Republic of	RC	4.9	6.4	4.7	7.1	5.3
Myanmar	RC	3	2	—	7	8.4
Norway	RC	1.7	2.1	1.3	1.6	2
Poland	RC	4.7	4.4	4.6	4.3	4.6
Sweden	RC	1.4	1.6	1.6	1.7	1.5
Trinidad and Tobago	RC	0.5	3.1	1.9	—	—
Ukraine	RC	8.9	8.4	8.3	9.3	8
United Kingdom	RC	0.7	0.6	0.72	—	—
United States	RC	4	4	4	4	—
Injuries and commuting accidents						
Croatia	CC	2.7	4.3	5	4.7	5.2
Cyprus	RC	5.4	5	6	5	—
Germany	CC	2.57	2.38	2.54	2.16	2.04
Hong Kong, China	RC	7.7	7.5	7.3	6.6	—
Lithuania	RC	9	10.9	9.6	8.7	6.6
Macau, China	RC	—	—	—	4.66	4.33
Romania	RC	7	9	7	8	7
Russian Federation	RC	12.9	12.4	11.9	12.4	10.9
Injuries and diseases						
Australia[d]	CC	2.1	2	2.1	2	2.1
Canada	CC	2.87	3.04	2.68	2.32	2.71
Kazakhstan	RC	10.4	10.3	11.3	8.7	8.2
Malta	CC	8.1	4	5.2	4.5	1.9
Injuries, diseases, and commuting accidents						
Bahrain	RC	5	10	8	7	5
Israel	CC	3.3	3	3	2.6	—
Kyrgyzstan	RC	8	5	5	—	—
Deaths per 100,000 workers insured						
Injuries only						
Austria	RC	5	4.6	3.9	3.9	—
Czech Republic	RC	4.2	3.7	3.4	4.1	3.8
France	CC	3.5	2.65	3.02	3.4	—
Portugal	RC	7	7	6	6.3	—
Slovakia	RC	3.91	3.72	4.6	4.1	4.2
Spain	RC	4.89	4.5	4.4	3.6	3.3
Injuries and commuting accidents						
Italy	CC	5	5	5	4	—
Slovenia	RC	2.6	2.6	3.8	5	—
Injuries and diseases						
Switzerland	CC	1.9	1.3	1.4	1.6	—
Turkey	RC	13.6	15.8	20.5	—	—
Zimbabwe	RC	—	6.2	7.5	6.3	—
Injuries, diseases, and commuting accidents						
Estonia	CC	5.71	3.95	4.3	3.2	3.2
Bulgaria	RC	6	5.8	7.2	7.1	—
Mexico	RC	11	11	10	9	10
Thailand	CC	11.66	18.7	10.1	9.1	—
Deaths per 1,000,000 hours worked						
Injuries only						
Japan	RC	0.01	0.01	0.01	0.01	—
Injuries and diseases						
Sri Lanka	RC	0.007	0.009	0.0135	0.012	0.008
Injuries, diseases and commuting accidents						
Jordan	RC	0.039	0.025	0.055	—	—
Korea, Republic of	CC	0.06	0.05	0.05	0.04	0.05

See source and limitations of data on page 194.
Note: Dash (—) indicates data not available.
[a]*Maximum period between accident and death for death to be counted.*
[b]*Types of workers included in the data.*
[c]*Workers covered by the statistics as a percentage of total employment; latest year available.*
[d]*Excluding Victoria and Australian Capital Territory.*
[e]*Includes reported cases (RC) and compensated cases (CC) of occupational fatalities.*

NATIONAL SAFETY COUNCIL

INJURY FACTS®

This appendix gives a brief explanation of some of the sources and methods used by the National Safety Council Statistics Department in preparing the estimates of deaths, injuries, and costs presented in this book. Because many of the estimates depend on death certificate data provided by states or the National Center for Health Statistics, it begins with a brief introduction to the certification and classification of deaths.

Certification and classification. The medical certification of death involves entering information on the death certificate about the disease or condition directly leading to death, antecedent causes, and other significant conditions. The death certificate is then registered with the appropriate authority and a code is assigned for the underlying cause of death. The underlying cause is defined as "(a) the disease or injury which initiated the train of morbid events leading directly to death, or (b) the circumstances of the accident or violence which produced the fatal injury" (World Health Organization, 1992). Deaths are classified and coded on the basis of a WHO standard, the *International Statistical Classification of Diseases and Related Health Problems*, commonly known as the International Classification of Diseases, or ICD (WHO, 1992). For deaths due to injury and poisoning, the ICD provides a system of "external cause" codes to which the underlying cause of death is assigned. (See pages 18-19 of *Injury Facts* for a condensed list of external cause codes.)

Comparability across ICD revisions. The ICD is revised periodically, and these revisions can affect comparability from year to year. The sixth revision (1948) substantially expanded the list of external causes and provided for classifying the place of occurrence. Changes in the classification procedures for the sixth, seventh (1958), and eighth (1968) revisions classified as diseases some deaths previously classified as injuries. The eighth revision also expanded and reorganized some external cause sections. The ninth revision (1979) provided more detail on the agency involved, the victim's activity, and the place of occurrence. The tenth revision, which was adopted in the United States effective with 1999 data, completely revised the transportation-related categories. Specific external cause categories affected by the revisions are noted in the historical tables.

The table at the end of this appendix (page 202) shows ICD-9 codes, ICD-10 codes, and a comparability ratio for each of the principal causes of unintentional injury death. The comparability ratio represents the net effect of the new revision on statistics for the cause of death. The comparability ratio was obtained by classifying a sample of death certificates under both ICD-9 and ICD-10, and then dividing the number of deaths for a selected cause classified under ICD-10 by the number classified to the most nearly comparable ICD-9 cause. A comparability ratio of 1.00 indicates no net change due to the new classification scheme. A ratio less than 1.00 indicates fewer deaths assigned to a cause under ICD-10 than under ICD-9. A ratio greater than 1.00 indicates an increase in assignment of deaths to a cause under ICD-10 compared to ICD-9.

The broad category of "accidents" or "unintentional injuries" under ICD-9 included complications and misadventures of surgical and medical care (E870–E879) and adverse effects of drugs in therapeutic use (E930–E949). These categories are not included in "accidents" or "unintentional injuries" under ICD-10. In 1998, deaths in these two categories numbered 3,228 and 276, respectively.

Under ICD-9, the code range for falls (E880–E888) included a code for "fracture, cause unspecified" (E887). A similar code does not appear in ICD-10 (W00–W19), which probably accounts for the low comparability ratio (0.8409). In 1998, deaths in code E887 numbered 3,679.

Beginning with 1970 data, tabulations published by NCHS no longer include deaths of nonresident aliens. In 2007, there were 866 such accidental deaths, of which 354 were motor vehicle-related.

Fatality estimates. The Council uses four classes and three venues to categorize unintentional injuries. The four classes are Motor Vehicle, Work, Home, and Public. Each class represents an environment and an intervention route for injury prevention through a responsible authority, such as a police department, an employer, a home owner, or a public health department. The three venues are Transportation, Work, and Home & Community.

Motor Vehicle. The Motor Vehicle class can be identified by the underlying cause of death (see the table on page 202).

Work. The National Safety Council adopted the Bureau of Labor Statistics' Census of Fatal Occupational Injuries figure, beginning with the 1992 data year, as the authoritative count of unintentional work-related deaths. The CFOI system is described in detail in Toscano and Windau (1994).

The 2-Way Split. After subtracting the Motor Vehicle and Work figures from the unintentional injury total (ICD-10 codes V01–X59, Y85–Y86), the remainder belong to the Home and Public classes. The Home class can be identified by the "place of occurrence" subclassification (code .0) used with most nontransport deaths; the Public class is the remainder. Missing "place of occurrence" information, however, prevents the direct determination of the Home and Public class totals. Because of this, the Council allocates nonmotor vehicle, nonwork deaths into the Home and Public classes based on the external cause, age group, and cases with specified "place of occurrence." This procedure, known as the 2-Way Split, uses the most recent death certificate data available from NCHS and CFOI data for the same calendar year. For each cause-code group and age group combination, the Motor Vehicle and Work deaths are subtracted and the remainder, including those with "place of occurrence" unspecified, are allocated to Home and Public in the same proportion as those with "place of occurrence" specified.

The table on page 202 shows ICD-10 cause-codes and CFOI event codes for the most common causes of unintentional injury death. CFOI event codes (BLS, 1992) do not match exactly with ICD cause codes, so some error exists in the allocation of deaths among classes.

State reporting system. Participating states send the Council tabulations of unintentional injury death data by age group, class, and type of event or industry. This is known as the Injury Mortality Tabulation reporting system. These data are used to validate current year estimates based on the most recent 2-Way Split and CFOI data.

Linking to current year. The benchmark data published by NCHS are usually two years old, while the

final CFOI data are usually one year old. Starting with the 2011 edition of *Injury Facts*, an exponential smoothing technique is used to make current year estimates. Exponential smoothing is a statistical technique to make short-term forcasts. In exponential smoothing (as opposed to in moving averages smoothing), older data is given progressively less relative weight (importance), whereas newer data is given progressively greater weight. The results of the exponential smoothing is then compared against the latest reported state data for validation.

Revisions of prior years. When the figures for a given year are published by NCHS, the 2-Way Split based on those figures and CFOI become the final estimate of unintentional injury deaths by class, age group, and type of event or industry. Subsequent years are revised by repeating the exponential smoothing and state data process described above. For example, in the current edition of *Injury Facts,* 2007 NCHS and CFOI data were used to produce final estimates using the 2-Way Split, the 2008 estimates were revised and the new 2009 estimates were made and validated with preliminary state data available in late summer 2010 together with 2009 preliminary CFOI data.

Nonfatal injury estimates. Starting with the 2011 edition of *Injury Facts*, the Council adopted the concept of "medically consulted injury" to define the kinds of injuries included in its estimates. Prior editions of *Injury Facts* used the definition of disabling injury. There is no national injury surveillance system that provides injury estimates on a current basis. The National Health Interview System, a household survey conducted by NCHS (see page 23), produces national estimates using its own definition of medically consulted injury (Adams, Heyman, Vickerie, 2009). A medically consulted injury as defined by NCHS is an injury serious enough that a medical professional was consulted. The Council uses the medically consulted injury estimates from the National Health Interview survey for its motor vehicle, home, and public injury estimates. In addition, the Occupational Safety and Health Administration defines injury or illness using criteria including "Medical treatment beyond first aid." The Council uses the total recordable case estimate defined by OSHA and published by the Bureau of Labor Statistics to estimate the number of workplace injuries. Because BLS's estimate excludes the self-employed, unpaid family workers, and federal government employees, the Council uses total employment estimates, as well as BLS nonfatal estimates, to calculate the total number of nonfatal medically consulted injuries.

Injury to death ratios. Because estimates for medically consulted injuries are not available for the current year, the Council used injury-to-death ratios to estimate nonfatal medically consulted injuries for the current year. Complete documentation of the procedure, effective with the 1993 edition, may be found in Landes, Ginsburg, Hoskin, and Miller (1990). The resulting estimates are not direct measures of nonfatal injuries and should not be compared with prior years.

Population sources. All population figures used in computing rates are estimates taken from various reports published by the Bureau of the Census, U.S. Department of Commerce, available at *www.census.gov*. *Resident* population is used for computing rates.

Costs (pp. 4-7). Procedures for estimating the economic losses due to fatal and nonfatal unintentional injuries were extensively revised for the 1993 edition of *Accident Facts®*. New components were added, new benchmarks adopted, and a new discount rate assumed. All of these changes resulted in significantly higher cost estimates. For this reason, it must be re-emphasized that the cost estimates should not be compared to those in earlier editions of the book.

The Council's general philosophy underlying its cost estimates is that the figures represent income not received or expenses incurred because of fatal and nonfatal unintentional injuries. Stated this way, the Council's cost estimates are a measure of the economic impact of unintentional injuries and may be compared to other economic measures such as gross domestic product, per capita income, or personal consumption expenditures. (See page 99 and "lost quality of life" [p. 201] for a discussion of injury costs for cost-benefit analysis.)

The general approach followed was to identify a benchmark unit cost for each component, adjust the benchmark to the current year using an appropriate inflator, estimate the number of cases to which the component applied, and compute the product. Where possible, benchmarks were obtained for each class: Motor Vehicle, Work, Home, and Public.

Wage and productivity losses include the value of wages, fringe benefits, and household production for all classes, and travel delay for the Motor Vehicle class.

For fatalities, the present value of after-tax wages, fringe benefits, and household production was computed using the human capital method. The procedure incorporates data on life expectancy from NCHS life tables, employment likelihood from BLS household survey, and mean earnings from the Bureau of the Census money income survey. The discount rate used was 4%, reduced from 6% used in earlier years. The present value obtained is highly sensitive to the discount rate; the lower the rate, the greater the present value.

For permanent partial disabilities, an average of 17% of earning power is lost (Berkowitz & Burton, 1987). The incidence of permanent disabilities, adjusted to remove intentional injuries, was computed from data on hospitalized cases from the National Hospital Discharge Survey and nonhospitalized cases from the National Health Interview Survey and National Council on Compensation Insurance data on probabilities of disability by nature of injury and part of body injured.

For temporary disabilities, an average daily wage, fringe benefit, and household production loss was calculated and then multiplied by the number of days of restricted activity from NHIS.

Travel delay costs were obtained from Council estimates of the number of fatal, injury, and property damage crashes and an average delay cost per crash from Miller et al. (1991).

Medical expenses, including ambulance and helicopter transport costs, were estimated for fatalities, hospitalized cases, and nonhospitalized cases in each class.

The incidence of hospitalized cases was derived from the NHDS data adjusted to eliminate intentional injuries. Average length of stay was benchmarked from Miller, Pindus, Douglass, and Rossman (1993b) and adjusted to estimate lifetime length of stay. The cost per hospital day was benchmarked to the National Medical Expenditure Survey.

Nonhospitalized cases were estimated by taking the difference between total NHIS injuries and hospitalized cases. Average cost per case was based on NMES data adjusted for inflation and lifetime costs.

Medical cost of fatalities was benchmarked to data from the National Council on Compensation Insurance (1989), to which was added the cost of a premature funeral and coroner costs (Miller et al., 1991).

Cost per ambulance transport was benchmarked to NMES data and cost per helicopter transport was benchmarked to data in Miller et al. (1993a). The number of cases transported was based on data from Rice and MacKenzie (1989) and the National Electronic Injury Surveillance System.

Administrative expenses include the administrative cost of private and public insurance, which represents the cost of having insurance, and police and legal costs.

The administrative cost of motor vehicle insurance was the difference between premiums earned (adjusted to remove fire, theft, and casualty premiums) and pure losses incurred, based on data from A.M. Best. Workers' compensation insurance administration was based on A.M. Best data for private carriers and regression estimates using Social Security Administration data for state funds and the self-insured. Administrative costs of public insurance (mainly Medicaid and Medicare) amount to about 4% of the medical expenses paid by public insurance, which were determined from Rice and MacKenzie (1989) and Hensler et al. (1991).

Average police costs for motor vehicle crashes were taken from Miller et al. (1991) and multiplied by the Council's estimates of the number of fatal, injury, and property damage crashes.

Legal expenses include court costs and plaintiff's and defendant's time and expenses. Hensler et al. (1991) provided data on the proportion of injured people who hire a lawyer, file a claim, and get compensation. Kakalik and Pace (1986) provided data on costs per case.

Fire losses were based on data published by the National Fire Protection Association in its journal. The allocation into the classes was based on the property use for structure fires and other NFPA data for nonstructure fires.

Motor vehicle damage costs were benchmarked to Blincoe and Faigin (1992) and multiplied by the Council's estimates of crash incidence.

Employer costs for work injuries is an estimate of the productivity costs incurred by employers. It assumes each fatality or permanent injury resulted in four person-months of disruption, serious injuries one person-month, and minor to moderate injuries two person-days. All injuries to nonworkers were assumed to involve two days of worker productivity loss. Average hourly earnings for supervisors and nonsupervisory workers were computed and then multiplied by the incidence and hours lost per case. Property damage and production delays (except motor vehicle-related) are not included in the estimates but can be substantial.

Lost quality of life is the difference between the value of a statistical fatality or statistical injury and the value of after-tax wages, fringe benefits, and household production. Because this does not represent real income not received or expenses incurred, it is not included in the total economic cost figure. If included, the resulting *comprehensive costs* can be used in cost-benefit analysis because the total costs then represent the maximum amount society should spend to prevent a statistical death or injury.

Work deaths and injuries. (p. 52). The method for estimating total work-related deaths and injuries is discussed above. The breakdown of deaths by industry division for the current year is obtained from CFOI. The estimate of nonfatal medically consulted injuries by industry division is made using the Survey of Occupational Injury and Illness' estimate of total recordable injury and illness after correcting for the exclusion of self-employed, unpaid family workers, and federal government employees (e.g., BLS, 2010).

Employment. The employment estimates for 1992 to the present were changed for the 1998 edition. Estimates for these years in prior editions are not comparable. The total employment figure used by the Council represents the number of people in the civilian labor force, age 16 and older, who were wage or salary workers, self-employed, or unpaid family workers, plus active-duty military personnel resident in the United

States. The total employment estimate is a combination of three figures—total civilian employment from the Current Population Survey as published in *Employment and Earnings*, plus the difference between total resident population and total civilian population, which represents active duty military personnel.

Employment by industry is obtained from an unpublished BLS table, "Employed and experience unemployed persons by detailed industry and class of worker, Annual Average [year] (based on CPS)."

Time lost (p. 55) is the product of the number of cases and the average time lost per case. Deaths average 150 workdays lost in the current year and 5,850 in future

years; permanent disabilities involve 75 and 565 days lost in current and future years, respectively; temporary disabilities involve 17 days lost in the current year only. Off-the-job injuries to workers are assumed to result in similar lost time.

Off the job (p. 56) deaths and injuries are estimated by assuming employed people incur injuries at the same rate as the entire population.

Motor vehicle (pp. 94-127). Estimates of miles traveled, registered vehicles, and licensed drivers are published by the Federal Highway Administration in *Highway Statistics* and *Traffic Volume Trends*.

SELECTED UNINTENTIONAL INJURY CODE GROUPINGS

Manner of injury	ICD-9 codes[a]	ICD-10 codes[b]	Comparability ratio[c]	OI & ICM[d] event codes
Unintentional injuries	E800–E869, E880–E929[e]	V01–X59, Y85–Y86	1.0305 (1.0278–1.0333)[f]	00–60, 63–9999
Railway accident	E800–E807	V05, V15, V80.6, V81(.2–.9)	n/a	44
Motor vehicle accident	E810–E825	V02–V04, V09.0, V09.2, V12–V14, V19.0–V19.2, V19.4–V19.6, V20–V79, V80.3–V80.5, V81.0–V81.1, V82.0–V82.1, V83–V86, V87.0–V87.8, V88.0–V88.8, V89.0, V89.2	0.9754 (0.9742–0.9766)	41, 42, 43 with source = 82, 83
Water transport accident	E830–E838	V90–V94	n/a	45
Air transport accident	E840–E845	V95–V97	n/a	46
Poisoning by solids and liquids	E850–58, E860–66	X40–X49	n/a	344
Poisoning by gases and vapors	E867–E869			341
Falls	E880–E888	W00–W19	0.8409 (0.8313–0.8505)	1
Fires and burns	E890–E899	X00–X09	0.9743 (0.9568–0.9918)	51
Drowning[g]	E910	W65–W74	0.9965 (0.9716–1.0213)	381
Choking[h]	E911–E912	W78–W80	n/a	382
Mechanical suffocation	E913	W75–W77, W81–W84	n/a	383, 384, 389
Firearms	E922	W32–W34	1.0579 (1.0331–1.0828)	0220, 0222, 0229 with source = 911[i]

Source: National Safety Council
Note: n/a means comparability ratio not calculated or does not meet standards of reliability or precision.
[a]WHO (1977)
[b]WHO (1992)
[c]Hoyert, Arias, Smith, et al. (2001). Table III
[d]BLS (1992)

[e]The National Safety Council has used E800-E949 for unintentional injuries. The code group in the table omits complications and misadventures of surgical and medical care (E870-E879) and adverse effects of drugs in therapeutic use (E930-E949).
[f]Figures in parentheses are the 95% confidence interval for the comparability ratio.
[g]Excludes transport
[h]Suffocation by ingestion or inhalation
[i]Struck by flying object where the source of injury was a bullet.

Adams, P.F., Heyman, K.M., Vickerie, J.L. (2009). Summary health statistics for the U.S. population: National health interview survey. 2008. *Vital and Health Statistics, Series 10, No. 243.* Hyattsville, MD: National Center for Health Statistics.

Berkowitz, M., and Burton, J.F., Jr. (1987). *Permanent Disability Benefits in Workers' Compensation.* Kalamazoo, MI: W.E. Upjohn Institute for Employment Research.

Blincoe, L.J., and Faigin, B.M. (1992). *Economic Cost of Motor Vehicle Crashes, 1990.* Springfield, VA: National Technical Information Service.

Bureau of Labor Statistics [BLS]. (1992). *Occupational Injury & Illness Classification Manual.* Itasca, IL: National Safety Council.

Bureau of Labor Statistics [BLS]. (2010, Oct. 21). *Workplace Injuries and Illnesses in 2009.* Press release USDL-10-1451.

Hensler, D.R., Marquis, M.S., Abrahamse, A.F., Berry, S.H., Ebener, P.A., Lewis, E.D., Lind, E.A., MacCoun, R.J., Manning, W.G., Rogowski, J.A., and Vaiana, M.E. (1991). *Compensation for Accidental Injuries in the United States.* Santa Monica, CA: The RAND Corporation.

Hoyert, D.L., Arias, E., Smith, B.L., Murphy, S.L., and Kochanek, K.D. (2001). Deaths: final data for 1999. *National Vital Statistics Reports, 49*(8).

Kakalik, J.S., and Pace, N. (1986). *Costs and Compensation Paid in Tort Litigation.* R-3391-ICJ. Santa Monica, CA: The RAND Corporation.

Landes, S.R., Ginsburg, K.M., Hoskin, A.F., and Miller, T.A. (1990). *Estimating Nonfatal Injuries.* Itasca, IL: Statistics Department, National Safety Council.

Miller, T., Viner, J., Rossman, S., Pindus, N., Gellert, W., Douglass, J., Dillingham, A., and Blomquist, G. (1991). *The Costs of Highway Crashes.* Springfield, VA: National Technical Information Service.

Miller, T.R., Brigham, P.A., Cohen, M.A., Douglass, J.B., Galbraith, M.S., Lestina, D.C., Nelkin, V.S., Pindus, N.M., and Smith-Regojo, P. (1993a). Estimating the costs to society of cigarette fire injuries. *Report to Congress in Response to the Fire Safe Cigarette Act of 1990.* Washington, DC: U.S. Consumer Product Safety Commission.

Miller, T.R., Pindus, N.M., Douglass, J.B., and Rossman, S.B. (1993b). *Nonfatal Injury Incidence, Costs, and Consequences: A Data Book.* Washington, DC: The Urban Institute Press.

Occupational Safety and Health Administration (2005). *OSHA recordkeeping handbook.* OSHA 3245-01R.

Rice, D.P., and MacKenzie, E.J. (1989). *Cost of Injury in the United States: A Report to Congress.* Atlanta, GA: Centers for Disease Control and Prevention.

Toscano, G., and Windau, J. (1994). The changing character of fatal work injuries. *Monthly Labor Review, 117*(10), 17–28.

World Health Organization. (1977). *Manual of the International Statistical Classification of Diseases, Injuries, and Causes of Death.* Geneva, Switzerland: Author.

World Health Organization. (1992). *International Statistical Classification of Diseases and Related Health Problems—Tenth Revision.* Geneva, Switzerland: Author.

The following organizations may be useful for obtaining more current data or more detailed information on various subjects in *Injury Facts*.

American Association of Poison Control Centers
515 King Street Suite 520
Alexandria, VA 22314
(703) 894-1858
www.aapcc.org
info@aapcc.org

Bureau of Labor Statistics
U.S. Department of Labor
2 Massachusetts Avenue, NE
Washington, DC 20212
(202) 691-5200
www.bls.gov
blsdata_staff@bls.gov

Bureau of the Census
U.S. Department of Commerce
4600 Silver Hill Road
Washington, DC 20233
(800) 923-8282
www.census.gov

Bureau of Justice Statistics
810 7th Street, NW
Washington, DC 20531
(202) 307-0765
www.ojp.usdoj.gov/bjs
askbjs@usdoj.gov

Research and Innovative Technology Administration
U.S. Department of Transportation
1200 New Jersey Avenue, SE
Washington, DC 20590
(800) 853-1351
www.bts.gov
answers@bts.gov

Centers for Disease Control and Prevention
1600 Clifton Road
Atlanta, GA 30333
(800) 232-4636
www.cdc.gov
cdcinfo@cdc.gov

Chemical Safety Board
2175 K Street, NW, Suite 400
Washington, DC 20037
(202) 261-7600
www.csb.gov
info@csb.gov

Data.gov
The purpose of Data.gov is to increase public access to high value, machine readable datasets.
www.data.gov

Eno Transportation Foundation
1250 I Street, NW, Suite 750
Washington, DC 20005
(202) 879-4700
www.enotrans.com

Environmental Protection Agency, U.S.
1200 Pennsylvania Avenue, NW
Washington, DC 20460
(202) 272-0167
www.epa.gov

European Agency for Safety and Health at Work
Gran Via, 33
E-48009 Bilbao, Spain
Phone: +34 944-794-360
Fax: +34 944-794-383
http://osha.europa.eu/en
information@osha.europa.eu

Federal Aviation Administration
U.S. Department of Transportation
National Aviation Safety Data Analysis Center
800 Independence Avenue, SW
Washington, DC 20591
(866) 835-5322
www.faa.gov

Federal Bureau of Investigation
935 Pennsylvania Avenue, NW
Washington, DC 20535-0001
(202) 324-3000
www.fbi.gov

Federal Highway Administration
U.S. Department of Transportation
1200 New Jersey Ave., SE
Washington, DC 20590
(202) 366-0660
www.fhwa.dot.gov
execsecretariat.fhwa@fhwa.dot.gov

Federal Motor Carrier Safety Administration
U.S. Department of Transportation
1200 New Jersey Ave., SE
Washington, DC 20590
(800) 832-5660
www.fmcsa.dot.gov

Federal Railroad Administration
U.S. Department of Transportation
1200 New Jersey Ave., SE
Washington, DC 20590
(202) 493-6024
www.fra.dot.gov

FedStats
Gateway to official statistical information available to the
public from more than 100 federal agencies.
www.fedstats.gov

Federal Transit Administration
1200 New Jersey Ave., SE
Washington, DC 20590
www.fta.dot.gov

Insurance Information Institute
110 William Street
New York, NY 10038
(212) 346-5500
www.iii.org

Insurance Institute for Highway Safety
1005 N. Glebe Road, Suite 800
Arlington, VA 22201
(703) 247-1500
www.iihs.org

International Hunter Education Association
2727 W. 92nd Ave., Suite 103
Federal Heights, CO 80260
(303) 430-7233
www.ihea.com
info@ihea.com

International Labour Office
4, rue des Morillons
CH-1211 Geneva 22
Switzerland
Phone: +41-22-799-6111
Fax: +41-22-798-8685
www.ilo.org
ilo@ilo.org

Mine Safety and Health Administration
1100 Wilson Boulevard, 21st Floor
Arlington, VA 22209-3939
(202) 693-9400
www.msha.gov

Motorcycle Safety Foundation
2 Jenner Street, Suite 150
Irvine, CA 92718-3812
(949) 727-3227
www.msf-usa.org

National Academy of Social Insurance
1776 Massachusetts Avenue, NW, Suite 400
Washington, DC 20036-1904
(202) 452-8097
www.nasi.org
nasi@nasi.org

National Center for Education Statistics
U.S. Department of Education
1990 K Street, NW
Washington, DC 20006
(202) 502-7300
http://nces.ed.gov

National Center for Health Statistics
3311 Toledo Road, Room 2217
Hyattsville, MD 20782
(800) 232-4636
www.cdc.gov/nchs

National Center for Injury Prevention and Control
4770 Buford Highway, NE
Atlanta, GA 30341-3724
(800) 232-4636
www.cdc.gov/injury/index.html
cdcinfo@cdc.gov

National Center for Statistics and Analysis
1200 New Jersey Avenue, S.E.
West Building
Washington, DC 20590
(202) 366-4198 or (800) 934-8517
www.nhtsa.dot.gov
NCSAweb@nhtsa.dot.gov

National Climatic Data Center
151 Patton Avenue
Asheville, NC 28801-5001
(828) 271-4800
www.ncdc.noaa.gov/oa/ncdc.html
ncdc.info@noaa.gov

National Collegiate Athletic Association
700 W. Washington Street
P.O. Box 6222
Indianapolis, IN 46206-6222
(317) 917-6222
www.ncaa.org

National Council on Compensation Insurance
901 Peninsula Corporate Circle
Boca Raton, FL 33487
(566) 893-1000
www.ncci.com

National Fire Protection Association
P.O. Box 9101
Batterymarch Park
Quincy, MA 02269-0910
(617) 770-3000 or (800) 344-3555
www.nfpa.org
custserv@nfpa.org

National Highway Traffic Safety Administration
U.S. Department of Transportation
1200 New Jersey Avenue, SE
Washington, DC 20590
(800) 877-8339

National Institute for Occupational Safety and Health
Clearinghouse for Occupational Safety and Health
    Information
4676 Columbia Parkway
Cincinnati, OH 45226
(513) 533-8383
www.cdc.gov/niosh
eidtechinfo@cdc.gov

National Spinal Cord Injury Association
1 Church Street #600
Rockville, MD 20850
(800) 962-9629
www.spinalcord.org
info@spinalcord.org

National Sporting Goods Association
1601 Feehanville Drive, Suite 300
Mt. Prospect, IL 60056
(800) 815-5422
www.nsga.org
info@nsga.org

National Transportation Safety Board
490 L'Enfant Plaza East, SW
Washington, DC 20594
(202) 314-6000
www.ntsb.gov

Occupational Safety and Health Administration
U.S. Department of Labor
Office of Statistics
200 Constitution Avenue, NW
Washington, DC 20210
(800) 321-OSHA (6742)
www.osha.gov

Prevent Blindness America
211 W. Wacker Dr., Suite 1700
Chicago, IL 60606
(800) 331-2020
www.preventblindness.org
info@preventblindness.org

Substance Abuse & Mental Health Service Administration
1 Choke Cherry Road
Rockville, MD 20857
(877) 726-4727
www.samhsa.gov

Transportation Research Board
500 5th Street, NW
Washington, DC 20001
(202) 334-2934
http://gulliver.trb.org

USA.gov
Gateway to federal, state, local, tribal, and international
government websites.
www.usa.gov

U.S. Coast Guard
2100 2nd Street, SW
Washington, DC 20593-0001
(800) 368-5647
www.uscgboating.org
uscginfoline@gcrm.com

U.S. Consumer Product Safety Commission
4330 East West Highway
Bethesda, MD 20814
(301) 504-7923
www.cpsc.gov
clearinghouse@cpsc.gov

World Health Organization
Avenue Appia 20
CH-1211 Geneva 27
Switzerland
Phone: +41-22-791-2111
Fax: +41-22-791-3111
www.who.int
info@who.int

Accident is that occurrence in a sequence of events that produces unintended injury, death, or property damage. *Accident* refers to the event, not the result of the event (see *Unintentional injury*).

Death from accident is a death that occurs within one year of the accident.

Disabling injury is an injury causing death, permanent disability, or any degree of temporary total disability beyond the day of the injury.

Fatal accident is an accident that results in one or more deaths within one year.

Home is a dwelling and its premises within the property lines including single-family dwellings and apartment houses, duplex dwellings, boarding and rooming houses, and seasonal cottages. Excluded from *home* are barracks, dormitories, and resident institutions.

Incidence rate, as defined by OSHA, is the number of occupational injuries and/or illnesses or lost workdays per 100 full-time employees (see formula on page 66).

Injury is physical harm or damage to the body resulting from an exchange, usually acute, of mechanical, chemical, thermal, or other environmental energy that exceeds the body's tolerance.

Medically consulted injury is an injury serious enough that a medical professional was consulted. For the motor vehicle, home and public venues, the Council uses the medically consulted injury estimates from the National Health Interview survey. The Council uses the total recordable case estimate, using OSHA's definition, published by the Bureau of Labor Statistics to estimate the number of workplace injuries. Because the BLS estimate excludes self-employed, unpaid family workers, and federal government employees, the Council extrapolates the BLS estimate to reflect the total worker population.

Motor vehicle is any mechanically or electrically powered device not operated on rails, upon which or by which any person or property may be transported upon a land highway. The load on a motor vehicle or trailer attached to it is considered part of the vehicle. Tractors and motorized machinery are included while self-propelled in transit or used for transportation. *Nonmotor vehicle* is any road vehicle other than a motor vehicle, such as a bicycle or animal-drawn vehicle, except a coaster wagon, child's sled, child's tricycle, child's carriage, and similar means of transportation; persons using these latter means of transportation are considered pedestrians.

Motor vehicle accident is an unstabilized situation that includes at least one harmful event (injury or property damage) involving a motor vehicle in transport (in motion, in readiness for motion, or on a roadway but not parked in a designated parking area) that does not result from discharge of a firearm or explosive device and does not directly result from a cataclysm. [See Committee on Motor Vehicle Traffic Accident Classification (1997), *Manual on Classification of Motor Vehicle Traffic Accidents*, ANSI D16.1-1996, Itasca, IL: National Safety Council.]

Motor vehicle traffic accident is a motor vehicle accident that occurs on a trafficway — a way or place, any part of which is open to the use of the public for the purposes of vehicular traffic. *Motor vehicle nontraffic accident* is any motor vehicle accident that occurs entirely in any place other than a trafficway.

Nonfatal injury accident is an accident in which at least one person is injured and no injury results in death.

Occupational illness is any abnormal condition or disorder other than one resulting from an occupational injury caused by exposure to environmental factors associated with employment. It includes acute and chronic illnesses or diseases that may be caused by inhalation, absorption, ingestion, or direct contact (see also pages 69 and 91).

Occupational injury is any injury such as a cut, fracture, sprain, amputation, etc., which results from a work accident or from a single instantaneous exposure in the work environment (see also page 69).

Pedalcycle is a vehicle propelled by human power and operated solely by pedals; excludes mopeds.

Pedestrian is any person involved in a motor vehicle accident who is not in or upon a motor vehicle or nonmotor vehicle. Includes persons injured while using a coaster wagon, child's tricycle, roller skates, etc. Excludes persons boarding, alighting, jumping, or falling from a motor vehicle in transport who are considered occupants of the vehicle.

Permanent disability (or permanent impairment) includes any degree of permanent nonfatal injury. It includes any injury that results in the loss or complete loss of use of any part of the body or in any permanent impairment of functions of the body or a part thereof.

Property damage accident is an accident that results in property damage but in which no person is injured.

Public accident is any accident other than motor vehicle that occurs in the public use of any premises. Includes deaths in recreation (swimming, hunting, etc.), in transportation except motor vehicle, public buildings, etc., and from widespread natural disasters even though some may have happened on home premises. Excludes accidents to persons in the course of gainful employment.

Source of injury is the principal object such as tool, machine, or equipment involved in the accident and is usually the object inflicting injury or property damage. Also called *agency* or *agent*.

Temporary total disability is an injury that does not result in death or permanent disability but that renders the injured person unable to perform regular duties or activities on one or more full calendar days after the day of the injury.

Total cases include all work-related deaths and illnesses and those work-related injuries that result in loss of consciousness, restriction of work or motion, or transfer to another job, or require medical treatment other than first aid.

Unintentional injury is the preferred term for accidental injury in the public health community. It refers to the *result* of an accident.

Work hours are the total number of hours worked by all employees. They are usually compiled for various levels, such as an establishment, a company, or an industry. A work hour is the equivalent of one employee working one hour.

Work injuries (including occupational illnesses) are those that arise out of and in the course of gainful employment regardless of where the accident or exposure occurs. Excluded are work injuries to private household workers and injuries occurring in connection with farm chores that are classified as home injuries.

Workers are all persons gainfully employed, including owners, managers, other paid employees, the self-employed, and unpaid family workers but excluding private household workers.

Work/motor vehicle duplication includes *work injuries* that occur in *motor vehicle accidents* (see *Work injuries* and *Motor vehicle accident*).